MANUAL OF CLINICAL PROBLEMS IN ASTHMA, ALLERGY, AND RELATED DISORDERS

WITH ANNOTATED KEY REFERENCES

MANUAL OF CLINICAL PROBLEMS IN ASTHMA, ALLERGY, AND RELATED DISORDERS
WITH ANNOTATED KEY REFERENCES

EDITED BY

DON A. BUKSTEIN, M.D.
Director, Division of Pediatric Allergy and Pulmonary Disease, Dean Clinic; Clinical Assistant Professor, Department of Family Medicine, University of Wisconsin Medical School, Madison

ROBERT C. STRUNK, M.D.
Associate Professor of Pediatrics, University of Colorado School of Medicine; Director, Clinical Services, Department of Pediatrics, National Jewish Hospital and Research Center/National Asthma Center, Denver

Foreword by Richard B. Johnston, Jr., M.D.
Professor and Vice Chairman, Department of Pediatrics, University of Colorado School of Medicine; Chairman, Department of Pediatrics, National Jewish Hospital and Research Center/National Asthma Center, Denver

LITTLE, BROWN AND COMPANY   BOSTON/TORONTO

Library of Congress Catalog Card No. 83-82938

ISBN 0-316-11473-1

Printed in the United States of America

HAL

CONTENTS

FOREWORD

What a genuine delight to see this book completed and to have the privilege of writing its foreword. This compilation of short reviews of pertinent literature was conceived by the pediatric postdoctoral fellows of the class of 1982 at the National Jewish Hospital and Research Center/National Asthma Center as a means of educating themselves in the major subjects of clinical allergy and immunology. Driven by the energy and enthusiasm of Don Bukstein and burnished by the critical input of Bob Strunk, the book grew into its present form. The chapters were constructed primarily by present and recently graduated postdoctoral fellows, but each section was reviewed by a member of the faculty and again by an outside authority. Because the reviewers recognized the unique character of the project, the reviews were universally thoughtful and constructively critical. Although these chapters should serve to introduce their subject to the relative beginner or to offer a quick review to those already knowledgeable in the field, they are not intended to furnish full details. Rather, it has been the hope of all concerned with this endeavor that this book might provoke its readers, as it has its authors, to truly educate themselves in the subject at hand.

Richard B. Johnston, Jr.

This manual reviews topics that reflect problems commonly encountered in the treatment of both children and adults in a primary care setting. These reviews are intended to provide the reader with a framework with which to approach these clinical problems and to direct the reader to the relevant literature that forms the basis for pathologic, diagnostic, and therapeutic understanding of the disease processes involved. Thus, the manual is designed to assist the nonspecialist in an understanding of allergy and related disorders. It is not meant to be a substitute for textbooks that cover allergic, pulmonary, and immunologic diseases comprehensively. Further, although a distinct approach to each problem is given, it is not a how-to manual for patient management in the usual sense.

This manual is a joint project of the fellows in training in allergy and clinical immunology at various institutions in Denver and is the result of their conscientious study. Each chapter has been reviewed by a recognized expert in the field.

Special thanks must be given to Drs. Hyman Chai and Richard B. Johnston, Jr., who have been dedicated to the completion of this manual. The authors are grateful to Ray S. Davis for his organizational assistance and advice. In order to complete this project, the editors and authors have relied greatly on the many resources that were made readily available by the National Jewish Hospital and Research Center/National Asthma Center, Denver. The authors wish to express their appreciation to Georgia Wheeler for her preparation of the typed manuscript and for her devotion to the completion of this project. The following medical faculty have provided their expertise, advice, and assistance: Mathea Allansmith, M.D., Harvard Medical School and Eye Research Institute of the Retina Foundation, Boston; Louis Barness, M.D., Tampa, Florida; Leonard I. Bernstein, M.D., University of Cincinnati College of Medicine, Cincinnati; S. Alan Bock, M.D., National Jewish Hospital and Research Center/National Asthma Center, Denver; Manon Brenner, M.D., National Jewish Hospital and Research Center/National Asthma Center, Denver; Jerome Buckley, M.D., National Jewish Hospital and Research Center/National Asthma Center, Denver; William Busse, M.D., University of Wisconsin Medical School, Madison; Hyman Chai, M.D., National Jewish Hospital and Research Center/National Asthma Center, Denver; Henry Claman, M.D., University of Colorado Health Sciences Center, Denver; Ernest Cotton, M.D., University of Colorado Health Sciences Center, Denver; Richard de Shazo, M.D., Tulane University School of Medicine, New Orleans; Elliot Ellis, M.D., State University of New York at Buffalo School of Medicine; J. Roger Hollister, M.D., National Jewish Hospital and Research Center/National Asthma Center, Denver; John Jenne, M.D., Hines, Illinois; Richard B. Johnston, Jr., M.D., National Jewish Hospital and Research Center/National Asthma Center, Denver; Nelson Jones, M.D., Denver; Charles Kirkpatrick, M.D., National Jewish Hospital and Research Center/National Asthma Center, Denver; Gary L. Larsen, M.D., National Jewish Hospital and Research Center/National Asthma Center, Denver; Philip Lieberman, M.D., University of Tennessee College of Medicine, Memphis; Robert Mason, M.D., National Jewish Hospital and Research Center/National Asthma Center, Denver; Kenneth Mathews, M.D., University of Michigan Medical School, Ann Arbor; Hugh Moffet, M.D., Madison, Wisconsin; William F. Morgan, M.D., Phoenix; Helen G. Morris, M.D., National Jewish Hospital and Research Center/National Asthma Center, Denver; Harold Nelson, M.D., Fitzsimons Army Medical Center, Aurora, Colorado, and University of Colorado School of Medicine, Denver; Robert Reisman, M.D., State University of New York at Buffalo School of Medicine; John E. Salvaggio, M.D., Tulane University School of Medicine, New Orleans; Alan

Schocket, M.D., University of Colorado School of Medicine, Denver; Guy Settipane, M.D., Providence, Rhode Island; Albert Sheffer, M.D., Harvard Medical School, Boston; Sheldon Siegel, M.D., UCLA School of Medicine, Los Angeles; Raymond Slavin, M.D., St. Louis University School of Medicine, St. Louis; Sheldon Spector, M.D., University of Colorado School of Medicine, Denver; Joseph Souhrada, M.D., National Jewish Hospital and Research Center/National Asthma Center, Denver; Robert C. Strunk, M.D., National Jewish Hospital and Research Center/National Asthma Center, Denver; Timothy Sullivan, M.D., University of Texas Health Sciences Center at Dallas, Dallas; William Weston, M.D., University of Colorado School of Medicine, Denver; Robert S. Zeiger, M.D., University of California, San Diego, School of Medicine, La Jolla, and Kaiser Permanente Medical Center, San Diego.

D.A.B.
R.C.S.

ALLEN D. ADINOFF, M.D.
Clinical Assistant Professor of Pediatrics, University of Colorado School of Medicine; Consultant Staff Physician, National Jewish Hospital and Research Center/National Asthma Center, University of Colorado Health Sciences Center, Denver

KARL M. ALTENBURGER, M.D.
Former Fellow, Division of Allergy and Clinical Immunology, National Jewish Hospital and Research Center/National Asthma Center, University of Colorado Health Sciences Center, Denver

NICK GEORGE ANAS, M.D.
Assistant Professor, Pediatrics, University of California, San Diego, School of Medicine, La Jolla; Co-director, Pediatric Intensive Care Unit, University Hospital, San Diego

FRANCINE G. ANDREWS, M.D.
Former Fellow, Division of Allergy and Clinical Immunology, National Jewish Hospital and Research Center/National Asthma Center, University of Colorado Health Sciences Center, Denver

B. LYN BEHRENS, M.D.
Former Fellow, Division of Allergy and Clinical Immunology, National Jewish Hospital and Research Center/National Asthma Center, University of Colorado Health Sciences Center, Denver

ROBERT BERKOWITZ, M.D.
Former Fellow, Division of Allergy and Clinical Immunology, National Jewish Hospital and Research Center/National Asthma Center, University of Colorado Health Sciences Center, Denver

RAJESH G. BHAGAT, M.D.
Former Fellow, Division of Allergy and Clinical Immunology, National Jewish Hospital and Research Center/National Asthma Center, University of Colorado Health Sciences Center, Denver

MANON BRENNER, M.D.
Assistant Professor of Pediatrics, University of Colorado School of Medicine, Denver

DON A. BUKSTEIN, M.D.
Director, Division of Pediatric Allergy and Pulmonary Disease, Dean Clinic; Clinical Assistant Professor, Department of Family Medicine, University of Wisconsin Medical School, Madison

FERNAN CABALLERO, M.D.
Former Fellow, Division of Allergy and Clinical Immunology, National Jewish Hospital and Research Center/National Asthma Center, University of Colorado Health Sciences Center, Denver

ROBERT D. COOK, M.D.
Former Fellow, Department of Clinical Immunology, University of Colorado School of Medicine, Denver

NANCY P. CUMMINGS, M.D.
Assistant Professor, Pediatrics, University of Colorado School of Medicine, Denver

KATHLEEN C. DAVIS, M.D.
Former Fellow, Division of Allergy and Clinical Immunology, National Jewish Hospital and Research Center/National Asthma Center, University of Colorado Health Sciences Center, Denver

RAY S. DAVIS, M.D.
Former Fellow, Division of Allergy and Clinical Immunology, National Jewish Hospital and Research Center/National Asthma Center, University of Colorado Health Sciences Center, Denver

PINKUS GOLDBERG, M.D.
Former Fellow, Allergy/Immunology, Fitzsimons Army Medical Center, Aurora, Colorado

GERALD L. GOLDSTEIN, M.D.
Former Fellow, Division of Allergy and Clinical Immunology, National Jewish Hospital and Research Center/National Asthma Center, University of Colorado Health Sciences Center, Denver

THOMAS B. HARPER, M.D.
Clinical Assistant Professor, Department of Pediatrics, Medical University of South Carolina, Charleston

JEFFREY H. HILL, M.D., Ph.D.
Former Fellow, Division of Allergy and Clinical Immunology, National Jewish Hospital and Research Center/National Asthma Center, University of Colorado Health Sciences Center, Denver

LINDEN HO, M.D.
Former Fellow, Division of Allergy and Clinical Immunology, National Jewish Hospital and Research Center/National Asthma Center, University of Colorado Health Sciences Center, Denver

MARK HOLBREICH, M.D.
Former Fellow, Division of Allergy and Clinical Immunology, National Jewish Hospital and Research Center/National Asthma Center, University of Colorado Health Sciences Center, Denver

SHMUEL KIVITY, M.D.
Former Fellow, Division of Allergy and Clinical Immunology, National Jewish Hospital and Research Center/National Asthma Center, University of Colorado Health Sciences Center, Denver

LELA A. LEE, M.D.
Instructor of Dermatology, University of Colorado School of Medicine, Denver

MICHAEL E. MARTIN, M.D.
Former Fellow, Division of Allergy and Clinical Immunology, National Jewish Hospital and Research Center/National Asthma Center, University of Colorado Health Sciences Center, Denver

UWE MANTHEI, M.D.
Former Fellow, Division of Allergy and Clinical Immunology, National Jewish Hospital and Research Center/National Asthma Center, University of Colorado Health Sciences Center, Denver

JAMES D. OGGEL, M.D.
Fellow, Division of Allergy and Clinical Immunology, University of Missouri—Kansas City School of Medicine; Attending Physician, Children's Mercy Hospital, Kansas City

PAUL S. RABINOWITZ, M.D., Cpt., MC
Chief, Allergy and Immunology Service, Ireland Hospital, Fort Knox, Kentucky

MARY SHIELDS, M.D.
Former Fellow, Division of Allergy and Clinical Immunology, National Jewish Hospital and Research Center/National Asthma Center, University of Colorado Health Sciences Center, Denver

ROBERT C. STRUNK, M.D.
Director, Clinical Services, Department of Pediatrics, National Jewish Hospital and Research Center/National Asthma Center; Associate Professor of Pediatrics, University of Colorado School of Medicine, Denver

GERI S. WOLFSON
Psychology Intern, Department of Psychology, Baylor College of Medicine, Houston

STEVEN A. WOOL, M.D.
Chief Resident, Family Practice, University of Arizona, School of Medicine, Tucson

EMERGENCIES

1. ANAPHYLAXIS
Paul S. Rabinowitz

Anaphylaxis is a systemic immediate hypersensitivity reaction that is potentially fatal if not recognized and treated. The reaction requires the cross-linking of two mast cell–bound or basophil-bound IgE molecules by an antigen. This results in membrane changes in mast cells and basophils, causing the cells to degranulate and release the mediators of anaphylaxis. For anaphylaxis to occur the individual must have been previously exposed to the antigen and have made a large amount of specific IgE antibody. On further exposure an immediate hypersensitivity reaction can then take place. In some cases mast cell and basophil degranulation occur without IgE as an intermediary; this is termed an *anaphylactoid reaction*. In these cases, prior sensitization is not necessary, and a reaction can occur on the first exposure. Substances that can induce an anaphylactoid reaction include the complement anaphylatoxins C3a and C5a, kinins, and a number of drugs, the most prominent of which are the opiates. Whether or not the reaction is IgE mediated, the clinical manifestations and treatment modalities are the same.

Penicillin and related antibiotics currently are the most frequent cause of anaphylaxis. It is estimated that there are 10 to 40 reactions per 100,000 injections, with an estimated 500 to 1000 deaths per year. Radiocontrast media most commonly cause anaphylactoid reactions, which occur in 1 to 2% of patients and result in as many as 500 deaths per year. Other causes of anaphylaxis include stinging insects, foods, heterologous antisera, hormones, vaccines, various antibiotics, nonsteroidal anti-inflammatory agents, enzymes, blood and blood products, and allergen extracts. Recently, exercise-induced anaphylaxis has been reported. In some patients, this type of anaphylaxis occurs only after eating. Postprandial exercise-induced anaphylaxis may be the result of mechanical, as well as immune, factors. There have been cases of idiopathic anaphylaxis, in which no etiology could be found. Curiously, atopic individuals probably are not at greater risk for developing anaphylaxis, although their reactions tend to be more severe.

The signs and symptoms of anaphylaxis usually occur within 30 minutes of exposure, although this may vary depending on the route of exposure. In general, intravenous dosing causes the most rapid (often occurring within seconds) and most severe reactions; reactions after oral administration tend to have a more delayed onset (hours) and tend to be much milder. The four organ systems most commonly involved are the skin, respiratory tract, gastrointestinal tract, and cardiovascular system. Skin manifestations may include diffuse erythema, pruritus, urticaria, and angioedema. Early signs in particular will often be seen at the injection site. Respiratory tract symptoms may include rhinitis, laryngeal edema with stridor and hoarseness, bronchospasm with wheezing, coughing, and dyspnea, and respiratory failure. Gastrointestinal tract involvement may include nausea, vomiting, diarrhea, and cramps. Cardiovascular findings may include hypotension, tachycardia and other arrhythmias, electrocardiographic indications of myocardial ischemia or injury, syncope, and, most serious, cardiac arrest. Other symptoms may include a "feeling of impending doom," uterine contractions, urinary incontinence, and seizures. Symptoms of anaphylaxis will usually subside within 1 to 2 hours whether or not treatment is administered. Occasionally, respiratory tract and cutaneous symptoms may persist for 1 or 2 days. Death is most commonly caused by severe hypoxia resulting from intractable laryngeal edema, cardiovascular collapse resulting from arrythmias, or shock resulting from increased vascular permeability and loss of plasma volume.

The mediators responsible for anaphylaxis are numerous. While histamine has been best studied, other mediators include the leukotrienes (slow-reacting substance of anaphylaxis), prostaglandins, kinins, platelet activating factor, and eosinophil and neutrophil chemotactic factors of anaphylaxis. Pathophysiologically, they are responsible for the increased capillary permeability, vasodilatation, smooth muscle constriction, increased glandular secretions, eosinophilia, and the neutrophil infiltrations that are found at autopsy.

Prior to instituting therapy in a patient suspected of having anaphylaxis, a vasovagal reaction—which occurs more commonly following an injection—should be ruled out. In a vasovagal reaction the patient exhibits pallor, bradycardia, and only mild hypotension, all of which should readily revert to normal upon lying down without medication. Such is not the case for anaphylaxis: here rapid therapeutic intervention is imperative.

Once the diagnosis of anaphylaxis has been made, pharmacologic management begins after ensuring a patent airway, spontaneous respiration, and an adequate heart rate. Epinephrine is the drug of choice and should be administered subcutaneously or intramuscularly in a dose of 0.01 ml/kg (to a maximum of 0.3–0.4 ml) at a 1 : 1000 dilution. If an injected drug or an insect sting is the suspected offender, applying a tourniquet proximal to the injection and injecting an additional dose of epinephrine into the site may prevent further absorption of the antigen. Hypotension should be treated aggressively with intravenous fluids and plasma expanders such as albumin or dextran when appropriate. Only when the patient remains hypotensive after such therapy should vasopressors, such as levarterenol, metaraminol, or dopamine, be employed. Persistent bronchospasm should be treated with IV aminophylline (see Chap. 30 for doses recommended for patients of different ages). Nasal O_2 (4–6 L/min) should also be used. Intractable laryngeal edema may require intubation or tracheostomy. Cardiac arrhythmias should be treated with the appropriate medication. With aggressive management, most patients will respond dramatically.

The precise value of antihistamines and corticosteroids in anaphylaxis is not clear. They are clearly not first-line drugs, and they will not reverse any of the immediate problems. However, they probably should be used to prevent protracted or recurrent symptoms. Diphenhydramine (25–50 mg IM or IV every 4–6 hours) and hydrocortisone (4–8 mg/kg every 4–6 hours) are usually recommended.

Prevention of anaphylaxis, of course, is most important. The following measures will help:

1. Take a thorough drug history prior to the use of any agent.
2. Administer a drug orally when possible.
3. If feasible, observe the patient for 30 minutes following drug administration.
4. If a history of drug sensitivity is obtained, skin test only if no alternative drug is available. If the skin test is positive, a desensitization protocol should be used.
5. If possible, obtain special preventive protocols if desensitization is not appropriate.
6. Teach patients who are predisposed to anaphylaxis to self-administer epinephrine.
7. Where appropriate, Medic Alert tags should be worn at all times by the patient.

Altman, L. C. Basic immune mechanisms in immediate hypersensitivity. *Med. Clin. North Am.* 65:941–957, 1981.
IgE, mast cells, basophils, and the mediators of immediate hypersensitivity are discussed in a straightforward manner.
Austen, K. F. Systemic anaphylaxis in the human being. *N. Engl. J. Med.* 291:661–664, 1974.
A concise review of the pathogenesis and treatment of anaphylaxis.

Bacal, E., Patterson, R., and Zeiss, C. R. Evaluation of severe anaphylactic reactions. *Clin. Allergy* 8:295–304, 1978.
In 10 of 21 patients a cause was found; the others were controlled with medication.
Barnard, J. H. Studies of 400 Hymenoptera sting deaths in the United States. *J. Allergy Clin. Immunol.* 52:259–264, 1973.
Autopsy findings are reviewed, with respiratory tract pathology most common.
Booth, B. H., and Patterson, R. Electrocardiographic changes during human anaphylaxis. *J.A.M.A.* 211:627–631, 1970.
Flattening or inversion of the T waves, elevation or depression of the ST segment, a nodal rhythm, and atrial fibrillation were the most common findings in the first 24 hours.
Editorial: Treatment of anaphylactic shock. *Br. Med. J.* 282:1011–1012, 1981.
The British point of view.
Golbert, T. M., Patterson, R., and Pruzansky, J. J. Systemic allergic reactions to ingested antigens. *J. Allergy* 44:96–107, 1969.
This article details anaphylactic reactions to foods and other ingested substances.
Kelly, J. F., and Patterson, R. Anaphylaxis: Course, mechanisms and treatment. *J.A.M.A.* 227:1431–1436, 1974.
A concise review of the pathogenesis and treatment of anaphylaxis.
Lockey, R. F., and Bukantz, S. C. Allergic emergencies. *Med. Clin. North Am.* 58:147–156, 1974.
A concise review of the pathogenesis and treatment of anaphylaxis.
Marney, S. R. Anaphylaxis and Serum Sickness. In H. F. Conn (Ed.), *Current Diagnosis*. Philadelphia: Saunders, 1982. Pp. 581–584.
An up-to-date review of treatment and prevention.
Novey, H. S., et al. Postprandial exercise-induced anaphylaxis. *J. Allergy Clin. Immunol.* 71:498–504, 1983.
Obeid, A. H., et al. Fluid therapy in severe systemic reaction to radiopaque dye. *Ann. Intern. Med.* 83:317–320, 1975.
Rapid saline infusion was necessary in two patients unresponsive to epinephrine.
Parker, C. Systemic Anaphylaxis. In C. W. Parker (Ed.), *Clinical Immunology*. Philadelphia: Saunders, 1980. Pp. 1208–1218.
A good summary of systemic anaphylaxis that includes a good discussion of causes and pathophysiology.
Sale, S. R., Greenberger, P. A., and Patterson, R. Idiopathic anaphylactoid reactions. A clinical summary. *J.A.M.A.* 246:2336–2339, 1981.
In 31 patients no etiology for their anaphylactoid reactions could be determined; in 16 of 18 patients, medications were effective in controlling or reducing the severity of symptoms. Reactions were always self-limiting and no medications were required in ten patients. There were no deaths. Remissions lasting more than 1 year occurred in seven patients.
Sheffer, A. L., and Austen, K. F. Exercise-induced anaphylaxis. *J. Allergy Clin. Immunol.* 66:106–111, 1980.
An entity distinct from cholinergic urticaria is described in 16 patients.
Smith, P. L., et al. Physiologic manifestations of human anaphylaxis. *J. Clin. Invest.* 66:1072–1080, 1980.
A thorough description of the pathophysiologic manifestations of anaphylaxis that occurred in three patients during immunotherapy for insect-sting hypersensitivity.
Wasserman, S. I. Anaphylaxis. In E. Middleton (Ed.), *Allergy: Principles and Practice* (2nd ed.). St. Louis: Mosby, 1983. Pp. 689–699.
A good summary of anaphylaxis in the current standard textbook on allergy.
Weiszer, I. Allergic Emergencies. In R. Patterson (Ed.), *Allergic Diseases: Diagnosis and Management*. Philadelphia: Lippincott, 1980. Pp. 374–394.
A good summary of allergic emergencies that includes a good discussion of treatment and prevention.

2. EMERGENCY ROOM MANAGEMENT OF ACUTE ASTHMA
Thomas B. Harper

When a patient appears in an emergency room or physician's office in obvious respiratory distress from an acute worsening of asthma, a physician first thinks of taking immediate action with various bronchodilator drugs. A few historical facts and physical findings elicited prior to any action, however, can be extremely helpful in assessing the severity of the attack and in avoiding problems that otherwise might be encountered in therapy. The previous severity and chronicity of the patient's asthma are important clues that can aid in determining the vigor of initial bronchodilator therapy and can possibly suggest the need for early intervention with systemic corticosteroids. In general, the shorter the duration of the present wheezing episode, the better the response to adrenergic bronchodilators will be. Frequent adrenergic inhaler use or abuse may indicate that the patient is not complying with other aspects of his or her prescribed asthma regimen (e.g., cromolyn or theophylline) and that he or she may be unresponsive, or even paradoxically responsive, to inhaled adrenergic agents. This response is much more likely if the inhaled drug was isoproterenol. A careful history of medications including doses, routes, and time of last dose is particularly pertinent for individuals using oral or inhaled adrenergic agents (for the reasons just mentioned) and for individuals using sustained-action theophylline preparations (whose prolonged presence in the body may delay emergency room use of intravenous aminophylline to avoid hazardous serum theophylline levels). Recent vomiting may explain why the patient is not receiving a desired effect from previously adequate oral bronchodilators; however, recent vomiting may also indicate theophylline toxicity in an individual who has ingested an excessive dose in an unsuccessful attempt to abort a worsening asthma attack.

A rapid but complete physical examination must include an assessment of general appearance—presence of cyanosis, use of accessory respiratory muscles, mental functioning, and so on. The presence and distribution of wheezing and breath sounds should be noted. Worsening asthma may be manifested by poor air exchange and minimal wheezing owing to poor air movement. Atelectasis of various lobes of the lung, particularly the right middle lobe, is a frequent complication of severe asthma and should be considered when breath sounds and wheezing are greatly diminished in any part of the chest. The degree of respiratory effort should be assessed initially and monitored; increasing severity of respiratory distress may be manifested either by increased respiratory effort (reflecting hypoxemia), or by decreased effort (indicating tiring). A rough correlate with the degree of severity of respiratory distress is the degree of prolongation of the expiratory phase of respiration, usually assessed by the inspiratory to expiratory, or I/E, ratio. The presence of a pulsus paradoxus (i.e., a fall in systolic blood pressure > 10 mmHg lower on inspiration than on expiration) is indicative of severe bronchospasm.

Several initial laboratory studies may be extremely helpful both in determining severity of the patient's asthma and in deciding what therapy should be initiated. If the patient has been receiving theophylline, a serum theophylline level can be useful, demonstrating patient noncompliance (very low or absent levels), inadequate dosage, or excessive usage of the drug. These levels are important in guiding initial administration of intravenous aminophylline when the patient has been receiving sustained-action theophylline preparations. A chest roentgenogram may show atelectasis, pneumomediastinum, pneumothorax, or pneumonia and should be performed in anyone with severe bronchospasm or with local inequality of breath sounds even without severe distress. Arterial blood gases are very important in determining the degree of obstruction and ventila-

Table 1. Alternatives for initial bronchodilator therapy

Drug	Route of administration	Dosage	Frequency
Epinephrine, aqueous (1 : 1000 solution)	Subcutaneous injection	0.01 ml/kg (max. 0.30 ml)	15 min × 2 (if needed)
Terbutaline sulfate* (1 mg/ml solution)	Subcutaneous injection	0.01 ml/kg (max. 0.25 ml)	10 min × 2 (if needed)
Isoproterenol HCl (1% solution)	Aerosol	0.005 ml/kg in 1–2 ml saline	30 min × 2 (if needed)
Isoethrine HCl (1% solution)	Aerosol	0.25–0.50 ml in 1–2 ml saline	30 min × 2 (if needed)
Metaproterenol sulfate (5% solution)	Aerosol	0.20–0.30 ml in 1–2 ml saline	30 min × 2 (if needed)

*Not approved for use in children less than 12 years of age or for aerosol use.

tion-perfusion imbalance, which is manifested primarily by decreased PaO_2. Decreased PaO_2 is associated with a decreased PCO_2 that is due to the increased respiratory rate in response to the hypoxia. As fatigue and progressive obstruction occur, ventilation becomes less effective—even though it may remain rapid—and the PCO_2 increases. Thus, an elevated or even "normal" $PaCO_2$ is an ominous sign. If the patient is cooperative and respiratory distress is not too severe, *spirometry* is also useful to quantitate the degree of obstruction and response to bronchodilators. In fact, pulmonary function testing is often more accurate than arterial blood gases as a guideline for determining whether or not hospitalization is necessary for a patient with acute severe asthma.

Initial intervention should be aimed at providing smooth muscle relaxation and improving arterial hypoxemia. Since some degree of arterial hypoxemia can be expected in every case of severe wheezing, O_2 should be used routinely. Administration of small amounts of humidified oxygen by Venturi mask (24–28%) or by nasal cannula (2 L/min flow) almost always improves hypoxemia without raising $PaCO_2$, even in adult patients with chronic obstructive lung disease and chronically elevated $PaCO_2$, who may hypoventilate when given higher concentrations of oxygen to breathe. Administration of oxygen should be continuous. "Mist tents" or ultrasonic nebulizers have not been shown to be of value.

Bronchodilator drugs may initially be administered by subcutaneous or aerosol routes. The subcutaneous route is preferred when the degree of bronchospasm is so severe that the patient has difficulty inhaling aerosol medication. Caution must be exercised when the patient has recently had large amounts of sympathomimetic bronchodilators or when the patient has a history of severe hypertension, cardiac arrhythmias, or recent symptomatic coronary artery disease. Acceptable alternatives for initial bronchodilator therapy are shown in Table 1.

If the patient demonstrates good reversibility with the initial bronchodilator therapy, extended bronchodilation may be provided by subcutaneous injection of 1) Sus-Phrine (1 : 200) 0.005 ml/kg or 2) terbutaline sulfate (1 mg/ml) 0.01 ml/kg. Most physicians administer Sus-Phrine only after the patient has had a significant improvement with the shorter-acting bronchodilators. In an attempt to ensure continued bronchodilation after initial treatment, most patients should be placed on an oral or inhaled beta$_2$-adrenergic agent and/or theophylline before being sent home. These drugs should be used regularly for 7 to 10 days after the

Table 2. Predictor index scoring system*

Factor	Value for score of 0	Value for score of 1
Pulse rate (beats/min)	<120	≥120
Respiratory rate (breaths/min)	< 30	≥ 30
Pulsus paradoxus (mmHg)	< 18	≥ 18
Peak expiratory flow rate (L/min)	<120	≥120
Dyspnea	Absent–mild	Moderate–severe
Accessory muscle use	Absent–mild	Moderate–severe
Wheezing	Absent–mild	Moderate–severe

*Score 0 or 1 for each factor as listed and add to give a total index of 0 to 7. The factor values used are those noted at presentation. A score of 4 or greater is very accurate in predicting the need for hospitalization.
Source: Fischl, M. A., Pitchenik, A., and Gardner, L. B. *New Engl. J. Med.* 305:783, 1981.

wheezing resolves because physiologic abnormalities persist for several days after the signs and symptoms of the acute attack have resolved and discontinuation of treatment too early may lead to relapse. The inclusion of a short, 3- to 4-day course of high-dose daily steroids (prednisone, 2 mg/kg/day, maximum 60 mg) following reversal of moderate to severe bronchospasm may also be indicated.

The patient should be considered to be in status asthmaticus and should be hospitalized for intensive bronchodilator and corticosteroid therapy if (1) the patient has a poor or transient response to initial bronchodilators, or if (2) it is apparent early in acute intervention that inhaled or injected bronchodilators are not reversing the acute process adequately, as reflected by persistent tachypnea, tachycardia, markedly abnormal peak expiratory flow rates and/or FEV_1 after treatment, moderate to severe dyspnea, accessory muscle use, and persistent wheezing. Many attempts have been made to quantify the response or lack of response to the early therapy for acute asthma. This assessment is best made using a multifactorial approach, predicting the risk of relapse and need for hospitalization. Table 2 demonstrates the use of such a predictive index.

Becker, A. B., Nelson, N. H., and Simons, F. E. F.   Inhaled salbutamol (albuterol) versus injected epinephrine in the treatment of acute severe asthma in children. *J. Pediatr.* 102:465–469, 1983.
One of many recent studies concluding that inhaled beta-2-agonists and subcutaneous epinephrine are equally effective. Increased adverse effects were seen in the group receiving epinephrine.

Ben-Zvi, Z., et al.   Acute asthma. *Am. Rev. Respir. Dis.* 127:101–105, 1983.
This report indicates that the time-honored tradition of serial epinephrine injections for acute asthma may be no more effective than a single epinephrine (Sus-Phrine) injection.

Chai, H., and Newcomb, R. W.   Pharmacologic management of childhood asthma. *Am. J. Dis. Child.* 125:757–765, 1973.
An earlier but still simple and practical outline of the treatment of asthma with drugs. The role of selective beta₂ agonists in the management of acute asthma is discussed briefly. The value of frequent objective measurement of lung function to guide pharmacologic therapy is stressed.

Children's Hospital Medical Center: *Manual of Pediatric Therapeutics.* Boston: Little, Brown, 1980. Pp. 45–49.
A short but fairly thorough review of acute asthma management, although the use of newer, beta₂-adrenergic agents is not mentioned.

Davis, W. J., et al.   Terbutaline in the treatment of acute asthma in childhood. *Chest* 72:614–617, 1977.
Terbutaline is an effective bronchodilator in acute asthma and is comparable in effect to epinephrine.

Fischl, M. A., Pitchenik, A., and Gardner, L. B.   An index predicting relapse and need for hospitalization in patients with acute bronchial asthma. *N. Engl. J. Med.* 305:783–798, 1981.
A predictive index based on (1) pulse, (2) respiratory rate, (3) presence of significant pulsus paradoxus, (4) pulmonary function testing, and (5) quantitation of dyspnea and wheezing was 95 to 96% accurate in predicting the risk of relapse and the need for hospitalization.

Gershel, J. C., et al.   The usefulness of chest radiographs in first asthma attack. *N. Engl. J. Med.* 309:336–339, 1983.
This article demonstrates that use of clinical signs improves the yield of chest radiographs in children with first asthma attacks.

Gross, N. J., et al.   Management of acute severe airways obstruction in the asthmatic patient. *ATS News* Fall, pp. 11–13, 1978.
A brief but concise overview of major aspects of acute asthma management.

Josephson, G. W., MacKenzie, E. J., Leitman, P. S., and Gibson, G.   Emergency treatment of asthma. A comparison of two treatment regimens. *JAMA* 242:639–643, 1979.
Subcutaneous epinephrine alone was found to be equivalent in effect to subcutaneous epinephrine plus IV aminophylline bolus for acute episodes of asthma.

Kelsen, S. G., et al.   Emergency room assessment and treatment of patients with acute asthma. Adequacy of the conventional methods. *Am. J. Med.* 64:622–628, 1978.
The best predictor of success of emergency room treatment for acute asthma is the degree of pulmonary function improvement achieved with initial therapy.

Lulla, S., and Newcomb, R. W.   Emergency management of asthma in children. *J. Pediatr.* 97:346–350, 1980.
The article rates risk factors for predicting hospitalization for severe asthma and emphasizes the importance of the use of pulmonary function testing to ascertain severity of asthma.

McFadden, E. F., Kiser, R., and deGroot, W. J.   Acute bronchial asthma. Relationship between clinical and physiologic manifestations. *N. Engl. J. Med.* 288:221–225, 1973.
The signs and symptoms of acute asthma do not necessarily reflect the severity of the physiologic alterations in lung functions during these episodes. Following acute asthma, pulmonary function abnormalities may last for prolonged periods of time, possibly as the result of continued peripheral airways obstruction.

Norwak, R. M., et al.   Arterial blood gases and pulmonary function in acute asthma. *J.A.M.A.* 249:2043–2046, 1983.
The authors conclude that patients with an FEV_1 of less than 25% predicted or a PEFR of less than 30% predicted probably should have an arterial blood gas.

Nowak, R. M., et al. Spirometric evaluation of acute bronchial asthma. *JACEP* 8:9–12, 1979.
Spirometry has an important place in evaluation of the asthmatic patient in the emergency room. Adult patients with initial FEV_1 of less than 0.60 L or an FEV_1 of less than 1.6 L after initial treatment require either hospitalization or close follow-up for the next 24 to 48 hours.

Pearlman, D. S., and Bierman, C. W.   Asthma (Bronchial Asthma, Reactive Airways Disorder). In C. W. Bierman and D. S. Pearlman (Eds.), *Allergic Diseases of Infancy, Childhood, and Adolescence.* Philadelphia: Saunders, 1980. Pp. 581–604.
A good discussion of the use of newer beta$_2$-adrenergic agents in acute asthma.

Rebuck, A. S., and Read, J.   Assessment and management of severe asthma. *Am. J. Med.* 51:788–798, 1971.
An earlier review of the authors' experience with severe asthma. Risk factors of severe asthma include: (1) disturbance of consciousness, (2) central cyanosis, (3) PaO_2 less than 60 mmHg, (4) any elevation of $PaCO_2$, (5) pulsus paradoxus, or (6) presence of pneumothorax or pneumomediastinum.

Rossing, T. H., et al.   Emergency therapy of asthma: Comparison of the acute effects of parenteral and inhaled sympathomimetics and infused aminophylline. *Am. Rev. Respir. Dis.* 122:365–371, 1980.
Short-acting sympathomimetics alone produce more rapid and potent bronchodilatation in

acutely ill asthmatics than IV methylxanthines alone. There is no disadvantage to using inhaled beta agonists rather than ones administered parenterally.

Rossing, T. H., Fanta, C. H., and McFadden, E. R.   A controlled trial of the use of single versus combined drug therapy in the treatment of acute episodes of asthma. *Am. Rev. Respir. Dis.* 123:190–194, 1981.

Combinations of sympathomimetics and aminophylline are more effective and no more toxic than epinephrine alone for initial treatment of acute episodes of asthma.

Simons, F. E. R., and Gillies, J. D.   Dose response of subcutaneous terbutaline and epinephrine in children with acute asthma. *Am. J. Dis. Child.* 135:214–217, 1981.

Subcutaneous terbutaline is no better than subcutaneous epinephrine in the treatment of acute asthma in children.

3. MANAGEMENT OF STATUS ASTHMATICUS
Thomas B. Harper

Initial Assessment
Status asthmaticus is an acute asthmatic crisis refractory to appropriate doses of inhaled or injected beta-adrenergic bronchodilators. Unresponsiveness to such adrenergic smooth muscle–relaxing agents probably represents the development of airway narrowing from a significant amount of airway edema, inflammation, and accumulation of mucus. Status asthmaticus must be treated rapidly with all available medical resources to prevent such complications as respiratory failure and to reduce the length of hospitalization. Attempts at providing "holding room treatment" for asthma resistant to adrenergic drugs—with oxygen, IV fluids, and bolus aminophylline—have met with variable success, but are not generally recommended as they frequently only delay hospital admission. The presence of atelectasis, pneumothorax, pneumonia, or a previous history of chronic corticosteroid use or respiratory failure are important factors in determining the mode and aggressiveness of acute intervention for status asthmaticus. As outlined in Chapter 2, the presence of these factors should be established with the appropriate history, physical examination, and preliminary laboratory data, including pulmonary function testing if possible. Every person hospitalized for the treatment of status asthmaticus should have at the least a chest roentgenogram, arterial or arterialized capillary blood gas studies, and pulmonary function testing (if possible) to provide baseline data for continuing respiratory status evaluation.

Initial Therapy
Varying degrees of arterial hypoxemia are present in every case of status asthmaticus, and the administration of continuous humidified oxygen therapy, via face mask or nasal prongs, is essential for all hospitalized patients. If the patient has chronic obstructive pulmonary disease, even with a history of hypoventilation with high concentration of oxygen, a 24 to 28% Venturi mask can be used with no risk of decreasing respiratory drive.

Controversy currently surrounds the use of beta-adrenergic bronchodilators in status asthmaticus, which is by definition "refractory" to the further administration of this class of bronchodilator. The safety of the patient is the physician's first concern, and particular care should be taken when considering the use of adrenergic agents in persons with hypertension, symptomatic coronary artery disease, or recent exposure to large amounts of sympathomimetic drugs. The inhaled beta-adrenergic drugs, as outlined in Table 1, may be used up to every 1 to 2 hours for the first few hours of therapy, thereafter repeated less frequently as the patient's pulmonary status improves. Pulse rates and electrocardiograms, obtained before and after aerosol treatment, can be used to monitor cardiovascular response in high-risk patients. (It should be noted that standard chest leads used to monitor rhythm are not adequate to detect myocardial ischemia that may result from the use of large amounts of adrenergic agents.) Aerosolized adrenergic drugs should be delivered by a standard nebulizer; positive pressure ventilators are to be avoided because of the possible complication of pneumothorax and pneumomediastinum. As beta-adrenergic drugs may actually decrease PO_2 by increasing ventilation-perfusion imbalances, nebulizers used for administration of the drugs should be driven by oxygen at a rate of 2 to 5 L/min.

Aerosolized atropine sulfate (0.05 mg/kg) causes minimal effects on tracheobronchial mucus viscosity and provides effective smooth muscle bronchodilation with a minimum of cardiovascular side effects in high-risk cardiovascular patients. In addition, this cholinolytic agent may be the only effective alternative in a person who has severe bronchospasm induced or exacerbated by beta adrenergic blocking agents, such as propranolol. See Chap. 33 for details on its use.

A peripheral IV line should be inserted for administration of medications and fluids. Previously, every patient in status asthmaticus was assumed to have some degree of dehydration, and large amounts of fluids, over and above homeostatic maintenance (approximately 1500 ml/m²/day), were routinely recommended. Recent studies, however, have shown that this recommendation may actually be hazardous because of the frequent finding of inappropriate antidiuretic hormone release and the potential for development of pulmonary edema. Intravenous solutions should be infused to maintain fluid and electrolyte homeostasis with extra amounts provided only if there is physical or laboratory evidence of dehydration. Serial urine specific gravities and blood electrolytes and BUN are useful as guidelines for determining initial and ongoing fluid requirements.

With the increased use of sustained-release theophylline preparations, a careful history of recent theophylline use is essential prior to administering IV aminophylline, in order to avoid dangerously high "overlap" serum levels (>20 µg/ml). A rough rule of thumb is to withhold aminophylline infusion temporarily (2–8 hr) if the patient has received a sustained-release theophylline preparation within the last 8 to 10 hours or a rapid-release theophylline preparation within the last 4 to 6 hours. Aminophylline may be given as an IV bolus of 4 to 5 mg/kg over 30 minutes every 6 hours, or, if equipment is available, by continuous IV infusion (0.9 mg/kg/hr for children and cigarette-smoking adults; 0.5–0.6 mg/kg/hr for other adults; see Chapter 30 for details on theophylline dosing). Serum theophylline levels are a useful guide to initial administration of aminophylline in patients who have previously received theophylline, and are essential to fine tune further aminophylline doses for maximum therapeutic benefit without toxicity. The development of signs of theophylline toxicity (i.e., CNS stimulation, headache, nausea, vomiting, arrhythmia, or seizure) requires immediate slowing of the aminophylline infusion and an immediate serum theophylline determination.

Systemically administered corticosteroids have been used routinely in status asthmaticus since the 1950s, when double-blind studies in England demonstrated their value. Most recent studies have shown that they restore in vivo responsiveness to catecholamines, enable more rapid restoration of normal PO_2, and significantly shorten hospital stay for status asthmaticus. Because of the significant delay in both onset of effect and maximum effect with corticosteroid therapy, however, it is imperative that patients in status asthmaticus receive these agents as soon as possible. Delaying the use of systemic corticosteroids until the patient's asthma is "sufficiently severe" can increase the risk of progression of severe status asthmaticus to impending or frank respiratory failure. Reasonable options for IV corticosteroid therapy include hydrocortisone hemisuccinate, 5 mg/kg every 6 hours, and methylprednisolone acetate, 1 mg/kg every 6 hours.

Additional Therapy

If increased tracheobronchial secretions appear to be a major problem, mobilization of these secretions may be assisted by postural drainage, preferably performed immediately after aerosol bronchodilator therapy. Postural drainage should not be implemented until initial bronchodilator, fluid, and corticosteroid therapy have provided enough bronchodilatation to allow effective mobilization of secretions into the larger airways. Atelectasis, a frequent complication of status asthmaticus, is usually caused by mucous plugging of a major or segmental bronchus and can be treated effectively by vigorous postural drainage of the affected side of the chest.

An intercurrent respiratory tract infection is much more likely to be caused by viral agents than by bacterial agents; therefore, the use of "routine" antimicrobial drugs should be avoided. Evidence of bacterial lung infection should be sought with chest roentgenogram and sputum stains and cultures, and when found, treated with the appropriate antimicrobial agent. The macrolide class of antibiotics, which contains the frequently used erythromycin, has been shown to impair theophylline metabolism and thus increase preexisting theophylline levels, at times into the toxic range.

Neither nonnarcotic nor narcotic sedatives should be used in status asthmaticus. They may mask clinical signs of hypoxemia and impair CNS respiratory center response to hypoxemia and hypercarbia. A variety of CNS depressants have been implicated in cases of status asthmaticus that have ended fatally. Agitation during status asthmaticus is probably due to hypoxemia and should be treated with oxygen. Agitation in a well-oxygenated patient is more appropriately treated by reassurance.

The mild acidosis that may develop in status asthmaticus is caused by impaired respiratory CO_2/HCO_3 buffering capacity and is usually adequately corrected by improving respiratory status. Severe respiratory acidosis (pH less than 7.20; base deficit over 5 mEq/L) can be transiently improved by administration of intravenous sodium bicarbonate as clinically indicated.

Ongoing Assessment

The institution of all the measures just described does not ensure automatic improvement of the acutely ill asthmatic patient; ongoing subjective and objective measurements of respiratory status (clinical score, arterial blood gases) must be closely followed. The recent development and use of transcutaneous O_2 and CO_2 skin electrode systems may provide excellent means by which the blood gas changes in acute asthma can be continuously monitored. Provided that ongoing studies with a given machine show good correlation between the transcutaneous O_2 and CO_2 readings and arterial blood gases, this equipment will be a valuable tool for simple, continuous, and noninvasive measurement of PO_2 and PCO_2. A simple pulmonary scoring system for quantitating the degree of severity on admission and serially thereafter, such as that outlined in Table 3, will enable independent observers to objectively assess the patient's condition and the ongoing response (or lack of one) to the specific therapy initiated.

Therapeutic Alterations with Improvement

As serial pulmonary status scores indicate significant patient improvement, serial pulmonary function testing can further quantitate the degree of improvement and response to therapy. With further improvement in the clinical status, arterial blood gases, and pulmonary functions the following changes in therapy should be considered in order of importance:

Table 3. Pulmonary scoring system[a]

SCORING OF RESPIRATORY EFFORT
1   Expiratory wheezing with tidal volume breathing
2   Inspiratory and expiratory wheezing with tidal volume breathing
3   Tidal volume wheezing with prolonged expiratory phase
4   No. 3 plus mild to moderate retractions (subcostal, lower intercostal)
5   No. 3 plus severe retractions (subcostal, intercostal, suprasternal; flaring ala nasi)

SCORING OF AIR ENTRY
G   Good (good inspiratory breath sounds)
F   Fair (slight to moderate decreased breath sounds)
P   Poor (markedly decreased breath sounds)

SAMPLE FLOW SHEET

| Date | Time | Respiratory rate | Pulmonary score | ABG[b] | | | Clincal comments/PFT[c]/ Theophylline levels |
				PO_2	PCO_2	pH	

[a]Score is expressed as single number/single letter (i.e., 2G, 3F, and so on).
[b]Arterial blood gases.
[c]Pulmonary function testing.

1. Gradually reduce the rate of O_2 administration.
2. Decrease the frequency of aerosol treatments.
3. Discontinue IV fluids, and change IV medications to comparable oral medications.

Intravenous aminophylline can be switched to an equivalent oral dose of aminophylline every 4 to 6 hours or to the patient's previous theophylline preparation and dose. If there is any possibility of wheezing recurrence or instability, resumption of a sustained-release preparation should be delayed. Intravenous corticosteroid therapy can safely be switched to oral prednisone (2 mg/kg/day) with subsequent rapid or slow tapering, depending on the previous history of the patient and the severity of the episode. Pulmonary function testing is also a useful guideline for discharging the patient from the hospital. For an uncomplicated episode of status asthmaticus in a patient without severe chronic pulmonary function impairment, FEV_1 should be greater than 50% of predicted before administration of an inhaled bronchodilator before the patient can be discharged. Other pulmonary function studies, including flows at lower lung volumes and static lung volumes such as residual volume, may take much longer to return to normal. Because physiologic abnormalities persist long after the episode of status asthmaticus has subsided clinically, bronchodilator therapy should be continued for at least 2 to 3 weeks. Thereafter, if the patient continues to have repeated problems with wheezing or demonstrates chronically decreased FEV_1, further evaluation, including studies of lung volumes and small airway function, may be indicated.

Bierman, C. W., and Pierson, W. E. The pharmacologic management of status asthmaticus in children. *Pediatrics* 54:245–247, 1974.

A brief summary of initial evaluation, therapy, and follow-up evaluation, with a pulmonary scoring system for assessing ongoing response to therapy.

Eggleston, P. A., Ward, B. H., Pierson, W. E., and Bierman, C. W.   Radiographic abnormalities in acute asthma in children. *Pediatrics* 54:442–449, 1974.

Chest x-ray abnormalities are noted in about 25% of cases of acute asthma (perihilar infiltrates, atelectasis, pneumomediastinum); therefore, chest x-rays should be included in any hospitalization for asthma.

Goldberg, P., et al.   Intravenous aminophylline therapy for asthma. A comparison of two methods of administration in children. *Am. J. Dis. Child.* 134:596–599, 1980.

There is a greater pulmonary response to continuous aminophylline infusion over a comparable bolus dose of aminophylline in asthmatic children.

Harfi, H., Hanissian, A. S., and Crawford, L. V.   Treatment of status asthmaticus in children with high doses and conventional doses of methylprednisolone. *Pediatrics* 61:829–831, 1978.

There are no additional advantages in giving massive doses of corticosteroid over conventional doses (equivalent to 30 mg/m^2 of methylprednisolone every 6 hours) in the treatment of severe acute asthma attacks.

Haskell, R. J., Wong, B. M., and Hansen, J. E.   A double-blind, randomized, clinical trial of methylprednisolone in status asthmaticus. *Arch. Int. Med.* 143:1324–1327, 1983.

The authors demonstrated a definite clinical benefit when high doses of steroid were used when compared to low doses. Three doses were compared, 4, 20, and 120 mg every 6 hours. Patients receiving the highest dose had significantly improved clinical scores, FEV_1s and arterial blood gases by 24–48 hours when compared to patients receiving the lowest dose.

Kattan, M., Gurwitz, D., and Levison, H.   Corticosteroids in status asthmaticus. *J. Pediatr.* 96:596–599, 1980.

The addition of corticosteroids to a regimen of inhaled beta$_2$-adrenergic drugs and intravenous aminophylline for status asthmaticus did not alter the degree of improvement over a similar regimen without corticosteroids. These authors concluded that corticosteroids did not increase the responsiveness of airways to beta$_2$ agents.

Kaushik, S. P., and Bahna, S. L.   Water and electrolyte balance during acute asthma (abstr.). *Ann. Allergy* 47:117, 1981.

Studies of water and electrolyte balance in 26 patients with status asthmaticus showed no evidence of inappropriate antidiuretic hormone. Serial serum osmolarities showed that significant dehydration was not a consistent finding in every patient.

Loren, M., Chai, H., Miklich, D., and Barwise, G.   Comparison between simple nebulization and intermittent positive-pressure in asthmatic children with severe bronchospasm. *Chest* 72:145–147, 1977.

Therapy with IPPB offers no advantage over simple nebulization in patients with severe, reversible airway obstruction.

Manson, J. I., and Thong, Y. H.   Immunological abnormalities in the syndrome of poliomyelitis-like illness associated with acute bronchial asthma (Hopkin's syndrome). *Arch. Dis. Child.* 55:26–32, 1980.

Report of a serious complication of status asthmaticus, flaccid lower motor neuron paralysis.

McFadden, E. R., and Lyons, H. A.   Arterial blood gas tension in asthma. *N. Engl. J. Med.* 278:1027–1032, 1968.

Age, history of asthma, and duration of acute asthma attack are unrelated to alterations in arterial blood gas values and to the severity of airway obstruction, thus indicating that serial arterial blood gas determinations are important for accurate reflection of the patient's respiratory status.

McKenzie, S. A., Edmunds, A. T., and Godfrey, S.   Status asthmaticus in children. *Arch. Dis. Child.* 54:581–586, 1979.

Another report noting poor correlation among clinical score, evidence for pulsus paradoxicus, and arterial blood gases. The authors also suggest the need for frequent use of arterial blood gases for accurate evaluation of severity.

Mitenko, P. A., and Ogilvie, R. I.   Rational intravenous doses of theophylline. *N. Engl. J. Med.* 289:600–603, 1973.

Pulmonary function improvement in acute asthma varied directly with the log of the serum theophylline concentration between levels of 5 to 20 μg/ml. The authors recommend a loading dose of 5.6 mg/kg, then 0.09 mg/kg/hour by continuous intravenous infusion.

Ormerod, L. P., and Stableforth, D. E.   Asthma mortality in Birmingham 1975–77: 53 deaths. *Br. Med. J.* 280:687–690, 1980.
   Studying the asthma-related deaths of 53 patients, these authors found the following related factors in 38 outpatient deaths: recent hospital or emergency room treatment for asthma (16%), unavailability of aerosol bronchodilators (45%), underuse of corticosteroids (66%), and lack of objective measurement of airflow obstruction (100%).
Petty, T. L.   Status Asthmaticus in Adults. In E. Middleton, Jr., C. E. Reed, and E. F. Ellis (Eds.), *Allergy: Principles and Practice* (2nd ed.). St. Louis: Mosby, 1983. Pp. 987–995.
   Complete discussion of pathophysiology and management of adult status asthmaticus. Recommendation of maintenance aminophylline infusion of 0.09 mg/kg/hour may be somewhat high for older individuals, particularly if they have heart or liver disease.
Pierson, W. E., Bierman, C. W., and Kelley, V. C.   A double-blind trial of corticosteroid therapy in status asthmaticus. *Pediatrics* 54:282–288, 1974.
   The addition of corticosteroids to conventional therapy for status asthmaticus (oxygen, aminophylline, adrenergic agents) enables significantly faster improvement in arterial hypoxemia.
Scoggins, C. H., Sahn, S. A., and Petty, T. L.   Status asthmaticus. A nine-year experience. *JAMA* 238:1158–1162, 1977.
   Mechanical ventilation for severe status asthmaticus is associated with a high rate of morbidity and should be instituted only when it is evident that maximal medical therapy will not be efficacious.
Shapiro, G. G., et al.   Double-blind study of effectiveness of a broad spectrum antibiotic in status asthmaticus. *Pediatrics* 53:867–872, 1974.
   The use of broad-spectrum antibiotics in children and adolescents with status asthmaticus and without clinical evidence of bacterial disease is of no benefit.
Shapiro, G. G., Simons, F., Pierson, W. E., and Bierman, C. W.   The Management of Status Asthmaticus. In C. A. Smith (Ed.), *The Critically Ill Child: Diagnosis and Management* (2nd ed.). Philadelphia: Saunders, 1977. Pp. 178–194.
   Excellent practical review of specifics of therapy for status asthmaticus. Newer specific beta$_2$ agents such as terbutaline were not available at the time this article was written and therefore are not included in the discussion.
Sheehy, A. F., DiBenedetto, R., Lefrak, S., and Lyons, H. A.   Treatment of status asthmaticus—a report of 70 episodes. *Arch. Intern. Med.* 130:37–42, 1972.
   Good correlation in this study of acute asthma between admission arterial blood gas findings (particularly a PCO$_2$ greater than 40 mm Hg) and the likelihood of developing severe asthma requiring mechanical ventilation.
Stalcup, S. A., and Mellins, R. B.   Mechanical forces producing pulmonary edema in acute asthma. *N. Engl. J. Med.* 297:592–596, 1977.
   This study demonstrates mean negative pleural pressures during the entire breathing cycle in patients with acute asthma, and suggests that vigorous fluid therapy in excess of homeostatic amounts favors the development of pulmonary edema.
Tremper, K. K., and Shoemaker, W. C.   Continuous CPR monitoring with transcutaneous oxygen and carbon dioxide sensors. *Crit. Care Med.* 9:417–418, 1981.
   Although there are no studies presently published on transcutaneous monitoring in acute asthma, this study in acutely ill patients demonstrates that transcutaneous sensors for PO$_2$ and PCO$_2$ correlate well with arterial puncture blood gases and provide accurate continuous information on tissue perfusion and oxygen delivery.
Westerfield, B. T., Carder, A. J., and Light, R. W.   The relationship between arterial blood gases and serum theophylline clearance in critically ill patients. *Am. Rev. Respir. Dis.* 124:17–20, 1981.
   Another article noting that theophylline clearance varies markedly for critically ill patients with pulmonary disease. They recommend an aminophylline infusion rate of 0.05 mg/kg/hour in all critically ill patients, with close monitoring of serum theophylline levels.

4. RESPIRATORY FAILURE

Thomas B. Harper

In general, respiratory failure is defined as the inability of the respiratory system to meet the metabolic needs of the body (i.e., to supply sufficient oxygen to the tissues and contribute to control of acid-base balance). Although there are many diverse disease processes that may ultimately lead to respiratory failure, this chapter considers only respiratory failure caused by severe, progressive, acute asthma.

Early identification of the acutely ill asthmatic patient at risk for development of respiratory failure is imperative for successful management. Successful management requires the presence of support personnel with ongoing experience in intensive care medicine and laboratory facilities available on a 24-hour basis. If these resources are not available, a patient at high risk for respiratory failure should be transferred to an appropriate facility as soon as possible. During transport, oxygen, IV fluids, and medications must be maintained and the patient should be attended by someone skilled in tracheal intubation and manual ventilation.

Clinical evaluations alone are unreliable in assessing ventilatory adequacy and in predicting the development of respiratory failure, even if clinical scoring systems are used. If clinical assessment is combined with the results of arterial blood gases, however, the potential for development of respiratory failure can usually be predicted accurately, and appropriate management undertaken. Such a combined scoring system as that developed by Wood and Downes is noted in Table 4.

Two types of respiratory failure have been described. Type I (rare in asthma), which is manifested by low PO_2 and normal or low PCO_2, may be caused by large intracardiac or intrapulmonary shunts or impaired alveolar diffusion. Type II, which is manifested by a low PO_2 and a high PCO_2, is due to alveolar hypoventilation usually caused by muscle weakness and/or tiring.

In status asthmaticus, ventilation-perfusion inequalities initially cause a reduced PO_2 that is accompanied by a reduced PCO_2 secondary to compensatory hyperventilation. As ventilation-perfusion abnormalities and generalized obstruction progress, however, the patient is ultimately unable to sustain adequate ventilation of the alveoli and the PCO_2 begins to rise to normal levels or above.

A diminished arterial PO_2 is always present in patients with respiratory failure; however, some patients in profound respiratory failure may have normal PO_2 if they are inspiring high concentrations of oxygen. All arterial blood gas determinations therefore must be interpreted with the concentration of inspired oxygen known.

Acute respiratory failure in adults and children caused by severe status asthaticus almost always requires mechanical ventilation. Intravenous infusion of isoproterenol has been used to improve respiratory status in some children and young adults, thus preventing mechanical ventilation. However, the vulnerability of the hypoxic myocardium to the effects of nonselective beta-adrenergic agents such as isoproterenol presents a significant hazard to older persons. Recently there have been reports of transient cardiac ischemia and even death from myocardial infarction in adolescents and adults during treatment of status asthmaticus with IV isoproterenol. Therefore, this therapeutic modality cannot be recommended for older adolescents and adults. The continuous IV infusion of salbutamol has been employed in a large number of asthmatic patients in Europe, where such selective beta$_2$-adrenergic drugs are considered the first choice in the treatment of severely ill asthmatic patients, even before aminophylline. Because salbutamol stimulates the myocardium much less than isoprotere-

Table 4. Criteria for diagnosis of respiratory failure

	Clinical asthma score*		
Criterion	0	1	2
Cyanosis (PO_2)	None (70–100)	In room air (< 70)	In 40% O_2 (< 70)
Inspiratory breath sounds	Normal	Unequal	Decreased to absent
Use of accessory muscles	Normal	Moderate	Maximal
Expiratory wheezing	None	Moderate	Maximal
Cerebral function	Normal	Depressed or agitated	Coma

*The criterion for impending respiratory failure is a clinical score of 5 or more (PCO_2 over 55) after routine therapy.
*The criterion for respiratory failure is a clinical score of 7 or more (PCO_2 over 65) after routine therapy.
Source: Modified from Wood and Downes, *J. Allergy Clin. Immunol.* 50:75–81, 1972.

nol and has fewer chronotropic effects, it may be safer to use in adolescent and adult patients with respiratory failure. Isoproterenol was used intravenously for many years before the complications of cardiac ischemia and death were recognized; therefore, the use of salbutamol in adolescents and adults must be approached with great caution. The unavailability of salbutamol in the United States (for IV use) presently eliminates this form of therapy from consideration in the treatment of impending or frank respiratory failure owing to status asthmaticus.

Although mechanical ventilation is the last resort for the severely ill asthmatic patient in respiratory failure, its use should be considered with enough forethought to allow intubation and initiation of artificial ventilation to be performed as an elective procedure, before respiratory arrest is imminent. The aims of mechanical ventilation are to allow the tiring patient to diminish the tremendous work of breathing during status asthmaticus and to restore adequate tissue oxygenation. Although mechanical ventilation is not without significant morbidity and mortality, a favorable outcome can result from attention to details, anticipation of potential problems, and an awareness of complications and how to deal with them.

Elective intubation immediately prior to mechanical ventilation usually does not require neuromuscular blocking agents such as pancuronium bromide. Occasionally, to facilitate cooperation from the extremely combative and anxious patient, these agents must be used. Once the patient is intubated and is being ventilated, sedatives may be given periodically to decrease anxiety and resistance to mechanical ventilation. Because both morphine sulfate and d-tubocurarine directly release histamine from mast cells and basophils, they probably should be avoided.

Mechanical ventilation is best accomplished with elective nasotracheal intubation and use of a volume preset, time-cycled respirator to overcome the increased resistance to air flow of asthmatic airways. Volume, rate, positive end expiratory pressure, and inspired oxygen concentration should be modified during the course of mechanical ventilation according to the patient's clinical response and serial arterial blood gases. Careful attention should be paid to suctioning, positioning of the patient, and to fluid and electrolyte balance. Enough supplemental humidified oxygen should be added to inspired air to maintain arterial oxygen tensions at or above 50 mmHg. As intravenous corticosteroids begin to reduce edema and inflammation in the airways and restore responsiveness to catecholamines, clinical improvement may be aided by serial aerosol treatments with selective beta$_2$-adrenergic agents supplied in line with inspired air and oxygen. The specifics of choosing a particular ventilator and providing ventilatory assistance, and of weaning the patient from the ventilator, are well covered by the annotated references on mechanical ventilation in respiratory failure following this chapter.

Cherniack, R. M.   Management and Intensive Care in Respiratory Failure. In A. P. Fishman (Ed.), *Pulmonary Diseases and Disorders*. New York: McGraw-Hill, 1980. Pp. 1636–1646.
An excellent discussion of theoretical and practical aspects of mechanical ventilation for acute respiratory failure.

Downes, J. J., Fulgencio, T., and Raphaely, R. C.   Acute respiratory failure in infants and children. *Pediatr. Clin. North. Am.* 19:423–445, 1972.
A comprehensive discussion of different diseases causing respiratory failure in children, with diagnostic criteria for respiratory failure owing to diseases of different organ systems (cardiac, respiratory, neurologic). Treatment is discussed in detail.

Flenley, D. C.   Blood Gas Abnormalities and Acute Respiratory Failure. In M. Stein (Ed.), *New Directions in Asthma*. Park Ridge Ill.: American College of Chest Physicians, 1975. Pp. 495–510.
An excellent, in-depth correlation of pathophysiology of respiratory failure in acute asthma and arterial blood gas alterations.

Klaustermeyer, W. B., DiBernardo, R. L., and Hale, F. C.   Intravenous isoproterenol: Rationale for bronchial asthma. *J. Allergy Clin. Immunol.* 55:325–333, 1975.
These authors found that when combined with adequate oxygenation and careful monitoring of heart rhythm and blood pressure, intravenous isoproterenol was safe even for adult asthmatic patients. Response to isoproterenol infusion (initiation or change in dose) was noted to be very rapid, within 2 to 5 minutes.

Kurland, G., Williams, J., and Lewiston, N. J.   Fatal myocardial toxicity during continuous infusion of intravenous isoproterenol therapy of asthma. *J. Allergy Clin. Immunol.* 63:407–411, 1979.
Report of a single case of cardiac arrest and death during intravenous isoproterenol continuous infusion. Postmortem examination showed multiple small areas of myocardial necrosis. This article points up the hazards of using nonselective adrenergic agents such as isoproterenol in hypoxic patients.

Levin, N., and Dillon, J. B.   Status asthmaticus and pancuronium bromide. *JAMA* 222:1265–1268, 1972.
The authors report on the advantages of a nondepolarizing neuromuscular blocking agent (pancuronium bromide) for use in initiating and maintaining paralysis during mechanical ventilation for respiratory failure caused by severe status asthmaticus. Advantages include no direct histamine release from mast cells and basophils and no significant cardiac effects.

Matson, J. R., Loughlin, G. M., and Strunk, R. C.   Myocardial ischemia complicating the use of isoproterenol in asthmatic children. *J. Pediatr.* 92:776–778, 1978.
Report of a case of chest pain associated with myocardial ischemia following use of recommended amounts of intravenous isoproterenol in a 14-year-old boy who apparently had no underlying coronary artery disease. Ischemic pattern was detected with a 12-lead electrocardiogram, but was not seen by chest leads used to monitor cardiac rhythm.

Newth, C. J. L.   Recognition and management of respiratory failure. *Pediatr. Clin. North Am.* 26:617–643, 1979.
A thorough overview of the pathophysiology of all forms of respiratory failure; however, the section on ventilator therapy is superficial.

Parry, W. H., Martorano, F., and Cotton, E. K.   Management of life-threatening asthma with intravenous isoproterenol infusions. *Am. J. Dis. Child.* 130:39–42, 1976.
This article relates these authors' considerable experience using intravenous isoproterenol for severe status asthmaticus. They found that this therapy was useful and only rarely attended by complications (arrhythmias, rebound bronchospasm). Although 27 of 34 severe asthmatic patients responded to this therapy and did not need mechanical ventilation,

their criteria for choosing participants was only a PCO_2 over 40 mmHg. Interestingly, all seven patients with initial pCO_2 over 65 years did not respond to intravenous isoproterenol and had to be mechanically ventilated.

Paterson, J. W.   Human pharmacology: Comparison of intravenous isoprenaline and salbutamol in asthmatic patients. *Postgrad. Med. J.* 47(suppl.):38–39, 1971.
Isoproterenol and salbutamol are equipotent as bronchodilators but salbutamol increases the heart rate one-seventh as much as isoproterenol.

Petty, T. L.   Status Asthmaticus in Adults. In E. Middleton, Jr., C. E. Reed, and E. F. Ellis (Eds.), *Allergy: Principles and Practice* (2nd ed.). St. Louis: Mosby, 1983. Pp. 987–995.
Good summary of major considerations in the management of patients with status asthmaticus who develop respiratory failure, particularly in regard to choice and use of mechanical ventilators.

Simons, F. E. R., Pierson, W. E., and Bierman, C. W.   Respiratory failure in childhood status asthmaticus. *Am. J. Dis. Child.* 131:1097–1101, 1977.
Retrospective review of 19 episodes of respiratory failure caused by severe status asthmaticus. Twelve of nineteen cases possibly could have been prevented with prompt or more appropriate medical therapy.

Simpson, H., Mitchell, I., Inglis, J. M., and Grubb, D. J.   Severe ventilatory failure in asthma in children. *Arch. Dis. Child.* 53:714–721, 1978.
Of 1225 admissions for severe asthma, 6 patients developed respiratory failure requiring mechanical ventilation and all survived. Each patient ventilated had been hospitalized an average of five times during the preceding year.

Warrell, D. A., et al.   Comparison of cardiorespiratory effects of isoprenaline and salbutamol in patients with bronchial asthma. *Br. Med. J.* 1:65–70, 1970.
Isoproterenol causes greater effects on pulmonary ventilation, pulmonary gas exchange, cardiac output, and heart rate than does salbutamol. The effects of salbutamol on heart rate were 10 times less than isoproterenol.

Westerman, D. E., Benatar, S. R., Potgieter, P. D., and Ferguson, A. D.   Identification of the high-risk asthmatic patient—experience with 39 patients undergoing ventilation for status asthmaticus. *Am. J. Med.* 66:565–572, 1979.
Important factors associated with the development of respiratory failure during the course of status asthmaticus included (1) long delays by patients before seeking attention, (2) incomplete assessment of acute asthmatic attacks, (3) underuse of corticosteroids prior to admission, and (4) sedation.

Wood, D. W., Downes, J. J., and Lecks, H. I.   The management of respiratory failure in childhood status asthmaticus. Experience with 30 episodes and evolution of a technique. *J. Allergy* 42:261–267, 1968.
An earlier article discussing criteria for respiratory failure and evolution of ventilatory techniques over several years at one institution. Volume-cycles ventilation with continual neuromuscular blockage (d-tubocurarine) were found most effective. Mean duration of ventilation was 23.9 hours, and major complications during ventilation were (1) mediastinal and subcutaneous emphysema, (2) pneumothorax, (3) cardiac arrest, (4) postextubation subglottic stenosis, and (5) sepsis.

Wood, D. W., Downes, J. J., Scheinkopf, H., and Lecks, H. I.   Intravenous isoproterenol in the management of respiratory failure in childhood status asthmaticus. *J. Allergy Clin. Immunol.* 50:75–81, 1972.
A description of these expert physicians' experience with the specifics of intravenous isoproterenol therapy for status asthmaticus. Of 19 children with status asthmaticus in confirmed respiratory failure, mechanical ventilation was avoided in 18 by using this technique.

LABORATORY DIAGNOSIS

5. IMMUNOGLOBULINS
Jeffrey H. Hill

Structure and Synthesis

Structural definition of antibody molecules began with the demonstration by Tiselius in the 1930s that the electrophoretic mobility of antibody molecules was in the gamma fraction of serum protein and led to the term *gamma globulin* as a synonym for *antibody*. By the 1960s, the term *immunoglobulins* began to replace *gamma globulins* because not all gamma globulins are antibody molecules. There are five classes of immunoglobulins, abbreviated IgM, IgG, IgA, IgE, and IgD.

All of the immunoglobulins have certain features in common (Fig. 1). All are composed of light chains (kappa or lambda, common to all immunoglobulin classes) and heavy chains (mu, gamma, alpha, epsilon, or delta, corresponding to the immunoglobulin class) in 1:1 ratios and are held together by disulfide bridges. All immunoglobulins have antigen binding sites (Fab regions) that are formed by portions of both heavy and light chains. In the area where antigen is bound, the amino acid sequence of the heavy and light chains is extremely variable and apparently accounts for both the specificity of individual antibody molecules and the heterogeneity of antigen binding by immunoglobulins as a whole. Antibody heavy chains are flexible and bend at a hinge region, which allows the antigen binding sites to alter their separation relative to each other and facilitates binding to multiple antigen molecules. Distant from their antigen binding sites, immunoglobulin molecules have regions of constant amino acid sequence (Fc regions) that mediate class-specific biologic activities such as complement activation, binding to phagocytes, or binding to mast cells.

Immunoglobulins are synthesized and secreted by stimulated lymphocytes of the B cell class. B cells have antigen-specific immunoglobulinlike surface receptors. When the appropriate "macrophage-processed" antigen is presented to those receptors by macrophages, the B cell increases production of a specific antibody, begins to secrete that antibody, and is then termed a *plasma cell*. IgG, IgA, and IgE production by plasma cells is significantly increased by the effects of "helper" T cell lymphocytes and decreased by "suppressor" T cell lymphocytes. IgM production appears to be T cell independent. Most plasma cells are found in lymphoid tissues such as lymph nodes, spleen, and Peyer's patches but they can produce antibody at nearly any site in the body.

Although the information necessary to produce immunoglobulin of any class and antigen specificity resides in the DNA sequences present in each B lymphocyte nucleus, it is generally accepted that a plasma cell secretes antibody molecules of a single class and specificity. Research is in progress to define the mechanisms by which a plasma cell becomes "committed" to the production of antibody of a single specificity.

Plasma cells are end-stage cells that die after a limited period of time. For unknown reasons, other antigen-stimulated B cells of the same clone or of similar antigenic specificity multiply and produce "expanded" clones of B cells that do not immediately begin secreting immunoglobulins. When appropriate antigen is presented to these cells at some time in the future, they can either become immunoglobulin-secreting cells (plasma cells) or once again multiply to further expand the B cell clone. By this means, immunologic "memory" can be conferred on the host for years.

Initial exposure to antigen results in detectable antibody levels in the circulation within 7 to 14 days (primary response). Specific antibody levels usually peak during the first month after immunization and then decline over the following weeks to months. The primary response consists mostly of IgM of relatively low affinity. Repeated antigenic exposure results in a detectable increase in circulat-

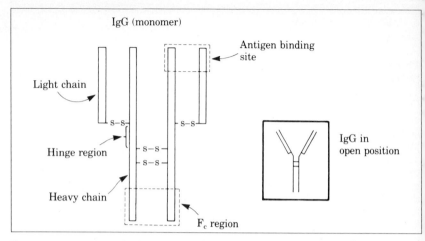

Fig. 1. Schematic diagram of IgG representing features that immunoglobulins have in common.

ing antibody within 48 hours of exposure, with a higher peak at about 1 week and more prolonged antibody production that declines over the following months to years (secondary, or anamnestic, response). The highest, most prolonged elevations in antibody production result from repeated antigen exposure 1 to 2 months apart. Successive immunizations result in the production of larger and larger amounts of increasingly higher-affinity IgG and decreasing amounts of IgM.

Immunoglobulin Classes

Although all immunoglobulins share the properties previously described, each of the five different classes of immunoglobulins has a unique set of properties that expands the range of host defenses.

IgM has a pentameric form with ten antigen binding sites (Fig. 2). IgM production is not T cell dependent, and the antibody is of relatively low affinity. IgM associated with antigen binds complement very effectively through the classical pathway, so much so that a single IgM molecule associated with antigen initiates complement activation. Phagocytes have receptors for the Fc portion of IgM-antigen-complement complexes that increase antigen recognition and phagocytosis. IgM accounts for 10 to 15% of the circulating antibody pool in the adult and relatively more in the child (Table 5). IgM composes a major portion of the antibody produced after a primary antigenic exposure and a decreasing portion with subsequent secondary exposures to antigen. IgM is the major class of antibody produced in response to polysaccharide-containing molecules independent of the number of antigenic exposures. A J chain is attached covalently to two mu chains in plasma cells at sites of external secretion of IgM antibody such as breast, nasal, lacrimal, and parotid glands and in the lamina propria of the intestinal tract. IgM with associated J chain is actively transported by epithelial cells to the luminal surface. This transport is accomplished by combination of IgM-associated J chain with secretory component (synthesized by epithelial cells) at the antiluminal epithelial cell membrane, with subsequent transcellular transport and luminal secretion of that complex from epithelial cells. Secretory component also prevents degradation of IgM in the intestine by the digestive enzymes. IgM composes 3 to 5% of luminal intestinal immunoglobulin and breast

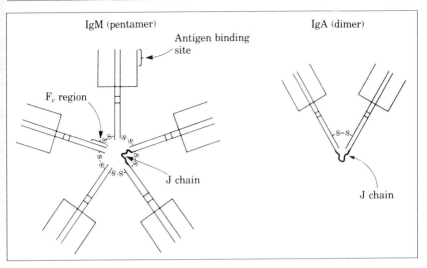

Fig. 2. Schematic diagrams of IgM and IgA.

milk immunoglobulin. IgM does not cross the human placenta; therefore, essentially all IgM in the circulation of the human neonate is of fetal-neonatal origin.

IgG is composed of two light and two heavy chains and has two antigen binding sites (see Fig. 1). IgG production can be enhanced by T helper cells or suppressed T suppressor cells. A significant IgG response to most antigens requires T cell help. The quantity and affinity of IgG antibody for specific antigens increases with multiple antigenic exposures. IgG has four subclasses designated IgG1, IgG2, IgG3, and IgG4. IgG1, IgG2, or IgG3 will activate the classical complement pathway if they are associated with antigen in such a manner that the Fc portions of at least two immunoglobulin molecules are closely and stably juxtaposed. Thus, IgG only activates complement when in high enough concentrations on surfaces, when in appropriate-sized immune complexes (see Chap. 39), or when aggregated. IgG accounts for 80 to 90% of circulating immunoglobulin in the adult and the majority of immunoglobulin in children (see Table 5). IgG is not actively transported into external secretions but a detectable amount apparently diffuses across epithelial membranes into external secretions. Free phagocytes and the fixed phagocytes of the liver, spleen, and lung have receptors for the Fc portion of antigen-associated IgG, which leads to improved recognition and enhanced phagocytosis of foreign protein and particles. IgG is actively transported into the fetus and nearly all IgG in the neonate is of maternal origin.

IgA occurs in monomeric, dimeric, and trimeric forms (see Fig. 2). IgA production is modulated by T cells in a manner similar to that of IgG. IgA does not activate complement by the classical pathway, but when aggregated IgA does activate the alternative pathway. This activation may or may not occur in vivo. IgA accounts for only 10 to 20% of circulating immunoglobulin, but accounts for greater than 80% of immunoglobulin found in the gastrointestinal tract and external glandular secretions. The primary roles of IgA appear to be neutralization of bacterial toxins in the fluids that bathe the mucous membranes and interference with the attachment of viruses and bacteria to epithelial cells, a step that must precede microbial penetration of the epithelial barrier. Similar to IgM,

Table 5. Normal immunoglobulin values

Age	IgG[a]	IgA[a]	IgM[a]
Cord blood	1086 ± 290 (740–1374)	2 ± 2 (0–15)	14 ± 6 (0–22)
1–3 months	512 ± 152 (280–950)	16 ± 10 (4–36)	28 ± 14 (15–86)
4–6 months	520 ± 180 (240–884)	22 ± 14 (11–52)	36 ± 18 (21–74)
7–12 months	742 ± 226 (281–1280)	54 ± 17 (22–112)	76 ± 27 (36–150)
13–24 months	945 ± 270 (290–1300)	67 ± 19 (9–143)	88 ± 36 (18–210)
25–36 months	1030 ± 152 (546–1562)	89 ± 34 (21–196)	94 ± 23 (43–115)
3–5 yr	1150 ± 244 (546–1760)	126 ± 31 (56–284)	87 ± 24 (26–121)
6–8 yr	1187 ± 289 (596–1744)	147 ± 35 (56–330)	108 ± 37 (54–260)
9–11 yr	1217 ± 261 (744–1719)	146 ± 38 (44–203)	104 ± 46 (27–215)
12–16 yr	1248 ± 221 (796–1647)	168 ± 54 (64–290)	96 ± 31 (60–140)
Adult	1274 ± 280 (564–1825)	227 ± 53 (59–311)	127 ± 46 (45–205)

[a]mg/dl (mean ± 1 standard deviation and range).
Source: data by Ellis, E. F., and Robbins, J. B. In T.R. Johnson, U. M. Moore, and J. E. Jeffries (Eds.), *Children are Different: Developmental Physiology* (2nd ed.). Columbus, OH: Ross Laboratories, 1978. P. 187.

IgA is actively secreted into external fluids by mechanisms involving the J chain and secretory component.

IgE has a structure similar to that of IgG and its production is modulated by T cells. IgE accounts for less than 1% of circulating immunoglobulin. The majority of IgE is bound to mast cells or basophils where its membrane concentration is relatively high. IgE associated with antigen does not activate complement, although aggregated IgE may activate complement through the alternative pathway. This activation has no known relevance in vivo. When one antigen molecule combines with two or more IgE molecules bound to basophils or mast cells, those cells release preformed, biologically active molecules from their granules into the extracellular milieu and begin to synthesize and secrete molecules that are not stored. Among other things, these molecules mediate increased vascular permeability (e.g., wheal-and-flare reactions), smooth muscle contraction (e.g., bronchoconstriction in an allergic person with asthma), and eosinophil chemotaxis (e.g., eosinophil influx into sites of parasitic infections).

IgD composes a very small portion of circulating immunoglobulin postnatally although it may represent 10 to 25% of circulating immunoglobulin in the second trimester of fetal life. The function of circulating IgD is not clear. IgD is present on the surface of the majority of nonantibody-secreting B cells. IgD may be very important as a "primitive" receptor for the uncommitted B cell and may play a significant role in determining the antigenic commitment of a naive B cell.

Immunoglobulin Deficiency

Immunoglobulin deficiency is the most common immunodeficiency. It can be inherited or acquired and has a relatively homogeneous presentation, even though its etiology is heterogeneous. Individuals with hypogammaglobulinemia can (1) lack B cells entirely, (2) have B cells that are unable to differentiate into immunoglobulin-secreting plasma cells, (3) lack T helper cells, or (4) have excessive numbers of T suppressor cells. The end effect in each of these cases is the inability of the host to manufacture adequate amounts of antibody to prevent infections. Hypogammaglobulinemic patients commonly have recurrent sinopulmonary infections and recurrent diarrhea. If the defect is severe enough, failure to thrive can occur in children, and chronic recurrent pyogenic pulmonary infections can result in bronchiectasis. Overwhelming bacterial infection can occur, but is not the usual presentation.

A presumed diagnosis can be made in adults who have an appropriate history and a total serum IgG less than 300 mg/dl. Further support can be gained by demonstration of deficient isohemagglutinin production (antibody to ABO blood group antigens), which indicates deficient specific IgM production, and inadequate antitetanus titers, which indicate deficient specific IgG production. Inadequate secondary responses to specific immunizations can also be demonstrated in individuals with hypogammaglobulinemia. To make the diagnosis of primary hypogammaglobulinemia, other causes, such as significant renal or intestinal protein losses, major intercurrent illnesses (particularly infections), and use of immunosuppressive drugs, must be ruled out. Each person's specific defect can be determined, if desired, through laboratory studies available in many academic medical institutions. Such information may assist in genetic counseling, as in the case where immunoglobulin deficiency is due to absence of B cells, a defect that is transmitted in an X-linked recessive pattern.

Diagnosis of hypogammaglobulinemia in young children is more difficult. Although the fetus is capable of making antigen-specific IgM and IgG by the end of the first trimester, the range of antigens that can evoke a response and the magnitude of that response seem to be restricted. In addition, T helper cells do not function well in the fetus and T suppressor cell activity is increased. Maternal IgG is actively transported across the placenta into the fetus, and essentially all IgG in the newborn is of maternal origin. Other immunoglobulins do not cross the placental barrier in significant amounts. Fetal concentrations of IgG reach approximately 600 mg/dl by 28 weeks' gestation and 1000 mg/dl by 36 weeks' gestation. In the preterm infant, repeated phlebotomy in the first few days of life may further decrease circulating IgG and render the neonate relatively hypogammaglobulinemic. IgG levels reach a nadir between 2 and 5 months after birth; adult levels are reached by 3 to 5 years of age. IgM reaches adult levels by 2 to 3 years of age, but IgA and IgE usually do not reach adult levels until adolescence. The diagnosis of hypogammaglobulinemia in children is made from a strong clinical history of recurrent or chronic infections, the demonstration of low immunoglobulin compared with age-matched controls (see Table 5), and deficient specific antibody titers and secondary antibody responses. The older the child, the more reliable are the results of these measurements. Isohemagglutinins are frequently low in normal children less than 1 year of age, and antitetanus titers can vary owing to varying immunization schedules.

"Transient hypogammaglobulinemia of infancy" is a poorly defined entity of low immunoglobulin levels in a child younger than 2 years of age with a history of usually non-life-threatening recurrent infections. In these children, specific antibody titers are usually low during infection but return to normal when the infection clears. With immunoglobulin measurements every 6 months and free use of appropriate antibiotics during febrile episodes, these children can usually be observed without immunoglobulin therapy. By 2 years of age, the child has usually experienced either a reduction of the recurrent minor infectious episodes with an increase of immunoglobulin into the normal range, or continued or increased recurrent infections with falling immunoglobulin levels and decreasing specific antibody titers consistent with true variable hypogammaglobulinemia.

Treatment of Hypogammaglobulinemia

Immunoglobulin therapy is aimed at elevating serum IgG to levels that decrease the morbidity of infections. That serum level is different for each patient, but most patients will have significantly decreased morbidity if serum IgG levels are maintained at levels greater than 300 mg/dl. Since the half-life of circulating immunoglobulin is approximately 3 weeks, reasonably constant levels are maintained by injections of immunoglobulins every 2 to 4 weeks. Until recently, the only immunoglobulin preparation available was administered intramuscularly. The recommended dosage of Ig is 100 mg/kg as a loading dose, followed by 100 mg/kg every 28 days (equivalent to 0.6 ml of the commercially available IM preparation per kg per month). Even in a small adult or average-sized adolescent, this dose every 2 weeks becomes large in volume (e.g., 15 ml intramuscularly every 2 weeks in a 50 kg person). In a large person, the injections can become limited by pain, available muscle mass, and patient compliance. Attempts to transfuse with plasma as an alternative immunoglobulin source have been limited by the immediate side effects of volume expansion and long-term risks of hepatitis, cytomegalovirus infection, and so on.

In the past, it was not possible to administer purified immunoglobulin intravenously. Available preparations contained immunoglobulin aggregates that caused complement activation, which was responsible for an anaphylactoid reaction with symptoms such as nausea, flushing, chills, arthralgias, abdominal cramping, anxiety, headache, hypotension, tachycardia, and (in rare cases) shock. Recently a preparation of human immunoglobulin for IV use has become commercially available. Immunoglobulin aggregation is prevented by mild reduction and alkylation of the disulfide bonds, and the preparation is stabilized with 10% maltose. When this preparation was given intravenously at a rate of 40 to 60 mg/kg/hr less than 5% of infusions resulted in even mild side effects, none of which required stopping or decreasing the rate of infusion. The IV preparation has been shown to decrease morbidity caused by hypogammaglobulinemia at least as well as the IM preparation, and it is possible that the increased amounts of immunoglobulin that can be given intravenously may result in much better control of disease symptoms than has previously been possible. Use of the IV preparation is currently limited by its high cost, the need for IV administration over several hours with close nursing observation, and the need for a readily available physician in the event of a systemic reaction.

Another method of administering immunoglobulin in large quantities has recently been described and may be useful in the future. The technique consists of a slow subcutaneous administration of the standard IM preparation by a portable slow infusion pump similar to that being used for constant insulin infusion.

Berger, M., Cupps, T. R., and Fauci, A. S.   Ig replacement therapy by slow subcutaneous infusion. *Ann. Intern. Med.* 93:55–56, 1980.
  This article describes the safety and efficacy of slow subcutaneous Ig infusion.
Litman, G. W., and Good, R. A.   Immunoglobulins. *Comprehensive Immunology* 5:1–381, 1978.
  An exhaustive discussion of immunoglobulin structure, function, and genetic control. An excellent reference for the basic immunologist but not for the clinician.
Nolte, M. T., Pirofsky, B., Gerritz, G. A., and Golding, B.   Intravenous immunoglobulin therapy for antibody deficiency. *Clin. Exp. Immunol.* 36:237–243, 1979.
  The authors found that 40% less infections occurred with IV Ig than with IM Ig therapy.

Ochs, H. D., et al.   Safety and patient acceptability of intravenous immune globulin in 10% maltose. *Lancet* 2:1158–1159, 1980.
  Double-blind prospective study showing adverse reactions to IV immunoglobulin administration during less than 5% of infusions.
Ochs, H. D., and Wedgwood, R. J.   Disorders of the Cell System. In E. R. Stiehm and V. A. Fulginiti (Eds.), *Immunologic Disorders in Infants and Children.* Philadelphia: Saunders, 1980. Pp. 239–285.
  Excellent discussion of clinical syndromes associated with primary B cell dysfunction resulting in deficient immunoglobulin production. This book is an excellent clinical resource on immunologic disorders.
Stiehm, E. R.   The B-lymphocyte System. In E. R. Stiehm and V. A. Fulginiti (Eds.), *Immunologic Disorders in Infants and Children.* Philadelphia: Saunders, 1980. Pp. 52–81.
  Excellent review of immunoglobulin synthesis, structure, and function and some clinical correlations.
Summary Report of a Medical Research Council Working Party. Hypogammaglobulinemia in the United Kingdom. *Lancet* 1:163–168, 1969.
  Prospective 10-year study of hypogammaglobulinemia and efficacy of immunoglobulin therapy at different doses. IM dosage is based on this article.

6. RADIOALLERGOSORBENT TEST
James D. Oggel and Don A. Bukstein

The radioallergosorbent test (RAST) was first described in 1967 by Wide and colleagues. It is a semiquantitative solid phase radioimmunoassay that allows for measurement of allergen-specific IgE in vitro. Whereas the paper radioimmunosorbent test (PRIST) measures total IgE antibody in a patient's serum, the RAST measures only that portion of the IgE that interacts with a specific allergen (e.g., ragweed pollen).

In this procedure selected allergens are first covalently linked to a cellulose or paper disk. An appropriate dilution of patient serum is added to the disk. IgE antibodies to that allergen present in the serum bind to the allergen on the disk. Unbound antibody, specifically other IgE molecules that are not specific for the tested allergen, are eliminated with subsequent washings. In the next step, radioactively tagged anti-human IgE antibody of the IgG class is mixed with the disk-allergen-IgE complex. The radiolabeled IgG antibody binds to the IgE molecules on the disk. After washing away the excess reagent, the disk-allergen-IgE-IgG complex is counted in a gamma counter, measuring the amount of radioactivity present. Hence, a semiquantitative measurement is derived that is related to the amount of allergen-specific IgE present in the patient's serum that bound to the disk. If there is a high quantity of allergen-specific IgE in the patient's serum, there will be a high count. If there is little allergen-specific IgE, the count will be correspondingly low. To be labeled positive, the tubes with the serum being tested should have radioactive counts at least three times higher than the tubes with the negative control serum. Figure 3 outlines this procedure. RASTs are available commercially to measure specific IgE antibodies against many inhalant allergens, a few foods, stinging insects, and the major determinant of penicillin—there is no RAST for antibodies to penicillin's minor determinants.

The comparative merits of skin tests and RASTs for routine diagnosis of specific allergens responsible for IgE-mediated disease have been the subject of much discussion recently. The following statements on this subject have been adapted by the American Academy of Allergy:

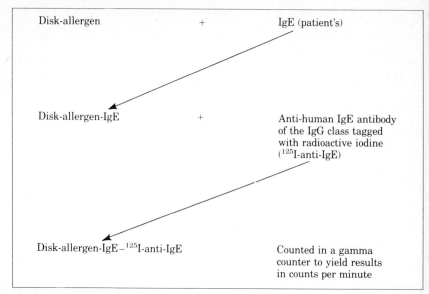

Fig. 3. Diagram of complex formation during RAST.

1. Optimally performed skin tests and RASTs both detect IgE antibody accurately and reproducibly.
2. Within the constraints of each method, both skin tests and RASTs yield information of a semiquantitative nature, but the RAST is less sensitive than skin tests.
3. Results of both tests usually correlate equally well with allergic symptoms and signs produced by exposure to the specific allergen tested.
4. Both tests can be used as grounds for instituting immunotherapy in an efficient and economic manner. Where the RAST is used as grounds for immunotherapy, a skin test with the planned initial dilution of immunotherapy solution should be done before starting immunotherapy to prove that the patient tolerates in vivo administration of this allergenic extract.
5. Skin tests appear to be superior to currently available RASTs in the diagnosis of certain life-threatening anaphylactic states where maximum sensitivity is important, particularly in the diagnosis of penicillin and Hymenoptera allergy.
6. The results of skin tests are more immediately available. While both tests can be initiated at the time of the patient's visit, the results of skin tests are available in about 45 minutes; RAST results are available in 2 to 3 days.
7. RAST is preferable to skin testing in certain conditions, where skin testing is unsatisfactory, particularly where there is dermatographia or widespread skin disease.
8. Skin tests are usually more cost effective than RASTs. Based on skin test and RAST charges from sources participating in the analysis, RAST cost two to six times more than skin tests per allergen tested.

Adkinson, N. F., Jr. The radioallergosorbent test: Use and abuses. *J. Allergy Clin. Immunol.* 65:1–4, 1980.
   This editorial discusses the appropriate use of the RAST.

Adkinson, N. F., Jr.   The radioallergosorbent test in 1981–limitations and refinements. *J. Allergy Clin. Immunol.* 67:87–89, 1981.
  This editorial places the RAST in perspective.
American Academy of Allergy: Statement by the Executive Committee. Position statement on use of radioallergosorbent and IgE tests in practice. *J. Allergy Clin. Immunol.* 66:431, 1980.
  This is an important position statement.
American Academy of Allergy.   Position statement. Skin testing and radioallergosorbent testing (RAST) for diagnosis of specific allergens responsible for IgE-mediated diseases. *J. Allergy Clin. Immunol.* 72:515–517, 1983.
  This position statement details the usefulness of both these studies.
Berg, T. L. O., and Johansson, S. G. O.   Allergy diagnosis with radioallergosorbent test. A comparison with results of skin and provocation tests in an unselected group of children with asthma and hay fever. *J. Allergy Clin. Immunol.* 54:209–221, 1974.
  Correlates provocation testing with the RAST.
Evans, R.   Advances in the Diagnosis of Allergy: RAST. *Proceedings of the First North American Conference on RAST.* Miami: Symposium Specialist, 1975.
  Monograph on various aspects and details of the RAST as used and understood.
Wide, L., Bennich, H., and Johansson, S. G. O.   Diagnosis of allergy by an in vitro test for allergen antibodies. *Lancet* 2:1105–1107, 1967.
  Classic article describing the RAST as currently used.
Yunginger, J. W., and Gleich, G. J.   The impact of the discovery of IgE on the practice of allergy. *Pediatr. Clin. North Am.* 22:3–15, 1975.
  Summarizes the RAST procedure and evaluates its accuracy and place in allergy practice.
Zimmermann, E. M., Yunginger, J. W., and Gleich, G. J.   Interference in ragweed pollen and honeybee venom radioallergosorbent tests. *J. Allergy Clin. Immunol.* 66:386–393, 1980.
  Describes an assay measuring existence of IgG antibodies in the serum of immunotherapy patients interfering with RAST accuracy.

7. SKIN TESTING
Robert C. Strunk and Don A. Bukstein

Identification of allergens responsible for precipitating respiratory, skin, or gastrointestinal symptoms is essential for the appropriate management of patients with allergic disease. As discussed in chapters 18, 20, and 23 a thorough history emphasizing cause and effect relationships between exposure to potential allergens and symptoms is the most important tool in this identification process. Allergy skin testing is the most useful laboratory adjunct to the history. When appropriately performed, it is the single most sensitive test for detecting specific allergic homocytotropic antibody (usually IgE, though occasionally IgG) in the skin. The results of the skin tests also reflect the presence of homocytotropic antibody in the blood and respiratory and gastrointestinal tracts.

Skin testing is generally performed for one of three reasons: (1) to clarify historical information and identify which of several possible allergens may be causing symptoms, (2) to detect allergens that may not be suggested by the history, and (3) to confirm the presence of specific IgE antibodies prior to initiation of hyposensitization. To yield useful information, skin tests must be performed by experienced technicians using valid antigens and good technique. Implicit in these guidelines is the recommendation that skin testing not be performed unless it can be done frequently by someone with the potential to become expert in the techniques necessary.

Immunologic Basis for Skin Testing

Allergy skin testing is used as a bioassay because it has the ability to specifically identify antibodies (immunoglobulin) capable of precipitating a type 1 immediate hypersensitivity reaction. The antibodies identified in skin testing have become attached to the surface of mast cells present in the skin. These antibodies are usually of the IgE class. Combination of antigen with the surface-bound IgE gives a signal to the mast cells that leads to the release of histamine and other mediators of the immediate hypersensitivity response. Histamine stimulates nerve endings, producing the itching sensation, and also causes the small capillaries in the area to dilate and leak plasma, thus resulting in the wheal-and-flare reaction. The patient feels an itching sensation within minutes, and the reaction generally progresses to its peak within 15 to 20 minutes. This immediate wheal-and-flare response may also be followed in 6 to 12 hours by a delayed (or late-phase) reaction, which is thought to be caused by the release of neutrophil chemotactic factor(s) from the mast cell and subsequent migration of neutrophils into the skin test site.

Antigen Selection

The history is always the most important guide in selection of skin tests. In a patient with specific seasonal symptoms that have recurred regularly over several years, the list of antigens used would be small and selection of the antigens would be directed by knowledge of the seasonal pattern of antigens in the area. When the history is not clear and skin testing is being done to detect allergens that might be relevant, the list of allergens may be much larger, but generally would not exceed 40 to 50 separate antigens. A list of the general categories of antigens is included in Table 6. Properly prepared extracts to food are among the most valid antigens. Skin tests for foods are done if there is any question of problem with these allergens, for it is important to sort out the nature of the complaints and to avoid unnecessary elimination of important food from a diet.

When respiratory symptoms occur alone without a suggestion of a relationship to the ingestion of foods, skin tests for foods are generally not useful. Along with the foods, pollen antigens are the most potent and therefore the most reliable

Table 6. List of suggested routine skin tests

Foods
Pollens
  Grasses
  Trees
  Weeds
Molds
  Alternaria
  Hormodendrum
  Aspergillus
  Helminthosporium
  Penicillium
Environmental agents
  House dust
  Mixed feathers (chicken, duck, goose)
  Dog
  Cat
  Mite
Histamine
Control (diluent)

skin-test reagents. It is essential to be familiar with pollens characteristic of the area in which the patient lives and to know how the prevalence of pollen varies with the seasons. There are several general rules that apply to the selection of pollen antigens for skin testing. Grasses tend to share antigens and most patients need to be tested with a maximum of only two to three different grasses. Rye grass contains the antigens present in most other grasses, however, timothy is relatively deficient in these antigens. Therefore, in parts of the country where these grasses are prevalent, both timothy and rye should be used for testing. Bermuda grass has unique antigens and does not share antigens with either rye or timothy; therefore, it needs to be tested separately. Pollen from trees and weeds varies widely in antigenicity and more antigens must be chosen from these classes.

Unlike the pollen antigens, mold antigens have a less well-defined seasonal pattern and the prevalence of a single mold within a particular time is not clearly distinguishable from the prevalence of other molds. Therefore, if mold antigens are suspected of being a problem, a larger number of molds must be selected. For most areas of the country, the five molds listed in Table 6 are important, however, a given section of the country may have molds unique to it and the list would then have to be expanded.

Environmental antigens cause the most problems. House dust is a mixture of antigens that varies widely from one part of the country to another and from one house to another. Commercial extracts are obtained only from a given part of the country and therefore may be totally irrelevant for a particular patient. In addition, the large number of antigens present in house dust tend to dilute any single antigen and make the testing less valuable. In general, dog and cat antigens are very prevalent in commercial housedust mixtures, and a positive house dust skin test is often due to a specific sensitivity to dog or cat dander. In general, dog, cat, and other animal dander extracts are not potent and a negative skin test does not mean that a patient is not sensitive to these animals. In addition to their lack of potency, it is widely suspected that there may be variation between species of dogs or cats or other animals and that species-specific extracts would be more appropriate. Not listed in Table 6 are a number of other environmental antigens that may be pertinent for a given location or a given patient. One example of such a group is insect antigens, especially cockroach, which can be extremely prevalent in certain areas and can be a major cause of allergic symptomatology.

Skin testing is also used for identification of patients sensitive to either Hymenoptera or penicillin (see Chaps. 40 and 44).

Skin-Test Techniques

Skin tests may be carried out by several different methods. These can be separated into two general categories: (1) epicutaneous techniques using concentrated solutions of the extracts (generally 1:10 or 1:20 weight-volume) either by abrading the skin and placing a drop of the extract onto the abrasion (scratch test), or by pushing the antigen into the skin with a sharp probe (puncture or prick test); and (2) intradermal testing using more dilute solutions (generally 1:1000 weight-volume) and injecting a small amount of the extract, generally 0.02 ml, into the dermis. The epicutaneous tests detect less antigen than the intradermal tests. But the epicutaneous tests correlate better with clinical sensitivity than do the intradermal tests, which identify patients who have no end-organ sensitivity when direct challenge tests are performed.

Epicutaneous tests are generally applied on the back unless the patient has experienced anaphylaxis, in which case the arms are used to allow application of a tourniquet if a reaction occurs. The patient lies prone and the back is cleansed with alcohol. After the alcohol has dried, skin responsiveness is ensured by a test with a histamine solution (Eli-Lilly, 1:1000) on the lower back where there is least reactivity, If no wheal occurs or if the wheal is less than 3 mm with little or no erythema, testing is abandoned until a later time. A small drop of a concentrated solution (generally 1:10 or 1:20) of each antigen is placed on the back by a corresponding number. The puncture or prick is made through the antigen drop using a sharp "testing" needle obtained from a surgical supply firm. The space between antigen drops should be 5 cm. The needle should be wiped with a clean alcohol sponge between punctures or pricks. In many patients there is an unpredictable degree of variability between duplicates using single antigens and either duplicate tests for single antigens should be done or the testing repeated if there is a discrepancy between the history and the skin-test results. The test results are read in 15 to 20 minutes, immediately after the antigens have been blotted (not rubbed) off with dry cotton balls. If reactions become intense before 20 minutes, the antigens may be removed to decrease absorption and decrease the intensity of the reaction. For testing in young children who have a difficult time remaining prone during the entire 20 minutes before the reaction can be read, the antigens can be removed immediately after all drops have been punctured and the child can then be allowed to play for the 20 minutes before the test results are read. Recent evidence has shown that the results obtained in this way are comparable to those obtained when the antigens are left on the skin for the entire 20 minutes.

Intradermal testing is done on the posterior and lateral regions of the upper arms or on the volar surface of the forearm. Sites should be low enough to permit proximal placement of a tourniquet. The area is cleansed and numbered as with prick testing. Short 30-gauge needles and a 0.5- or 1.0-ml syringe are used. The syringe should never be reused for a different antigen even after sterilization because of the possibility of contamination of a new antigen with the old antigen. Enough solution is injected to produce a definite but very small bleb (of approximately 3 mm in diameter). This generally requires approximately 0.02 ml. If air is injected by mistake, or if bleeding or leaking of the solution occurs, the test should be repeated at another site. Intradermal tests are useful in supplementing the results of the epicutaneous tests that have been negative. This is especially important when the history suggests that there is a definite sensitivity to an allergen that has been negative in the epicutaneous tests. This most commonly occurs for antigens that are of weak potency or poorly characterized, such as the environmental allergens or molds. Intradermal skin tests can also be useful in young children, less than 3 years of age, who do not have large amounts of IgE in their skin and thus may have negative epicutaneous tests though they have clinical sensitivity.

Assessment of the reaction is most appropriately done by measuring the long and short diameters of the wheals and recording a mean diameter. Wheals are also graded as 1 + to 4 +, but this method is less precise and interpretation varies from practitioner to practitioner. It is important to measure the wheals and only note excessive flares, because flares without wheals generally do not correlate with clinical symptoms. The results of any antigen skin test must always be compared with a test performed with diluent alone to take into consideration the skin's reaction to the trauma of the testing (often an indication of dermatographism). In general it is not possible to say that a meaningful test should always be a particular size and that anything below that size is not meaningful. Tests must be always interpreted in light of the clinical history and a positive test (wheal with allergen larger than the wheal with diluent) should never be disregarded. It is true, however, that larger positive skin tests tend to be more closely related to clinical symptoms than small positive tests.

Large positive skin tests can continue to itch intensely for several hours. Applying topical adrenaline-epinephrine nasal solution, 1:1000, to positive reactions after the results have been recorded can reduce this problem. Any systemic reaction following skin testing should be treated with aqueous epinephrine,

1:1000, followed by an antihistamine. A tourniquet is applied above the test site if the site has been on the arm. The patient should always be kept in the office for at least 1 hour following testing to ensure that no serious immediate reactions occur. Analysis of late-phase responses should be done by observing the patient's skin-testing sites at a 6- and 24-hour interval following the testing. This can be especially important for mold antigens.

Factors Affecting Results

Numerous factors can affect the results of skin testing in a particular patient; therefore, it is extremely important that the practitioner keep in mind the possibility of an inaccurate result. The first factor is age. Patients at the extremes of the age groups (younger than 2 years of age and older than 70) tend to have decreased skin reactivity to both histamine and specific allergens to which clinical sensitivity is known to occur. A second factor is the circadian rhythm by which the skin responds to an allergen. Skin responses are increased in the afternoon and late evening and lowest in the morning. The differences are not extremely large, however, and it is unlikely that testing in the morning would result in a negative skin test to an allergen for which there is a definite clinical sensitivity. Interpretation of wheal size in relation to possible clinical sensitivity can be altered by this phenomenon. The third factor is the effect of drugs on skin reactivity. Antihistamines clearly affect skin-test results. The effect of some antihistamines can last for as long as 4 days after the last dose of antihistamine has been taken. In general, patients should be tested only after they have been off all antihistamines for 48 hours, unless the antihistamine is hydroxyzine, in which case the interval should be at least 96 hours. Other drugs commonly used in the treatment of allergic disease, such as beta$_2$ sympathomimetics, theophylline, and prednisone, have been shown not to affect the results of skin tests when given in usual doses for short periods of time. However, these studies have not demonstrated that drugs used in combination or over long periods of time do not suppress skin reactivity to some extent; therefore, the patient should be on the minimal amount of drug necessary to control symptoms at the time the skin tests are done. Finally, the location on the skin will alter the result to a given allergen. In general, the lower part of the back is least reactive and the volar area of the forearm is more sensitive than the radial area. In addition, the area of the forearm near the cubital crease produces larger reactions than the area near the styloid process.

Many parents and patients dread skin testing as a major ordeal or expense. A clear description of the minimal discomfort associated with epicutaneous testing, and the slight transient pain of a few required intradermal tests will reassure them. Parents should also be told that skin testing is not necessarily followed by injection therapy. Patients should receive a printed sheet advising avoidance of premedication and describing the possible appearance of delayed reactions. These instructions should be reinforced verbally.

Abramowitz, P. W., Perez, M. M., Johnson, C. E., and McLean, J. A.   Effect of theophylline, terbutaline and their combination on the immediate hypersensitivity skin test reaction. *J. Allergy Clin. Immunol.* 66:123–128, 1980.
   A combination of theophylline and terbutaline had no effect on skin-test results.
Barbee, R. A., Lebowitz, M. D., Thompson, H. C., and Burrows, B.   Immediate skin-test reactivity in a general population sample. *Ann. Intern. Med.* 84:129–133, 1976.
   An interesting look at allergen skin-test reactivity in a community population sample and its correlation with age, histamine skin reactions, and total IgE.
Bocks, S. A., Lee, W. Y., Remigio, L. K., and May, C. D.   Studies of hypersensitivity reactions to foods in infants and children. *J. Allergy Clin. Immunol.* 62:327–334, 1978.
   Demonstration that the clinical impression of food allergy can be supported by the presence

of positive skin tests to food extracts that correlate very well with reproduction of symptoms on double-blind food challenge.

Brown, W. G., Halonen, M. J., Kaltenborn, W. T., and Barbee, R. A.   The relationship of respiratory allergy, skin test reactivity, and serum IgE in a community population sample. *J. Allergy Clin. Immunol.* 63:328–335, 1979.
The authors showed that prick skin-test reactivity correlates with both total and specific IgE and allergic symptomatology, but intradermal reactions in the absence of prick reactivity do not correlate with either clinical or immunologic evidence of allergy.

Bruce, C. A., Rosenthal, R. R., Lichtenstein, L. M., and Norman, P. S.   Diagnostic tests in ragweed-allergic asthma. A comparison of direct skin tests, leukocyte histamine release, and quantitative bronchial challenge. *J. Allergy Clin. Immunol.* 53:230–239, 1974.
Outlines the usefulness of diagnostic tests in predicting clinical sensitivity to a specific allergen.

Cavanaugh, M. J., Bronsky, E. A., and Buckley, J. M.   Clinical value of bronchial provocation testing in childhood asthma. *J. Allergy Clin. Immunol.* 59:41–47, 1977.
Information derived from bronchial provocation can be predicted with a high degree of accuracy from a puncture test with 5-mm wheal.

Chipps, B. E., Talamo, R. C., Mellits, E. D., and Valentine, M. D. Immediate (IgE-mediated) skin testing in the diagnosis of allergic disease. *Ann. Allergy* 41:211–215, 1978.
Showed that intradermal end-point titration skin tests seemed to be much more specific than prick or scratch method. There was a relatively better correlation between prick and intradermal tests than between scratch and intradermal skin tests.

Chipps, B. E., et al.   Effect of theophylline and terbutaline on immediate skin tests. *J. Allergy Clin. Immunol.* 65:61–64, 1980.
No changes in intradermal end-point titration skin tests were seen with theophylline or terbutaline therapy.

Cook, T. J., et al.   Degree and duration of skin-test suppression and side effects with antihistamines. A double-blind controlled study with five antihistamines. *J. Allergy Clin. Immunol.* 51:71–77, 1973.
All antihistamines of the five major groups suppressed allergy skin tests. Longest duration of suppression was 4 days (hydroxyzine) and the shortest was 2 days (diphenhydramine). Side effects of the antihistamines did not parallel the effectiveness in suppressing skin-test reactivity.

Galant, S. P., and Maibach, H. I.   Reproducibility of allergy epicutaneous test techniques. *J. Allergy Clin. Immunol.* 51:245–250, 1973.
The authors compared the various epicutaneous techniques in terms of variability and reproducibility, and found that variability was large for each of the epicutaneous techniques. The variability was less when the same region of the back was used. The middle region of the back was most sensitive and the bottom region the least. There was good reproducibility for all epicutaneous tests during the 4-week period of the study.

Hagy, G. W., and Settipane, G. A.   Prognosis of positive allergy skin tests in an asymptomatic population. A three-year follow-up of college students. *J. Allergy Clin. Immunol.* 48:200–211, 1971.
Many patients have positive skin tests without evidence of clinical sensitivity.

Imber, W. E.   Allergic skin testing: A clinical investigation. *J. Allergy Clin. Immunol.* 60:47–55, 1977.
The effects of skin-test method, concentration, diluent, manufacturer, and mixtures of various antigens on skin test to inhalant antigens were tested.

Indrajana, T., Speiksma, F. T. M., and Voorhorst, R.   Comparative study of the intracutaneous, scratch and prick tests in allergy. *Ann. Allergy* 29:639–650, 1971.
The mean wheal size of various concentrations of intradermal, prick, and scratch tests were compared and showed that concentrations gave reactions of equal size.

Murphree, J. T., and Kniker, W. T.   Correlation of immediate skin test responses to antigens introduced by Multi-Test[R] and intracutaneous routes. *Ann. Allergy* 43:279–285, 1979.
Skin-test responses administered by Multi-Test were comparable to those obtained from the same antigens applied intradermally in aqueous dilutions of 1:1000 or 1:1500 wt/vol.

Nelson, H. S.   The clinical relevance of IgE. *Ann. Allergy* 49:73–75, 1982.
An excellent review article outlining the usefulness of IgE determination, cutaneous skin tests, and RAST testing.

Reddy, P. M., et al.   Reappraisal of intracutaneous tests in the diagnosis of reaginic al-
lergy. *J. Allergy Clin. Immunol.* 61:36–41, 1978.
*This study concluded that a negative prick skin test (with 1 : 50 wt/vol antigen solution) and
a positive intradermal test (1 : 1000 wt/vol) do not indicate the presence of reaginic allergy.*
Shapiro, G., Bierman, C. W., Furukawa, C. T., and Pierson, W. E.   Allergy skin testing:
Science or quackery? *Pediatrics* 59:495–498, 1977.
A discussion of the value and limitations of skin testing.
Sheldon, J. M., Lovell, R. G., and Matthews, K. P.   *A Manual of Clinical Allergy.* Philadel-
phia: Saunders, 1967. Pp. 507–532.
Best description of different skin-testing techniques.
Siraganian, R. P., and Hook, W. A.   Histamine Release and Assay Methods for the Study
of Human Allergy. In M. R. Rose and H. Friedman (Eds.), *Manual of Clinical Immunol-
ogy* (2nd ed.). Washington D.C.: The American Society for Microbiology, 1980. Chapter
80. Pp. 1480–1507.
The most authoritative review of various methods used to investigate human allergy.
Smith, A., Mansfield, L. E., deShazo, R. D., and Nelson, H. S.   An evaluation of the
pharmacologic inhibition of the immediate and late cutaneous reaction to allergen. *J.
Allergy Clin. Immunol.* 65:118–121, 1980.
*Study of H_1 and H_2 antihistamines on skin tests. The results suggested a synergistic
activity of the H_1 and H_2 blocker combination on both immediate and late reactions. The
late cutaneous response was not affected by H_1 blockers alone, but was markedly reduced
by the combination.*
Voorhorst, R., and vanKreiken, H.   Atopic skin test re-evaluated. I. Perfection of skin
testing technique. *Ann. Allergy* 31:137–142, 1973.
Voorhorst, R., and vanKreiken, H.   Atopic skin test re-evaluated. II. Variability of skin
testing done in octuplicate. *Ann. Allergy* 31:195–204, 1973.
Voorhorst, R., and vanKreiken, H.   Atopic skin test re-evaluated. III. The wheal : flare
ratio, the log-dose response curve and the bioassay of allergen extracts. *Ann. Allergy*
34:77–86, 1975.
This series of three articles provides a detailed review of skin-testing procedures.

8. PULMONARY FUNCTION TESTS
Rajesh G. Bhagat

Pulmonary function testing is an integral and crucial step in the evaluation of
patients with asthma and other chronic pulmonary disorders. This chapter discusses the pulmonary function tests commonly used in the diagnosis and assessment of various pulmonary diseases, with special emphasis on asthma.

The commonly measured pulmonary function tests are (1) static lung volumes
and capacities, (2) spirometry, (3) flow volume curves, (4) airway resistance, (5)
compliance, and (6) arterial blood gas.

Static lung volumes and capacities reflect the anatomic dimensions of the
lung. By definition a volume is a unit that cannot be further divided. A capacity is
composed of two or more volumes.

The following four lung volumes are measured in pulmonary function laboratories (Fig. 4):

1. Tidal volume (V_T) is the amount of air inhaled (or exhaled) with a normal
   inspiratory (or expiratory) effort.
2. Inspiratory reserve volume (IRV) is the additional amount of air that can be
   inhaled following a normal inspiratory effort.
3. Expiratory reserve volume (ERV) is the amount of air that can be exhaled
   with maximal effort following normal expiration.
4. Residual volume (RV) is the amount of air remaining in the lungs following
   maximal expiration.

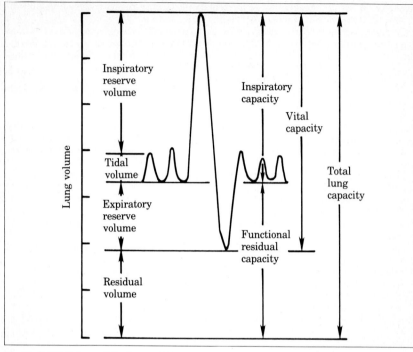

Fig. 4. Subdivisions of the lung volumes.

The four capacities measured in pulmonary function laboratories are as follows (see Fig. 4):

1. Total lung capacity (TLC) is the amount of air contained in the lungs following maximal inspiration. It is equal to the sum of all four lung volumes.
2. Inspiratory capacity (IC) is the additional amount of air that can be inhaled following normal expiratory effort. IC = IRV + V_T.
3. Functional residual capacity (FRC) is the amount of air remaining in the lungs following normal expiration. FRC = ERV + RV.
4. Vital capacity (VC) is the amount of air that can be expelled from the lungs when exhalation begins at the maximal inspiratory level and proceeds to the maximal expiratory level. VC = IRV + V_T + ERV.

With the exception of FRC, all the measurements are dependent on the subject's maximal inspiratory and expiratory efforts and the strength of respiratory muscles.

FRC, TLC, and RV are measured by body plethysmography or gas dilution techniques, techniques usually accessible only to pulmonary physiologists. FRC is first measured by one of the two techniques. TLC and RV are then calculated from the FRC and maximal inspiration and maximal expiration, respectively. The gas dilution methods often underestimate lung volumes in patients with obstructive lung disease, as they only measure the lung volume that communicates freely with the upper airways. Body plethysmography, on the other hand, gives accurate measurements of lung volumes. V_T, ERV, IC, and VC can be determined by means of a spirometer.

Lung volumes (RV, FRC, TLC) are abnormally increased in obstructive lung disease such as asthma. The exact mechanism of this hyperinflation is unknown although it is thought to be caused by (1) an increase in the volume of gas trapped beyond closed airways with the resultant overexpansion of the involved lung units and (2) the decreased ability of the lung to deflate during expiration because of reversible changes in the elastic property of the lungs secondary to longstanding airflow obstruction. In contrast, in purely restrictive lung diseases lung volumes are abnormally decreased. Thus, the measurement of lung volumes not only provides a sensitive index of airways obstruction, but also differentiates a purely restrictive lung disease from an obstructive lung disease.

Spirometry

Although a spirometer can measure tidal volume, expiratory reserve volume, inspiratory capacity, and vital capacity, only those spirometric indices that assess the patient's ventilatory ability during a maximum forced exhalation are evaluated in most patients with an obstructive lung disease such as asthma. These indices are as follows (Fig. 5):

1. Forced vital capacity (FVC), which is the amount of air forcefully exhaled following a maximal inspiratory effort.
2. Forced expiratory volume in 1 second (FEV_1), which is the amount of air forcefully exhaled in the first second of the FVC maneuver.
3. Maximal midexpiratory flow rate (MMEFR or FEF25–75%), which is the rate of flow of air during the middle half of the forced vital capacity maneuver (i.e., between 25 and 75% of vital capacity).

Different types of spirometers are commercially available. In its simplest form (Fig. 6) a mouthpiece is attached to a tube through which air passes into a lightweight bell that is inverted over a water bath. Air movement into and out of the mouthpiece causes the bell to rise or fall; the corresponding movement of an attached pen registers the change in volume on a graph-paper drum rotating at a constant speed.

Initially the patient is seated comfortably, nose clips in place, lips sealed around the mouthpiece. The patient is first instructed to carry out a few normal inspiratory and expiratory maneuvers (i.e., tidal volume breathing) followed by a maximal inspiration, and is then urged to completely expire all the air from the lungs as rapidly as possible. A graph of expired volume against time is obtained (see Fig. 5). From the graph, FEV_1 and VC can be measured easily. MMEFR can be calculated by the following formula:

$$MMEFR = \frac{\frac{1}{2} \, VC}{MET}$$

MET = time required to exhale the middle half of vital capacity.

Spirometric measurements are effort dependent; therefore, coaching of the patient is absolutely essential to get valid measurements. The spirometric measurements are usually carried out in triplicate and the best of the three measurements is considered in the patient's evaluation.

The spirometric measurements are then compared with the "predicted values" available for the patient's height, age, sex, and race. It is a common practice to accept measurements within a certain range (such as ± 2 standard deviations of the predicted mean) as normal. By comparing the patient's lung function with predicted values, the degree of lung function abnormalities can be assessed in most patients. Although the mean predicted values for various pulmonary functions are derived from a large population of normal persons of a specific height, age, sex, and race, they may not be indicative of normal in any individual patient. This suspicion can be elicited by the presence of a marked dichotomy

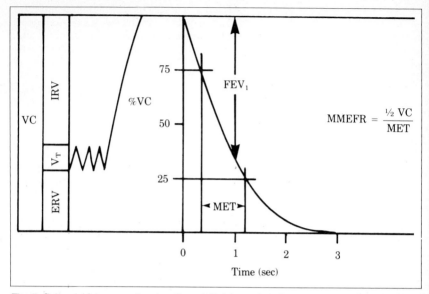

Fig. 5. Spirographic curve showing the subdivisions of vital capacity (VC) and a forced expiratory vital capacity (FVC) maneuver. IRV = inspiratory reserve volume; V_T = tidal volume; ERV = expiratory reserve volume; FEV = forced expiratory volume in 1 second; MET = midexpiratory time; MMEFR (FEF25 – 75%) = maximal midexpiratory flow rate or forced expiratory flow rate from 25 to 75% of VC.

between the patient's clinical status and predicted values of pulmonary functions obtained at the same time. In such cases the patient's previous best postbronchodilator values, obtained during an asymptomatic state, should be used as "normal" values for comparison.

FVC measures lung volume and reflects, among other things, the degree of difficulty the patient has in distending the lungs and chest wall. Normal subjects should expire their whole vital capacity in less than 3 seconds and about three quarters of it in 1 second. In general, FVC between 65 and 80% of predicted values signifies mild impairment, between 50 and 65% signifies moderate impairment, and less than 50% signifies severe impairment. An abnormally low FVC can be indicative of either a restrictive pulmonary defect resulting from internal scarring or inflammation of lungs, pleural diseases, and chest wall diseases (e.g., kyphoscoliosis), or an obstructive pulmonary disorder such as asthma. A less than maximal effort during the forced expiratory maneuver can also produce abnormally low FVC. This last possibility is a common cause of lower FVC in children.

The measurement of FEV_1 reflects the resistance to air flow in the tracheobronchial tree during the first second of the FVC maneuver. The assessment of the degree of abnormality in FEV_1 can be carried out by comparing the patient's FEV_1 with the predicted value of FEV_1. The criteria used for judging mild, moderate, and severe impairment are similar to those described for FVC.

A lower than expected FEV_1 may indicate obstruction to airflow or restrictive diseases of the lung or chest wall. Thus, a lower than expected FVC or FEV_1 cannot distinguish between the restrictive and obstructive diseases. The distinction between these two pathologic entities can be made by measuring lung volumes by body plethysmography. This differentiation can also be carried out by evaluating the FEV_1/FVC ratio. The FEV_1 for normal individuals is 75% of FVC.

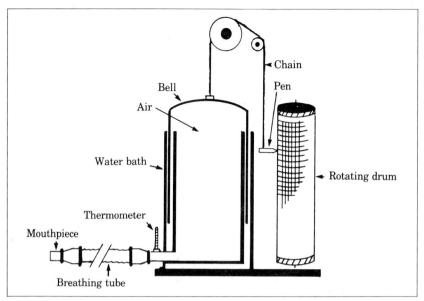

Fig. 6. Belltype spirometer. Movement of air through the breathing tube results in movement of the bell. The output signal is a mechanical pen that marks a drum rotating at a constant speed.

In obstructive ventilatory defects the reduction in FEV_1 is proportionately higher than the reduction in FVC; therefore, the FEV_1/FVC ratio is reduced. In a purely restrictive defect both FVC and FEV_1 are reduced, but lung emptying as judged by FEV_1 may not be reduced to the same degree as the FVC, or may even be normal. Therefore, the FEV_1/FVC ratio is 75% or higher. In addition to restrictive disease of the lung, the FEV_1/FVC ratio may be normal or elevated in patients with respiratory muscle weakness or obesity, and during a submaximal forced expiratory effort.

MMEFR measurements (i.e., FEF25–75%) correlate well with the FEV_1, but it may be a more sensitive measure of airways obstruction in some cases. The normal range of values for MMEF is extremely wide, and there would have to be a substantial reduction in this parameter to be certain of abnormality. In clinical practice determinations of FEV_1, FVC, and FEV_1/FVC ratio are sufficient for evaluation of airways obstruction in most instances.

In addition to assessing the nature and degree of ventilatory defect (obstructive or restrictive), spirometry can also be used to assess the presence or absence of reversibility following inhaled bronchodilator therapy. If the baseline FEV_1 increases by 20% or greater following administration of an inhaled bronchodilator, then the patient has a component of reversible airways obstruction. Such reversibility of FEV_1 is not observed in purely restrictive diseases or emphysema. Thus, spirometry is helpful in establishing the diagnosis of reversible airways disease in most instances. (The interpretation of lack of reversibility should be made with caution, because in some cases aggressive round-the-clock bronchodilator treatment or a course of high-dose steroid therapy can often reverse, at least partially, obstructive pulmonary disease that initially appears irreversible following inhaled bronchodilator therapy.)

In treating patients with obstructive airways disease, it is necessary to verify the amount of reversibility by means of spirometry. When a patient's spirometric indices return to the normal range, the patient's asthma often becomes more stable and, in some cases, oral steroids can be stopped and bronchodilator use can be reduced. Thus, spirometry can be used as an objective method first to monitor the effectiveness of the treatment, and then to guide the physician in timing and tapering of steroids and bronchodilators.

It is now well known that spirometric abnormalities identify patients at risk for postoperative complications following all forms of major surgery. Thus, spirometry helps in optimal preoperative evaluation of patients with lung diseases undergoing surgery.

Generally, a significantly lower than expected FEV_1 and MMEF for a given age, height, sex, and race suggest airflow limitations during expiration. However, these flows can appear normal even in a patient with significant airways obstruction because of the effect of the lung volumes on flows. The rate of airflow is greatest at high lung volume and falls as the volume diminishes. Therefore, a patient with significant airways obstruction and elevated lung volumes may have FEV_1 and FEF25–75% closer to the predicted value than would be expected based on the degree of obstruction. In addition, if there is a premature cessation of effort prior to achieving residual volume, there will be an artifactual increase in the values of these parameters at even lower lung volume. On the other hand, FEV_1 and FEF25–75% will be lower than expected at any volume if the patient does not exhale as hard and as fast as possible. Therefore, the spirometric measurements should be interpreted with reference to the lung volume at which they are achieved, the degree of effort involved in maximal expiration, and the completion (or incompletion) of the forced expiratory maneuver.

In summary, once the spirometric data are obtained, the physician should consider the following questions before correct interpretation of the spirometric abnormalities can be done:

1. Are the results normal or abnormal?
2. What type of abnormality is present?
3. Is the abnormality reversible?
4. Over what period of time has the abnormality developed and progressed?
5. Is there need for additional studies (e.g., lung volumes, flow volume curves, and so on)?

Flow-volume tracing is a relatively recent innovation that assesses the patient's ventilatory capacity during both inspiratory and expiratory maneuvers. During the procedure instantaneous flow rates are recorded against the corresponding lung volume to construct a flow-volume curve in the inspiratory and expiratory phases of respiration (Fig. 7). The flow is measured by a pneumotachygraph and the volume (i.e., vital capacity) can be measured by linking a spirometer into the system beyond the pneumotachygraph. An x-ray recorder or an oscilloscope can be used to obtain a display. The highest flow rates are obtained during the first part of the forced expiratory maneuver. After approximately one-third of the vital capacity has been exhaled, the flow-volume curve peaks and proceeds down toward residual volume. In pulmonary physiology laboratories flow-volume tracings are constructed by plotting flow versus absolute lung volume (i.e., TLC and RV) instead of vital capacity. Generation of such a tracing requires the use of body plethysmography; hence, is not readily available to practicing physicians.

Although flow-volume tracings, like spirograms, are markedly sensitive to dynamic events, they have many of the disadvantages discussed in the section on spirometry. They are influenced not only by the resistance to airflow within the tracheobronchial tree, but also by the degree of distensibility of the lungs, the absolute volume of air in communication with bronchi, the strength of the respiratory muscles, and the motivation of the patient.

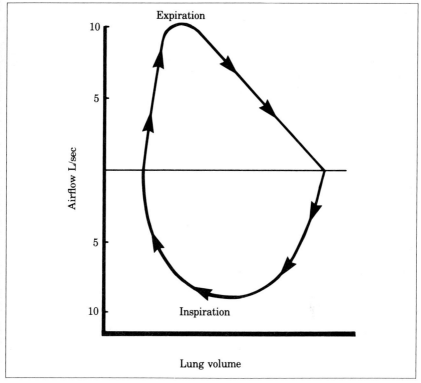

Fig. 7. Maximal expiratory and inspiratory flow-volume loop.

Flow-volume tracings, however, have the following distinct advantages over spirometry:

1. PEFR achieved during a forced expiratory maneuver can be measured.
2. Air flow related to a specific point in lung volume can be assessed.
3. More subtle abnormalities of airways obstruction can be revealed merely by observing the shape of the curve near the residual volume. In normal subjects the descending portion of the curve is linear or concave toward volume axis, while in patients with chronic airways obstruction (e.g., asthma) and smokers, this portion of the curve is convex toward volume axis (Fig. 8), suggesting airways obstruction. These abnormalities are seen in patients without symptoms and are exaggerated in patients with symptomatic airways obstruction.
4. The displacement of the flow-volume curve toward higher lung volumes in asthmatics compared with normal individuals indicates presence of hyperinflation (see Fig. 8). Such a displacement is revealed only if flow is plotted against TLC and not against VC. Because the measurement of TLC requires the use of body plethysmography, such a displacement of the flow-volume tracing is not obtained when commonly available pulmonary function devices are used to obtain flow-volume tracings in clinical practice.
5. A pattern suggestive of restrictive lung disease may be evident on flow-volume tracing. It is characterized by low flow rates in absolute terms but normal or slightly high flow when corrected for lung volume (see Fig. 8).
6. Superimposition of flow-volume curves obtained before and after inhalant bronchodilator therapy can help in evaluating the efficacy of the bron-

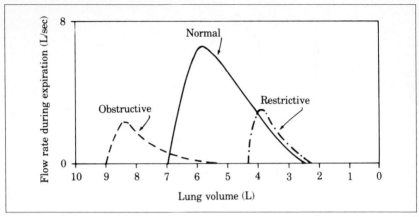

Fig. 8. Schematic representation of typical maximal expiratory flow-volume curves from a normal subject and from patients with restrictive and obstructive lung disease. Airways obstruction results in low expired flows both in absolute terms and relative to the lung volume. In contrast, restrictive disease results in low flow in absolute terms, but normal or slightly high flows when corrected for lung volume.

chodilator on various regions of the tracheobronchial tree. Exclusively large airways can be measured by changes observed in peak flow; a mixture of large and peripheral airways can be measured by changes in flows at 50% of VC and in flows toward very low lung volumes in patients with reactive airways disease (Fig. 9).

7. Provided maximal effort is ensured, an inspiratory flow-volume tracing can be particularly useful in evaluating obstruction within the trachea or large bronchi. In the latter condition there is marked reduction of both inspiratory and expiratory flow with a characteristic alteration of the shape of both the inspiratory and expiratory loops (Fig. 10).

When using spirometry alone in an office, even with measurements as often as twice a week, it is often difficult to follow the course and variability of chronic airflow obstruction and to fully define the many potential triggering factors, because lung function varies so widely over short periods of time. Although completeness of pulmonary function testing is important in diagnostic evaluation and in determining the effectiveness of various treatments on lung volume in general, the most important factor in any pulmonary function test used as a measurement in asthma is the frequency with which it is performed. A simple test performed frequently provides a much clearer picture of the patient's asthmatic state over a period of time than sophisticated measurements performed at longer intervals. A portable device called a **peak flowmeter** can be used by patients on a daily or twice daily basis to follow the course and variability of airflow obstruction in the home or work environment. It measures the maximal flow rate during a forced expiratory maneuver. Because this device measures only one effort-dependent parameter of pulmonary function it cannot be used to assess overall respiratory status. Serial measurements of PEFR, however, provide a profile of variability of airways obstruction with time, a distinct characteristic of asthma.

Many types of peak flowmeters are commercially available. The Wright peak flowmeter is the most accurate of these and can be used in the physician's office or in the hospital during recovery from status asthmaticus, and will help to assess a

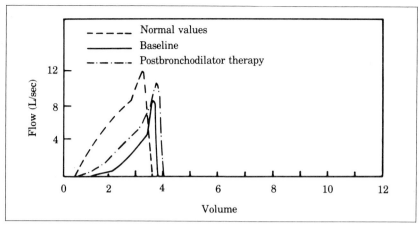

Fig. 9. Maximal expiratory flow-volume curves in a patient with asthma before and after administration of an inhaled bronchodilator. Dashed line represents the normal curve for the patient's age, sex, and height.

patient's response to the therapeutic regimen. The Mini-Wright peak flowmeter, on the other hand may be less accurate, but it is inexpensive, lightweight, and compact and therefore can be used at home or in the work place to follow the course of the disease.

The technique of measurement of PEFR by means of peak flowmeters is relatively simple and can be easily learned by children. The patient is asked to take a deep breath and then to blow as hard as possible into the mouthpiece. Unlike the spirometer, the peak flowmeter does not require complete emptying of the lungs, a potential cause of bronchospasm, and can be used repeatedly with little risk. In addition, the results with a peak flowmeter may be more reproducible than spirometry in young children, who often will not completely empty their lungs during spirometry. Moreover, PEFR correlates closely with spirometric measurements of FEV_1; therefore, peak flow measurements are a reasonable substitute for spirometry in young children.

Airway resistance is a measure of resistance to air flow through the central airways and is measured by body plethysmography. It is assessed by first determining the pressure required to overcome airflow resistance and the resultant rate of air flow. Airway resistance is then calculated by the following formula:

$$\text{Resistance} = \frac{\text{Pressure}}{\text{Flow}}$$

The **measurement of compliance** is helpful in evaluating the elastic behavior, or distensibility, of lungs. It can be calculated by measuring the change in pressure (P) across the lung that occurred as a result of change in the volume (V)

$$\text{Compliance} = \frac{V}{P}$$

Lung compliance is reduced in restrictive lung diseases, whereas in patients with emphysema the compliance is increased. In obstructive diseases, the lung compliance is normal. Lung compliance is not routinely measured during evalua-

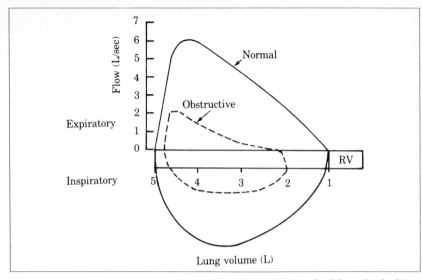

Fig. 10. Inspiratory and expiratory flow-volume relationships in a healthy individual (solid line) and in a patient with upper airways obstruction (dotted line). RV = residual volume.

tion of patients with chronic lung disease in the physician's office because of the complexity of measurements and requirements of trained personnel.

Arterial blood gas measurements are generally normal in asymptomatic asthma. It is essential, however, to monitor the patients with status asthmaticus by serial arterial blood gas determinations. In the initial stages of status asthmaticus there is hypoxemia, hypocapnia, and respiratory alkalosis. Hypoxemia occurs as a result of alteration in ventilation-perfusion ratios; hypocapnia and respiratory alkalosis occur as a result of hyperventilation. As the status of the patient worsens, there is progressively increased retention of CO_2 that may result in "normal" PCO_2. The onset of hypercapnia and respiratory acidosis is an ominous sign indicating impending respiratory failure. Therefore, aggressive management must be instituted in a patient with status asthmaticus and "normal" PCO_2 in order to prevent respiratory failure and to avoid mechanical ventilation.*

A discussion of sophisticated tests of small airway functions, such as frequency dependence of dynamic compliance, the single-breath nitrogen test, closing volume, and so on, is beyond the scope of this chapter.

American Thoracic Society.   ATS statement–Snowbird workshop on standardization of spirometry. *Am. Rev. Respir. Dis.* 119:831–838, 1979.
Makes recommendations on instrumentation standards for spirometer to provide guidelines for diagnostic purposes as well as to ensure comparison of results from one laboratory to another.
Cherniack, R. M.   Pulmonary Function Testing. Philadelphia: Saunders, 1972.
This article is an excellent short reference on pulmonary function testing.

*Arterial PO_2 can be monitored continuously by analysis of oxygen diffusing from the skin heated to 44°C. In small infants analysis is usually carried out by placing the electrode on the skin overlying the abdominal or thoracic aorta. In an older child the medial surface of the forearm is generally used. In general, transcutaneous PO_2 values correlate well with arterial PO_2 values.

Cherniack, R. M.   Pulmonary Function Testing. In T. L. Petty and R. M. Cherniack (Eds.), *Seminars in Respiratory Medicine,* Vol. 4, 1983.
   An excellent brief review of various aspects of pulmonary function tests with strong emphasis on correlation of clinical status and the abnormalities observed in various pulmonary functions.
Gardner, R. M., Hemkinson, J. L., and West, B. J.   Evaluating commercially available spirometers. *Am. Rev. Respir. Dis.* 121:73–82, 1980.
   This study evaluated many commercially available spirometers and found that if a spirometer meets ATS requirements, it makes no difference which device is used to record spirogram.
Henry, R. L., Mellis, C. M., South, R. T., and Simpson, S. J.   Comparison of peak expiratory flow rate and forced expiratory volume in one second in histamine challenge studies in children. *Br. J. Dis. Chest* 76:167–171, 1982.
   The authors observed good correlation between the percentage fall from baseline FEV_1 and PEFR following inhalation of histamine in asthmatics. The authors suggested that change in FEV_1 in asthmatic patients correlates with changes in PEFR; therefore, PEFR measurements can be substituted for FEV_1 measurements in bronchial provocation studies.
Hyatt, R. E., and Black, L. F.   The flow volume curve. A current perspective. *Am. Rev. Respir. Dis.* 107:191–199, 1975.
   Reviews measurement and usefulness of flow-volume curves.
Kraemer, R., Meister, B., Schaad, U. B., and Rossi, E.   The reversibility of lung function abnormalities in children with perennial asthma. *J. Pediatr.* 102:347–350, 1983.
   The authors conclude that a subgroup of asthmatic children with hyperinflation only may be at risk for irreversible loss of elastic recoil of the lungs.
McFadden, E. R., and Lyons, H. A.   Arterial blood gas tension in asthma. *N. Engl. J. Med.* 278:1027–1032, 1968.
   A study explaining the pathophysiologic mechanisms underlying abnormalities in arterial blood gas during acute attacks of bronchospasm.
Miller, R. D., and Hyatt, R. E.   Evaluation of obstructing lesions of trachea and larynx by flow-volume loops. *Am. Rev. Respir. Dis.* 108:475–481, 1973.
   The article classifies the abnormalities in flow-volume loop according to site of obstruction.
Morrill, C. G., et al.   Calibration and stability of standard and mini-Wright Peak Flow Meters. *Ann. Allergy* 46:70–73, 1981.
   The authors compared the Wright and Mini-Wright peak flowmeters and observed that peak flow readings varied from actual flow in both the devices but the variation from actual flow was greater for the Mini-Wright peak flowmeter.
Polgar, A., and Promadhat, V.   Pulmonary function testing in children: Techniques and standard. Philadelphia: Saunders, 1971.
   Presents a complete reference text in the field, both in the discussion and in the outline of many clinical applications.
Tisi, G. M.   State of the art: Preoperative evaluation of pulmonary function. *Am. Rev. Respir. Dis.* 119:293–310, 1979.
   Comprehensively reviews the validity, indications, and benefits of preoperative evaluation of pulmonary functions.

9. BRONCHIAL INHALATION CHALLENGE PROCEDURES
Don A. Bukstein

Reactivity is of fundamental importance in the regulation of airways patency. In asthma, the airways reactivity is characteristically increased. The increase in reactivity is in part due to the response to certain inhaled antigens. This is termed *antigen-induced,* or *specific, bronchial reactivity. Nonspecific bronchial reactivity* is the term used to indicate the responsiveness of the airways to chemical mediators such as histamine and acetylcholine, or methacholine (the synthetic analogue of acetylcholine). Although both specific and nonspecific hyperreactivity are important in asthma, their relative contributions are likely to vary from one patient to another.

Some controversy exists in the literature as to whether there is a significant correlation between the level of nonspecific bronchial hyperreactivity and the severity of asthma. In general, the degree of bronchial reactivity correlates with the severity of asthma.

Inhalation challenges with pharmacologic and antigenic substances are employed to detect this airways hypersensitivity and hyperreactivity clinically. Guidelines for these challenges have been recently published by the Subcommittee on Bronchial Inhalation Challenges, Assembly of Allergy and Clinical Immunology of the American Thoracic Society (ATS). These guidelines form the basis for many of the recommendations outlined in this chapter.

Pharmacologic challenge of the airways with histamine or methacholine is used to confirm a diagnosis of hyperreactive airways when other more conventional studies (such as reversal of airways obstruction with inhaled bronchodilators or induction of airways obstruction with exercise testing) have been inconclusive. In addition, it may be helpful to confirm the diagnosis of asthma in patients with less usual presentations, such as cough alone without obvious wheezing. In this situation, although spirometry may be normal, methacholine challenge produces bronchoconstriction. A positive test can convince the patient, parent, or physician of the need for specific avoidance of or compliance to a regimen of therapy. Contraindications for challenge with pharmacologic agents include (1) well-documented asthma with demonstrated reversibility of bronchospasm by bronchodilators; (2) symptoms of asthma at the time the challenge is to be administered; (3) pulmonary function impairment beyond that normally observed in an individual patient; and (4) a bronchospastic response to diluent.

Antigenic challenge is used to identify specific antigens suspected of causing acute or delayed airways obstruction. Patients with a strong history of responses to identifiable antigens and with positive skin tests to the antigen do not fall into this group. Rather, patients who have historical and immediate skin-test data that are inconclusive in identifying precipitants to respiratory difficulty will have the most benefit from investigations of this nature. Antigenic challenge may also help to evaluate the efficiency of therapy in lessening pulmonary reactivity to significant antigens. The contraindications for antigenic challenges to the airway include a history of strong responses to identifiable antigens as well as all those listed for pharmacologic agents.

Pharmacologic agents commonly used in inhalation challenges are methacholine and histamine. Methacholine is a parasympathomimetic drug that produces its effect in the airways by stimulating acetylcholine receptors on bronchial smooth muscle cells. Histamine, on the other hand, produces bronchospasm by less well-defined mechanisms. Some experimental work has suggested that the parasympathetic nervous system is involved; other studies have not supported this and have instead implicated the H_1 histamine receptor as being mechanistically important. Additional work is needed to define all the mechanisms involved in producing bronchoconstriction caused by histamine.

Antigenic aerosols may also be used to challenge the airways when clinically indicated. The bronchospasm elicited by inhalation of aerosolized antigens is produced by reaction of the antigen with IgE antibody bound to basophil-like cells present in the airways and subsequent release of chemical mediators. With more concentrated solutions (greater than 1:1000 on a weight/volume basis), bronchospasm may also be caused by irritation of the airways and may be unrelated to immunologic sensitivity to the allergen. For antigen challenges, the potency and stability of the antigenic extracts are of major importance; therefore, use of lyophilized extracts from a lot standardized by an approved method of assessing potency of allergenic extracts is necessary. (See Chai and colleagues, 1975 for more details.)

The many factors that can influence the response to bronchial challenge must be considered in order to obtain reliable, interpretable studies. The factors are detailed in the article by Chai and colleagues (1975). Responsiveness may be decreased by treatment of patients with bronchodilators, antihistamines, and cromolyn. Infection with natural rubeola will also decrease the response to challenge. Increased responsiveness is noted after acute viral respiratory tract infections, after recent antigenic challenges, and after both rubeola and influenza vaccination. Other factors affecting the response to inhalation challenges include the characteristics of the nebulizer and delivery system, the patient's breathing pattern, and the rate of drug or antigen administration. Therefore, all these variables need to be standardized in a laboratory to ensure reproducibility of results and meaningful comparisons between patients. There are no published data on the reproducibility of the methacholine challenge over a period of years, nor on serial challenges in patients whose asthma has changed from severe to a more mild form over a period of time.

Methods of Bronchial Inhalation Challenge
The method of bronchial inhalation challenge is as follows:

1. Patients to be tested should be free of signs and symptoms of airways obstruction, and they need to be interviewed and examined on the day of testing before challenge. Because viral upper respiratory tract infections may increase bronchial reactivity in otherwise normal individuals (see Empey and colleagues, 1976), patients should have no history of such infections within the previous 6 weeks.

2. Drugs that may alter the response to inhalation challenges should be stopped prior to challenge, if this can be tolerated by the patients. The one absolute requirement is that antihistamines be discontinued for tests involving antigenic agents and histamines. Antihistamines may effect the bronchial challenge itself, and will alter the results of intradermal skin tests needed to determine the starting dilution of antigen employed for challenge. The ATS recommended time intervals for discontinuing the various drugs before challenge are meant to be used as a guideline (Table 7), and may have to be altered under certain clinical circumstances. In patients for whom discontinuing medications for the recommended time periods is impossible, the minimum time they should be off any one medication is one dosing interval. For example, a patient taking a sustained-release theophylline preparation every 12 hours should be tested 12 hours after the last dose of medication, or just before the next prescribed dose.

3. Smoking and drinking of cola drinks, chocolate, tea, or coffee should be discontinued 6 hours prior to testing. Exercise and exposure to cold air should also be avoided in the immediate study period.

4. Before antigen challenge on the day of the challenge, intradermal skin tests should be performed. During the first inhalation challenge to an allergen, the initial antigen concentration used should be the one that produces approximately a 5-mm wheal (minus diluent control) on intracutaneous injection. Antigen skin tests should include diluent (nonreacting) and histamine (positively reacting) controls. If the histamine skin test is negative before a challenge, consideration should be given to possible interference of the test from oral antihistamines and the challenge should be rescheduled.

5. Antigens to be used in a challenge are serially diluted in 0.9% NaCl containing 0.4% phenol. Most antigens used for bronchial provocation testing come from the allergen extract companies as 1:10 wt/vol; therefore, typical dilutions for

Table 7. Guidelines for periods of time medications are
withheld for various drugs, as outlined by the ATS committee

Drug	Time interval (hr)
Inhaled bronchodilators	
Isoproterenol	4
Isoetharine	6
Metaproterenol	8
Terbutaline	12
Salbutamol	12
Atropine	10
Injected bronchodilators	
Epinephrine	4
Terbutaline	12
Oral bronchodilators	
Liquid theophylline preparations	12
Short-acting theophylline preparations	18
Aminophylline preparations	18
Intermediate-acting theophylline preparations	24
Terbutaline	24
Long-acting theophylline preparations	48
Other	
Antihistamines	48
Cromolyn sodium	48
Lodoxamine	48
Hydroxyzine	96

challenge range from 1:1000 to 1:100,000 (the latter is used for the initial challenge). More dilute solutions might be used, depending on the results of the intradermal skin testing.

6. Histamine and methacholine are also serially diluted for challenges. For histamine, a solution of 10 mg/ml in saline is obtained from the pharmacy. Serial dilutions are made in the saline-phenol diluent to obtain concentrations of 10, 5, 2.5, 1.0, 0.5, 0.25, 0.06, and 0.03 mg/ml of histamine. Before making methacholine into a solution, methacholine chloride (Mecholyl) powder should be stored within a larger container of anhydrous crystals in the freezer compartment of the refrigerator. For testing, the powder is added to the saline-phenol solution to produce a solution with 25 mg/ml of methacholine. Subsequently, dilutions are made from this stock solution of 25 mg/ml to obtain solutions containing 10, 5, 2.5, 1.25, 0.62, 0.31, 0.15, and 0.075 mg/ml of Mecholyl. For patients with a history of rapid deterioration in lung function, an even lower dose of methacholine may be used as the starting concentration. All solutions are made the day of the challenge and refrigerated until immediately before use when they are warmed to 37° C. Stock solutions of Mecholyl (25 mg/ml) remain active for at least 4 months from the date of preparation.

7. The equipment used to administer the inhalation challenge should conform to certain guidelines. In order to prevent excessive loss and sedimentation of large aerosol particles ($> 5~\mu$) in the generation and delivery systems, and to minimize inhalation of particles less than $0.2~\mu$, the diameter of inhaled particles should range between 0.3 and $4~\mu$. No matter which units are employed, the same nebulizer should be used in any one bronchial challenge and with repeated challenges in the same patient because of considerable variations between mass-produced units. If a dosimeter is used in which nebulization is automatically triggered by the onset of inspiration, aerosol generation is adjusted to 0.5 to 0.6

seconds after the initial inspiration, followed by further inspiration of at least 0.5 seconds. The slow inspiration should start from functional residual capacity (FRC) with the patient holding his or her breath for 2 to 5 seconds after the slow inhalation to near total lung capacity (TLC). The subject should take a total of five consecutive, slow deep breaths at each concentration, with tests of lung function assessed 1 to 5 minutes after histamine or methacholine, or 10 minutes after antigen challenge. In the absence of a dosimeter, the most practical way to administer the aerosol is by a continuous high-flow method in which subjects inhale all of their air from a large airflow source containing the challenge material in known concentrations. Again, five slow inhalations from FRC to near TLC, with breath-holding near TLC in between breaths, is probably the most effective way of administering the test solution. In younger children who cannot reproducibly inhale to near TLC, inhalation of ten tidal breaths of graded doses of aerosol is an acceptable alternative.

8. The inhalation of pharmacologic or antigenic agents proceeds from the most dilute to the more concentrated solutions, with clinical examination of the chest and lung function tests done before and after diluent (control), and before and after each concentration of challenge solution. As noted in step 7, five inhalations of a solution are administered followed by lung function tests to determine if a response has occurred. If no clinical or lung function response can be documented, five inhalations of the next concentration of agent are inhaled. This process continues until clinical or pulmonary function response dictates discontinuing the test, or until the most concentrated solution is inhaled without effect (methacholine = 25 mg/ml; histamine = 10 mg/ml; antigen = 1:1000 wt/vol). Once a positive response has been obtained, the cumulative dose of drug or antigen delivered to subjects is most easily assessed employing inhalation units where 1 inhalation unit of a pharmacologic bronchoconstrictor agent is equal to 1 breath of solution with 1 mg of drug/ml. For antigen challenge, 1 inhalation unit is equal to 1 breath of a 1:5000 wt/vol dilution of antigen. In assessing inhalation responses, inhalation units per five breaths as well as the cumulative dose of inhalation units may be recorded for future reference in determining bronchial sensitivity. More details of determining cumulative doses of pharmacologic and antigenic inhalation challenges are given in Rosenthal (1979).

9. Pulmonary function must be assessed before any challenges are performed, after five inhalations of the saline-phenol diluent, and after each series of five inhalations of increasing concentrations of pharmacologic mediators or antigens. Ideally, both spirometric and plethysmographic tests should be employed. Regardless of the tests employed changes should exceed 2 standard deviations or coefficients of variation for repeated measures for that test before statistically significant changes can be established. Common minimum acceptable changes in various lung functions indicative of a positive bronchial provocation include

TEST	CHANGE FROM BASELINE (%)
Vital capacity	-10
FEV_1	-20
FEF25–75%	-25
Peak expiratory flow rate	-25
SGaw	-40
FRC	$+25$

Where FEV_1 is the forced expiratory volume in 1 second, FEF25–75% is the maximal midexpiratory flow rate; SGaw is specific conductance; and FRC is functional residual capacity.

Before challenge baseline lung function as assessed by the FEV_1 should be at least 80% of the best previous value, with the patient free of symptoms of airways obstruction. After inhalation of the saline-phenol diluent the FEV_1 should not decrease more than 10% from the baseline value. After an inhalation challenge, if the FEV_1 falls less than 10% and no other lung function deteriorates by 2 standard deviations, the next higher dilution should be used. When any function shows a response at least one-half of that considered to indicate a positive response (e.g., a 10–19% fall in FEV_1), then the same concentration of challenge solution is repeated. When a positive response is noted after methacholine or histamine, as defined by a 20% decrease in FEV_1, the test is concluded. A positive response after antigen inhalation should be sustained for 20 minutes. All positive challenges should be reversed with an inhaled bronchodilator. In addition, all patients subjected to antigen challenge should be monitored for 2 to 12 hours for late asthmatic responses that may occur in the absence of an early response.

Safety Precautions

Adequate ventilation and exhaust fans should be available so that all aerosols generated during the challenge procedure are evacuated. The technicians performing the challenges should be certified in cardiopulmonary resuscitation. For challenges in young pediatric patients, the physician must be in attendance. For challenges in adult patients, the physician must be present while initial tests of lung function are assessed so it may be decided if the patient is stable enough for challenge. In addition, the physician should be in attendance during the initial challenge to any inhaled agent to which a patient has a history of a marked pulmonary response. The physician must be readily available in the event that a severe adverse reaction occurs. Resuscitation equipment in the form of a fully equipped and closely monitored resuscitation cart must be immediately available. Oxygen and injected bronchodilators must be available at all times.

A significant complication of bronchial provocation testing with allergens is the development of recurrent nocturnal asthmatic reactions, which can last for several nights with normal daytime function. About 25 percent of asthmatics who have a positive immediate response to allergen challenge will develop an additional fall in flow rates 1 to 12 hours after their immediate reaction. The late reaction may also occur in the absence of an immediate reaction. This late fall in flow rate is referred to as "late-onset asthma" and is usually not recurrent. This type of late reaction to allergen inhalation has been shown to increase nonspecific bronchial reactivity to histamine and methacholine.

Bronchial Provocation Testing in Occupational Asthma

Bronchial provocation tests may be the only way to prove a causal relationship between the development of respiratory symptoms and an inhaled substance, especially those found under various working conditions. In tests of this kind the suspected offending agent may be delivered by aerosol nebulizer or face mask, as a dust diluted in lactose powder or a vapor in a closed environment. By controlling the amount of agent inhaled, and by measuring respiratory function in a standardized way after exposure (as outlined for histamine, methacholine, and antigens), one can (1) define patterns of bronchial reactivity, (2) examine patients for changes in that reactivity with time, and (3) study the effects of various therapeutic agents. Limitations of such testing include a lack of information obtained by the studies relating to mechanism (immunologic vs nonimmunologic). In addition, useful information about the potential offending agent (in terms of quantity of dust, vapor, or fume present in the work place) is commonly not available to serve as useful data to construct the challenge. For considerations concerned with such testing and recommendations for specific substances, the reader is referred to a recent symposium by Rosenthal (1979).

Boushey, H. A. Holtzman, M. J. Sheller, J. R., and Nadel, J. A.   State of the art. Bronchial hyperreactivity. *Am. Rev. Respir. Dis.* 121:389–413, 1980.
Suggests that the reactivity, both specific and nonspecific, may be inducible because of a genetic predisposition.

Cavanaugh, M. J., Bronsky, E. A., and Buckley, J. M.   Clinical value of bronchial provocation testing in childhood asthma. *J. Allergy Clin. Immunol.* 59:41–47, 1977.
Skin testing correlates very well with bronchial provocational testing in childhood asthma.

Chai, H., et al.   Standardization of bronchial inhalation challenge procedures. *J. Allergy Clin. Immonol.* 56:323–327, 1975.
The standard recommendations concerning bronchial inhalation challenges.

Corrao, W. M., Braman, S. S., and Irwin, R. S.   Chronic cough as the sole presenting manifestation of bronchial asthma. *N. Engl. J. Med.* 300:633–637, 1979.
Excellent study illustrating the use of provocation inhalation challenge in making the diagnosis of reactive airways disease in patients with chronic cough and normal spirometry.

Cropp, C. J. A., et al.   Guidelines for bronchial inhalation challenges with pharmacologic and antigenic agents. *American Thoracic Society News* 6:11–19, 1980.
A recent review with specific recommendations on preparation and performance of both pharmacologic and antigenic inhalation challenge.

Empey, D. W., et al.   Mechanisms of bronchial hyperractivity in normal subjects after upper respiratory tract infection. *Am. Rev. Respir. Dis. 113:131–139, 1976.*
Bronchial hyperreactivity is increased in normal subjects for several weeks after viral upper respiratory tract infections.

.Rosenthal, R. R. (Ed.).   Workshop proceeds on bronchoprovocation techniques for the evaluation of asthma. *J. Allergy Clin. Immunol.* 64:561–692, 1979.
Additional recommendations concerning the usefulness of bronchial inhalation challenges as both a diagnostic and investigational tool.

Simmonsson, B. G., Jacobs, F. M., and Nadel, A.   Role of autonomic nervous system and the cough reflex in the increased responsiveness of airways in patients with obstructive lung disease. *J. Clin. Invest.* 46:1812–1818, 1967.
Pioneering studies in the basic autonomic mechanisms responsible for increased airway reactivity in patients with obstructive airway disease.

Woenne, R., Kattan, M., Orange, R. P., and Levison, H. L.   Bronchial hyperreactivity to histamine and methacholine in asthmatic children after inhalation of SCH 1000 and chlorpheniramine maleate. *J. Allergy Clin. Immunol.* 62:119–124, 1978.
The effects of anticholinergic agents and antihistamines on airway reactivity are explored.

DEVELOPMENT AND EPIDEMIOLOGY

10. ALLERGY AND GENETICS
Steven A. Wool and Don A. Bukstein

Obtaining a comprehensive family history is an integral and time-honored part of the evaluation of an allergic patient. The earliest scientific studies of the association between allergy and heredity date back to those of Cooke and VanderVeer in 1916. Their work was based on the analysis of a large number of pedigrees of patients both with and without symptoms of allergy. Their results revealed a strong correlation between allergic symptoms and a positive family history. As was the practice of the times, allergy was proposed to be inherited along simpler mendelian terms. Subsequent population studies confirmed the association between allergic symptoms and a positive family history, but could not reach agreement on a particular model of inheritance.

In contrast to pedigree studies, twin studies, the other major form of genetic analysis, have emphasized the importance of nongenetic factors in the expression of allergy. The concordance for allergic disorders was as high for fraternal twins as for identical twins, suggesting that common environmental exposures or other nongenetic factors are at least as important as the genetic factors. It is now generally accepted that susceptibility to allergy is inherited along multiple genetic loci, but the clinical expression is dependent on both environmental stimuli and the strength of the genetic message.

Research in the areas of the immunoglobulin IgE and the major histocompatibility system, as expressed through human leukocyte antigens (HLA), have had important implications for the study of the genetics of allergy. This research has provided a basis to empirically study the relationship between defined genetic markers and clinical evidence of allergy. With this information better understanding can be obtained concerning the interaction of genetic and environmental factors in the immune response.

Extended analysis of this subject is beyond the scope of this brief discussion. The interested reader is encouraged to examine many of the recent reviews noted in the annotated references. Noted here are a few of the major studies in this field as well as the prospects for future investigation.

IgE has been studied as a marker of atopic disease because of its unique role as the primary mediator of the allergic response. Since its characterization in the late 1960s, numerous studies have appeared. In general elevated serum IgE levels have shown a significant correlation with the presence of allergy; however, the predictive value in an individual patient is weak because there is a wide overlap in the ranges of values in normal persons and allergic persons. There are also multiple limitations in the assessment of IgE levels in allergic populations. In particular the definition of allergy is often based on clinical history as opposed to objective measurements. Within recent years, many investigators have attempted to circumvent this problem by defining the study populations with skin-test reactivity or radioallergosorbent test (RAST) screening.

The basis for the inheritance of high or low IgE levels is unknown. The major hypothesis is that two alleles determine the serum level of IgE, and that elevated IgE levels are inherited as a recessive trait. Although attractive, this theory has been difficult to prove. Marsh (1981) proposed the concept of a single regulatory site. A second genetic site could be responsible for recognizing certain environmental stimuli, and a person would respond with either high or low levels of IgE depending on genetic predisposition. The mode of genetic control, however, could exist at many other levels such as the release of IgE from plasma cells, cellular recognition of antigens, or cellular interaction with other immunologic factors such as T-lymphocytes.

A recent study in Sweden illustrates a potential role of IgE in the evaluation of the allergic patient. IgE screening was done on the cord blood of a large number of newborns (1701 of 1884 over a 13-month period). The parents later filled out questionnaires about family history of allergy and the development of allergic symptoms in their child. Results were evaluated without knowing the original IgE levels. There was an extremely high correlation between elevated IgE levels at birth and the development of clinical allergy. The correlation between family history and symptoms did not increase the significance of IgE's predictive capability. Follow-up studies of the infants with high IgE levels documented that levels at 18 to 24 months had remained elevated. The longer the patient was followed, the stronger the correlation between IgE levels and clinical allergy became. Serum IgE levels were recommended as a predictive test of atopy in a high-risk population. In the absence of the strong family history of atopy, however, the yield from monitoring of serum IgE concentrations was small. In addition, measures thought to be effective in preventing or delaying allergic disease should probably be instituted for newborns with a strong family history of allergy regardless of the level of IgE. Thus, monitoring IgE levels in newborns is of questionable value at this time.

The major histocompatibility locus (HLA) has been used to study genetic patterns in many diseases. The HLA system is a group of antigens determined by four genetic loci (areas) on human chromosome 6. The four genetic loci are highly polymorphic and closely linked. Three of the gene products (A, B, and C) are defined serologically, and a fourth (D) is defined by mixed lymphocyte culture. The different alleles for each loci are almost always expressed; therefore, each person has two identifiable antigens for each of the four genetic loci.

HLA is useful clinically in its ability to predict transplant compatibility. Although other loci are important, HLA has the greatest predictive capability. Because transplant rejection is mediated through the immune system and HLA compatibility predicts this response, the HLA system may be important in immune regulation in general. In fact, evidence has identified a probable role for the HLA system in the regulation of the T-lymphocyte function. The combination of the identifiable genetic pattern of the HLA system and its probable relation to immunoregulation has made HLA a useful model with which to study the genetic determination of immune function in different disease states.

As with IgE, the data concerning HLA and different diseases have been extensive. There have been strong associations among HLA and various disorders of the immune response such as the rheumatic diseases, myasthenia gravis, and Grave's disease. Studies relating allergy to HLA, however, have not been as successful. Because of the clinical diversity of patients with allergic symptoms, results of initial studies were highly variable. Within recent years the use of well-defined clinical subsets and objective measurements of allergy (skin test, RAST) has improved the quality and reproducibility of many studies.

A positive correlation has been noted between the presence of HLA A1, B8 haplotype and a history of infantile eczema and asthma, as opposed to a history of asthma or hay fever without eczema. This same haplotype has been associated with an increased frequency of other diseases, such as celiac disease, chronic active hepatitis, and myasthenia gravis. Another study was unable to identify a particular HLA haplotype in ten families in which at least two members had asthma. The study, however, showed a linkage between HLA in individual families and the development of either asthma or positive skin-test reactivity, thus implying a value of HLA in determining the risk to development of atopy and perhaps asthma in a single member of a large family. As discussed previously, the tendency to have high or low levels of IgE is inherited. Attempts to link the level of IgE to HLA have been unsuccessful.

Currently HLA testing cannot be recommended for routine genetic screening for allergy. As a clinical tool, it is useful for assessing susceptibility to only a few diseases. Certain predominant HLA haplotypes may determine a "hyperresponsiveness" of the immune system. As with IgE, these haplotypes may have been selected through evolution at the expense of increasing the risk of atopic disease.

As a model of disease, allergy is unique in that it has both a well-documented familial association and a relatively extensive body of information concerning its immunologic expression. Identification of the mechanisms of interaction between genetic and environmental factors responsible for allergy would provide valuable insight into the pathogenesis and treatment of allergic disease. Despite the many advances noted, the genetics of allergy remains at a conceptual level.

Barbee, R. A., Halonen, M., Lebowitz, M., and Burrows, B.   Distribution of IgE in a community population with age, sex, and allergen skin test reactivity. *J. Allergy Clin. Immunol.* 68:106, 1981.
Presents a brief discussion of IgE and its relationship to skin-test reactivity.

Bias, W. B., Marsh, D. G., and Platts-Mills, T. A. E.   Genetic Control of Factors Involved in Bronchial Asthma, Hay Fever, and Other Allergic States. In S. D. Litwin (Ed.) *Genetic Determanants of Pulmonary Disease,* Vol. 11. New York, Marcel Dekker: 1978. Pp. 127–148.
Contains much of the same information as in the Marsh, Meyers, and Bias but more explicitly described with the use of diagrams.

Blumenthal, M. N., Mendell, N., and Yumis, E.   Immunogenetics of atopic diseases. *J. Allergy Clin. Immunol.* 65:403–405, 1980.
Presents brief but very informative review of the recent developments and problems with investigation in the field of immunogenetics. Outlines the limitations and future prospects of the study of immunogenetics of allergy.

Brady, R. E., et al.   The association of an HLA "asthma associated" haplotype and immediate hypersensitivity in familial asthma. *J. Immunogenet.* 8:509–517, 1981.
Study referred to in text, which revealed that the inheritance of HLA in different families correlated with asthma as well as tests of immediate hypersensitivity, thus implying the control of asthma resides on chromosome 6.

Croner, S., Kjellman, N. M., and Erickson, R. A.   IgE screening in 1701 newborn infants and the development of atopic disease during infancy. *Arch. Dis. Child.* 57:364–368, 1982.
Recent study referred to in text that illustrates the predictive capability of IgE in determining susceptibility to atopy.

Johansson, S. G. O.   Raised levels of a new immunoglobulin class (IgND) in asthma. *Lancet* 2:951–953, 1967.
Presents one of the first reports of the association of IgE with allergy.

Levine, B. B. Genetics of atopic allergy and reagin production. *Clin. Allergy* 3(suppl.):539–558, 1973.
Excellent review of some of the early studies of the use of IgE and HLA in the study of the genetics of allergy.

Marsh, D. G., Meyers, D. A., and Bias, W. B.   The epidemiology and genetics of atopic allergy. *N. Engl. J. Med.* 305:1551–1559, 1981.
State-of-the-art discussion concerning the genetics of allergy. Very comprehensive with an excellent bibliography. A must for anyone further interested in this topic.

Masala, C., and Bonni, S.   Studies of Atopic Twins. In A. Gaetano and G. Mellillo (Eds.), *Respiratory Allergy.* Italy: Masson Italia Editoria, 1980. Pp. 37–49.
Recent twin study confirming many of the earlier works illustrating the important environmental factors at work in allergy.

McDevitt, H. O.   Regulation of the immune response by the major histocompatibility system. *N. Engl. J. Med.* 303:1514–1517, 1980.
Excellent, brief discussion of the presumed role of HLA in immune regulation and its association with susceptibility to disease.

Merrett, T. G., Merrett, J., and Cookson, J. B.   Allergy and parasites: The measurement of total and specific IgE levels in urban and rural communities in *Rhodesia. Clin. Allergy* 6:131–134, 1976.
An interesting study relating elevated IgE levels to parasitic diseases and the subsequent increased risk of asthma. It also discusses the potential protective effect of elevated IgE.

Nye, L., Merrett, T. G., Landon, J., and White, R. J.   A detailed investigation of circulating IgE levels in a normal population. *Clin. Allergy* 5:13–24, 1975.
Studies IgE in the normal population.

Orgel, H. A., Hamburger, R. N., and Bazaral, M.   Development of IgE allergy in infancy. *J. Allergy Clin. Immunol.* 56:296–307, 1975.
Study presenting the evidence that elevated IgE levels often predict the development of clinical allergy.

Schaller, J. G., and Hansen, J. A.   HLA relationships to disease. *Hosp. Pract.* 16:41–49, 1981.
Excellent, easy-to-read discussion concerning HLA. Good starting point for someone interested in learning about HLA.

Sibbald, B., Horn, M. E. C., Brain, E. A., and Gregg, I.   Genetic factors in childhood asthma. *Thorax* 35:671–674, 1980.
Presents recent family study of the prevalence of asthma and atopy in a general practice.

11. EPIDEMIOLOGY AND NATURAL HISTORY OF ASTHMA AND ALLERGIC DISEASE
Linden Ho

Asthma is recognized as a significant cause of illness and disability. Attempts to accurately determine its incidence, prevalence, and natural history, however, have been complicated by a lack of uniform criteria in defining the disease. The protean nature of asthma itself may be partly to blame. In adults, there is significant overlap with chronic bronchitis and emphysema; in children "recurrent bronchitis," "asthmatic bronchitis," or single episodes of wheezing not leading to frank asthma defy strict categorization. Another methodologic problem has been the heterogeneity of populations studied by various investigators, for example, in terms of geographic distribution or age. Little data exist concerning the incidence of asthma in whole populations. There are, however, numerous prevalence studies. The estimated cumulative prevalence (i.e., all persons with symptoms, past or present) in school-aged children in the United States, is 2.8 to 4.7%. Among college students in the United States, the comparable range is 4.0 to 7.1%; in adult populations, the prevalence is 3.6 to 4.4%. Striking geographic variation in asthma prevalence occurs. For example, asthma is relatively rare in the New Guinea Highlands, in the American Indian and Eskimo populations, and in parts of west Africa. In contrast, the prevalence of asthma in the genetically inbred population of Tristan da Cunha exceeds 30%. Differences in prevalence have also been documented between different racial groups in the same areas, but the relative roles of environment versus race remain unclear.

Certain characteristics are associated with an increased incidence of asthma. The male predominance in childhood asthma is well known. Under the age of 10 years, boys outnumber girls by two to one in age-specific prevalence of asthma. During adolescence and mid-adult life, an increase in new cases among females tends to equalize the ratio. After age 65, there is again a male predominance, though slight. An even more important factor appears to be a positive family history for atopic disease (i.e., asthma, allergic rhinitis, or eczema). Various studies have shown that asthma occurs with increased frequency in first-degree relatives of asthmatic patients compared with those of normal controls. In one study the risk was 31% versus 11%. In another analysis of hay fever and asthma in almost 6000 students at the University of Washington, the empiric risk for developing either condition was clearly related to a family history of atopy. If both parents had hay fever or asthma, 58% of the offspring were affected. If only one parent was atopic, 38% of offspring were affected. Only 12.5% of children developed symptoms when both parents were normal.

The inheritance of atopic diseases is thought to be multifactorially determined. Twin studies have confirmed the genetic component of asthma, demonstrating a concordance of 19% for asthma between monozygotic twins, and 4.8% concordance between dizygotic twins. The lack of 100% concordance suggests that although a susceptibility to the development of asthma may be inherited, the person may not manifest disease without the participation of certain environmental triggers.

The epidemiology of asthma is clearly related to that of the other atopic diseases, allergic rhinitis, and eczema. It has been reported that 78% of extrinsic asthmatic patients also have hay fever; conversely, 38% of patients with hay fever have episodes of asthma. Persons with allergic rhinitis have been shown to have increased bronchial reactivity to methacholine and histamine inhalation challenges in the absence of overt asthma. In addition, the risk of a person with allergic rhinitis developing asthma in later years has been investigated in at least two studies and is estimated to be 5 to 10%. Associated atopic disease may also adversely affect the outcome of asthma and will be discussed later. The basic underlying relationship between the atopic states remains to be elucidated.

Our understanding of the natural history of asthma is based on numerous retrospective reports, but only a handful of well-controlled, prospective studies. The majority of persons appear to develop asthma during childhood. Surveys of school-aged children in Houston, Denver, and Aberdeen, Scotland, during the 1960s revealed that more than half of the asthmatic patients were less than 5 years old at the onset of symptoms. In a general population in rural Iowa, 76% of patients with asthma became symptomatic before the age of 20. Those patients developing asthma after age 20 tended to have "intrinsic" asthma (i.e., with negative skin tests) whereas younger asthmatic patients tended to be allergic. In most asthmatic patients symptoms appear to improve over time. One well-done, 20-year follow-up of 449 children found that 21% were free of asthma symptoms. Three prospective studies exist in the literature and report similar outcomes. One of these examined 331 asthmatic children in Melbourne, Australia, at the ages of 7, 14, and 21 years. Most subjects improved during adolescence but 45% of these individuals had relapsed by age 21. In the final analysis, 30% were completely asymptomatic and the majority of the remainder were significantly improved. Risk factors for an adverse outcome in this and other studies taken together were the severity of asthma at initial evaluation, associated allergic rhinitis or positive family history of atopy, and perhaps artificial milk feeding as an infant. These prospective studies have not yet been carried out into later adult life. In addition, the prognosis of adult-onset asthma is not well described; those with the intrinsic type associated with nasal polyps, sinusitis, and aspirin idiosyncrasy may have a severe progressive course. Although the overall outcome for asthma is favorable, even those patients who are asymptomatic have been shown to have significant, occult pulmonary function abnormalities reflecting persistent small airways obstruction. Complete remission in terms of totally normal pulmonary physiology may therefore be rare.

Mortality attributable to asthma is a relatively infrequent occurrence and is more often seen in adults than in children. The rates also vary among countries. In the United States mortality caused by asthma in the general population is about 1.0 to 2.0 per 100,000; for children, it is less than 0.5 per 100,000. During the mid-1960s, a striking increase in asthma mortality was observed in England and Wales. This increase was subsequently attributed in part to the local marketing of an isoproterenol hand-held nebulizer five times more concentrated than available elsewhere in the world. No such increase in deaths was seen in the

United States. In the past few decades mortality has tended to decrease, probably as a result of increased recognition and improved management of asthma. Analysis of the etiology of deaths in asthmatic patients suggests that the most important contributing factor is a delay in appropriate therapy for status asthmaticus and extreme bronchial hyperreactivity.

In conclusion, asthma is a relatively common atopic condition whose epidemiology is influenced by both genetic and environmental circumstances. The general prognosis is favorable although a minority of individuals develop refractory disease, and those who become asymptomatic may persist in having mild, residual pulmonary function abnormalities.

Blair, H.   Natural history of childhood asthma. 20-year follow-up. *Arch. Dis. Child.* 52:613–619, 1977.
Presents a 20-year prospective study in a private practice.
Broder, I., Higgins, M. W., Mathers, K. P., and Keller, J. B.   Epidemology of asthma and allergic rhinitis in a total community: Tecumseh, Michigan. IV. Natural history. *J. Allergy Clin. Immonol.* 54:100–110, 1974.
This article presents an often-quoted whole population study.
Cohen, C. Genetic aspects of atopy. *Med. Clin. North Am.* 58:25–42, 1974.
Discusses various models of inheritance in atopy and risk data for genetic counseling.
Kuzemko, J.   Natural history of childhood asthma. *J. Pediatr.* 97:886–892, 1980.
A review of natural history studies and factors that influence prognosis.
Marsh, D., Meyers, D. A., and Bias, W. B.   The epidemiology and genetics of atopic allergy. *New Engl. J. Med.* 305:1551–1559, 1981.
Focuses on genetic aspects of immune responses that control allergy.
Martin, A. J., McLennan, L. A., Landau, L. I., and Phelan, P. D.   The natural history of childhood asthma to adult life. *Br. Med. J.* 280:1397–1400, 1980.
In one of the best natural history studies available, children were evaluated at ages 7, 14, and 21 years.
Smith, J. M.   Incidence of atopic disease. *Med. Clin. North Am.* 58:3–24, 1974.
Smith presents a nicely written and organized review.
Stolley, P. D.   Asthma mortality. Why the United States was spared an epidemic of deaths due to asthma. *Am. Rev. Respir. Dis.* 105:883–890, 1972.
Relates increased mortality rates to highly concentrated isoproterenol aerosol nebulizer in England and Wales.
Taussig, L., Smith, S. M., and Blumenfeld, R.   Chronic bronchitis in childhood: What is it? *Pediatrics* 67:1–5, 1981.
Chronic bronchitis in childhood may have considerable overlap with asthma.

12. BREAST-FEEDING AND ALLERGIC DISEASE
Nancy P. Cummings

The prevention of allergic diseases in children by breast-feeding infants has been recommended for at least 40 years, however, controversy still exists as to whether allergic diseases can be prevented, or even delayed, by breast-feeding infants at high risk. Although many studies have suggested beneficial effects from breast-feeding, parental history of allergic disease remains the best predictor of subsequent development of allergic disease in children.

Early studies found that children who had a family history of atopy, but had avoided cow's milk in infancy, had less atopic dermatitis than siblings who had received cow's milk. Other studies have suggested that if breast-feeding is not possible, children with an atopic background should be given a soy-based formula rather than cow's milk. Matthew (1977), Chandra (1979), and Kjellman (1979) all studied children with a strong family history of atopy and found significant benefit in the prevention of atopic dermatitis, otitis media, and respiratory infections when there was at least 6 months of breast-feeding; children who had received formula had an increased incidence of atopic disease, as well as markedly elevated serum IgE levels. In another study 50% of a group of infants fed cow's milk, but only 18% of the group fed a soy-based formula, developed allergic rhinitis.

During the past decade, many studies have confirmed these findings while others have failed to show a decreased risk for the development of atopic disease in breast-fed infants. However, all the studies that fail to confirm that dietary elimination of cow's milk in infancy reduces the risk for development of atopic diseases have had limitations. For example, cow's milk was often eliminated for less than 6 months, and various solid foods, such as egg, veal, chicken, beef, and wheat, were not restricted. In general, studies that have demonstrated a benefit have used a much stricter regimen than those failing to show a benefit.

Although many studies exist both for and against the prevention of allergies by breast-feeding, use of preventive measures appears to be prudent in the infant who is at risk of developing asthma or other allergic diseases. Breast-feeding should be recommended for 6 months with dietary avoidance of cow's milk, beef, veal, eggs, chicken, and wheat for the first 9 months. If the mother cannot nurse, a soybean formula is preferable to cow's milk, although allergy to soy protein can also occur. A nursing mother should be advised to limit her own intake of highly allergenic foods because cow's milk hypersensitivity has been found in nursing infants of mothers who consumed large amounts of cow's milk, probably due to passage of cow's milk protein into the breast milk. Furthermore, during episodes of acute gastroenteritis, ingestion of highly allergenic foods by the infant should be avoided because absorption of potential allergens is probably enhanced when the gastrointestinal tract is injured. Strict environmental control for the infant's room should also be maintained to reduce sensitization to aeroallergens (e.g., dust and molds), although no definitive studies have confirmed that this will be beneficial. Even if all the aforementioned preventive measures fail to prevent the development of allergies in infants at high risk, these measures may at least help delay the onset or lessen the severity of allergic diseases.

In addition to the potential benefits in the prevention of allergies, many studies have confirmed that human milk is nutritionally and immunologically superior to commercial formulas and cow's milk. Nutritionally, human milk protein is qualitatively and quantitatively ideal for the infant, whereas cow's milk protein is more difficult for the infant to digest and absorb. Lipids in human milk are also better absorbed by the infant, and some studies have suggested that adults who were strictly breast-fed as infants have significantly lower serum cholesterol levels. Immunologically, human milk—and particularly colostrum—contains macrophages, lymphocytes, immunoglobulins, complement, lysozyme, lactoperoxidase, lactoferrin, lactobacillus (bifid) growth factor, and interferon. All of these elements appear to provide suckling neonates with added protection from viral and bacterial pathogens at a time when they are just beginning to develop their own immune competence.

Chandra, R. K.   Prospective studies of the effect of breast-feeding on the incidence of infection and allergy. *Acta. Paediatr. Scand.* 68:691–694, 1979.
Thirty infants breast fed for the first 2 months of life had less eczema and wheezing and lower IgE than controls.
Halpern, S. R., et al.   Development of childhood allergy and infants fed breast, soy, or cow milk. *J. Allergy Clin. Immunol.* 51:139–151, 1973.
In 1753 infants fed either breast, soy, or cow's milk until age 6 months, the development of atopic disease was similar.

Hide, D. W., and Guyer, B. M.   Clinical manifestations of allergy related to breast and cow milk feeding. *Arch. Dis. Child.* 56:172–175, 1981.
Eczema and rhinitis were present equally in breast-fed and cow's milk-fed infants, but breast-feeding protected against asthma and bronchitis.

Kjellman, N.-I. M., and Johansson, S. G. O.   Soy vs. cow's milk in infants with a biparental history of atopic disease: Development of atopic disease and immunoglobulins from birth to 4 years of age. *Clin. Allergy* 9:347–358, 1979.
Two-thirds of children with a biparental history of atopy fed either soy or cow's milk developed atopic disease.

Kramer, M. S., and Morroz, B.   Do breast feeding and delayed introduction of solid foods protect against subsequent atopic eczema? *J. Pediatr.* 98:546–550, 1981.
In 636 patients followed in a dermatology clinic, a review of feeding history showed breast-feeding and delayed introductioun of solids did not protect against atopic dermatitis.

Kuroume, T., et al.   Milk sensitivity and soybean sensitivity in the production of eczematous manifestations in breast-fed infants with particular reference to intrauterine sensitization. *Ann. Allergy* 37:41–46, 1976.
Three cases of milk sensitivity and two of soybean sensitivity suggest both prenatal and postnatal sensitization may be involved in infantile eczema.

Matthew, D. J., et al.   Prevention of eczema. *Lancet* 1:321–324, 1977.
Infants of allergic parents on an allergen-avoidance regimen from birth to 6 months had less eczema at 6 months and 1 year of age.

Saarinen, U. L., Backman, A., Kajosaari, M., and Siimes, M. A.   Prolonged breast feeding as prophylaxis for atopic disease. *Lancet* 2:163–166, 1979.
Prolonged breast-feeding resulted in lower incidence of atopic disease particularly in babies with a family history of atopy. Thirty neonates fed breast milk for the first 2 months were followed for 24 months and had less eczema, wheezing, and lower serum IgE than controls.

EYES, EARS, NOSE, AND THROAT

13. OCULAR ALLERGIES
Pinkus Goldberg

The eyes, as well as the nose and skin, often make first contact with the environment; therefore, ocular mucosa frequently serve as the site of allergenic exposure. The eyelids, conjunctiva, and cornea generally suffer the initial insult. Pruritus, photophobia, and excess lacrimation are prominent symptoms, and—when accompanied by edema, redness, conjunctival injection, or dermatitis—are indicative of an ongoing allergic process. Bilateral signs and symptoms, mucoid secretions, and the presence of eosinophils on Wright's staining of conjunctival material confirm the diagnosis of ocular allergy. In contrast to infectious eye disease, allergic disease tends to be chronic (episodes last several weeks) and the course waxes and wanes. In children "allergic facies" and in particular bilateral periocular puffiness and darkening ("allergic shiners") point to an allergic etiology. Frontal headaches and facial discomfort of allergic causation may at times be prominent manifestations. Air pollutants, chemical exposure at home or work, toiletries, cosmetics, contact lenses, aerosols, and bacterial antigens as well as IgE-mediated hay fever and other atopic disorders account for the majority of ocular allergies.

Aeroallergen-induced conjunctivitis has environmental and/or seasonal fluctuations (hay fever) and is often associated with rhinitis. Usually both eyes suffer from pruritus, excessive lacrimation, vascular injection, a feeling of "pressure" behind or in the eyes, and edematous lower lids, all without photophobia. Symptoms can be unilateral. Symptoms generally begin immediately after exposure and may greatly exceed the nasal reactions. This disease is IgE mediated and increased levels of histamine and other allergic mediators are present in the tears during symptomatic periods. Conjunctival edema (chemosis), redness, and mucopurulent fluid containing eosinophils along with a characteristic symptom-exposure history point to the diagnosis. The cornea remains clear and free of disease; thus, there is no photophobia or other signs of corneal involvement. Immediate hypersensitivity skin testing should be positive to the pollen, mold, dander, or house dust thought to be the cause of the allergic disease.

Treatment includes avoidance of offending allergens as well as administration of oral antihistamines—best given in large doses at bedtime to avoid drowsiness as much as possible. Soothing solutions such as sterile, buffered, isotonic boric acid solutions either with or without local decongestants such as naphazoline hydrochloride (0.025%) or tetrahydrozoline (0.05%) are often helpful. Topical antihistamines are highly sensitizing and should be avoided. Although cromolyn solutions for ophthalmic uses are not currently marketed or approved by the FDA, research studies have shown beneficial effects when used in allergic conjunctivitis. Steroids are of value in severe cases but should be used with extreme caution, and probably only after consultation with an ophthalmologist to ensure absence of disease that may be exacerbated by their use. Immunotherapy for the appropriate aeroallergen may be beneficial in reducing symptoms, if the allergen can be clearly identified.

Vernal conjunctivitis is also thought to be atopic in character. Like allergic conjunctivitis, vernal conjunctivitis is seasonal and is associated with elevated IgE levels in tears and profuse lacrimal eosinophilia. It occurs in both childhood and adulthood. Between the age of 6 and puberty males are most often affected, but by young adulthood both sexes are involved equally. Although it can be seen in temperate climates, vernal conjunctivitis is often a disease of warm climates and is generally worse in spring and summer. Patients experience intense pruritus, photophobia, and ocular foreign body sensations. "Cobblestone" giant papillary hypertrophy of the superior tarsal conjunctiva is the most common presentation, but limbic (corneal sclera junction) region and even corneal ulcerations have been reported. Punctate whitish yellow eosinophilic accumulations (Trantas' dots) in the limbal region are pathognomonic; their presence parallels the activity of the disease.

Vernal conjunctivitis may be treated with topical vasoconstrictors and cold compresses. Topical corticosteroids, 2 to 4% disodium cromoglycate solutions, and mucolytics for the thick mucoid lacrimation often prove beneficial. Spontaneous improvement by young adulthood is commonplace.

"**Contact lens–associated giant papillary conjunctivitis**" mimics vernal conjunctivitis with similar signs and symptoms and is believed to be caused by adherence of material to the contact lens or the thimerosal in the soft lens soaking solution. A similar environmental insult is hypothesized for vernal conjunctivitis. Treatment involves discontinuing the use of the contact lens or a change in soaking solutions.

Stimuli ranging from Hymenoptera venoms to any common airborne allergens can initiate **immediate hypersensitivity reactions.** Involved sites include the conjunctiva, cornea, lid margins (blepharitis), and the eyelids—where urticaria and angioedema may be seen. Blepharitis may be induced by allergic reactions, often to infective organisms such as *Staphylococcus aureus*. These reactions to pathogenic organisms may result in phlyctenulosis (small vesicles) on the cornea and conjunctiva. *S. aureus, Candida,* and *Coccidioides* are the most frequently implicated organisms inducing these vesicles. Treatment of blepharitis requires good lid hygiene and ophthalmologic follow-up care. Vigorous treatment is needed with antibiotics and topical corticosteroids for the conjunctival disease.

One of the more commonly encountered allergic disorders is **contact dermatoconjunctivitis.** Like contact dermatitis elsewhere, cell-mediated delayed hypersensitivity is responsible for the clinical manifestations experienced by the patient. After initial antigen sensitization, the interval between repeat exposure and clinical disease is usually 24 hours. Neomycin, penicillin, atropine, local anesthetics, and numerous other sensitizers have been implicated in disease production. IgE-mediated reactions are of minor importance and the histology is notable for the many lymphocytes and neutrophils in the lesions. Pruritus, photophobia, and tearing are prominent symptoms, accompanied by erythema, vesiculation, edema, crusting, and scaling on the eyelids and facial skin. A reaction originating on the periocular skin, such as that elicited by cosmetics, often spares the eye, while ophthalmic drug reactions result in conjunctivitis and adjacent dermatitis, sometimes following the natural flow of tears down the skin. Also, contact conjunctivitis usually develops less vascular injection than pollen or dander-induced inflammation. Whenever corneal involvement is present, contactant-induced keratitis and punctate erosions are usually most severe over the lower corneal surface.

Diagnosis is often confirmed by patch testing, and primary treatment consists of avoidance of the offending agent, cleansers, and other irritants. Acute oozing lesions may be dried with dressings containing Burow's solution; topical corticosteroids are valuable in treating the more chronic drier stages of dermatitis.

Conjunctivitis associated with atopic dermatitis is another category of atopic disorder. Here, the eyelids may be thickened, lichenified, or fissured, or have weeping lesions. Patients experience ocular itching far exceeding that observed in conjunctivitis associated with hay fever. In contrast to vernal conjunctivitis, giant papillae appear primarily on the lower eyelids. Corneal ulcerations, superficial keratitis, vascularization, and stromal opacification may occur. Keratoconus (ectatic protuberant cornea), retinal detachments, anterior and posterior "atopic" cataracts, and an increased incidence of staphylococcal and herpetic infections may be encountered. Corneal involvement with the potential for visual loss can be suspected if the patient has photophobia. Four percent cromolyn sodium eyedrops 4 times daily have relieved symptoms as have topical corticosteroids, but long-term corticosteroid therapy and sensitizing chemicals such as neomycin should be avoided. To help reduce the severe itching associated with this disease crushed ice compresses or oral aspirin may be tried.

In treating these disorders, the adverse effects of **corticosteroid therapy** are well known and should always be a consideration. Topical corticosteroids may enlarge a simple epithelial herpetic infection into the severe corneal dendritic form of the disease. In addition, topical and systemic corticosteroids can significantly increase intraocular pressure and precipitate glaucoma.

Many other hypersensitivity disorders of the eye may occur including those thought to be allergic, cytotoxic (sympathetic ophthalmia), immune complex mediated, and cell mediated.

Allansmith, M. R., Baird, R. S., and Greiner, J. V. Contact Lens-associated Giant Papillary Conjunctivitis as a Model for Vernal Conjunctivitis. In A. M. Silverstein and G. R. O'Connor (Eds.), *Immunology and Immunopathology of the Eye*. New York: Masson Publishing, 1979. Pp. 346–349.
This important topic is presented in a concise and informative manner.

Anderson, J. A., and Leopold, I. H. Antiproteolytic activities found in human tears. *Ophthalmology* 88:82–84, 1981.
Inhibitory properties of human tears are compared in normals, atopics, and those with blepharitis.

Ashton, N., and Cook, C. Allergic granulomatous nodules of the eyelid and conjunctiva. *Am. J. Ophthalmol.* 87:1–28, 1979.
An extensive discussion of granuloma formation as a manifestation of localized immune complex disease is well covered.

Chumbley, L. C. *Ophthalmology in Internal Medicine*. Philadelphia: Saunders, 1981. Pp. 108–116, 201–203.
Corticosteroid side effects and atopic ocular diseases are discussed with the internal medicine patient in mind.

Cohen, E. J., and Allansmith, M. R. Ocular Allergy. In E. Middleton, C. E. Reed, and E. F. Ellis (Eds.), *Allergy: Principles and Practice* (2nd ed.). St. Louis: Mosby, 1983. Pp. 1379–1388.
Excellent overview of allergy and immunology of ocular disorders.

Friday, G. A., et al. Treatment of ragweed allergic conjunctivitis with cromolyn sodium 4% ophthalmic solution. *Am. J. Ophthalmol.* 95:169–174, 1983.
Cromolyn sodium 4% solution was shown to be a safe and effective way to control ragweed allergic conjunctivitis.

Lyle, W. M., and Hopkins, G. A. The unwanted ocular effects from topical ophthalmic drugs, their occurrence, avoidance and reversal. *J. Am. Optom. Assoc.* 48:1519–1523, 1977.
The treatment of acute rises in intraocular pressure and other drug-induced ocular reactions are discussed.

Marsh, R.J., Towns, S., and Evans, K. F. Patch testing in ocular drug allergies. *Trans. Ophthalmol. Soc. (U.K.)* 90:278–280, 1978.
Patients with ocular drug reactions showed a high rate of positive patch tests to the suspected drugs.

Shnider, H. A. The eye—part 2. *J. Am. Optom. Assoc.* 49:399–404, 1978.
The diagnosis and treatment of ocular allergies are presented in an easily understood format.

Shnider, H. A. The contact lens—part 3. *J. Am. Optom. Assoc.* 49:811–815, 1978.
The diagnosis and treatment of contact lens–induced reactions are thoroughly presented. "The presence of allergy is not sufficient by itself to contraindicate contact usage."

Weiss, A. Immunologic Diseases of the Eye. In C. W. Parker (Ed.), *Clinical Immunology*, Vol 2. Philadelphia: Saunders, 1980. Pp. 1145–1175.
Immunology from transplantation to uveitis is nicely discussed.

Wilson, F. M. Zd. Adverse external ocular effects of topical ophthalmic medications. *Surv. Ophthalmol.* 24:57–88, 1979.
All the nonopthalmologist would want to know about the subject.

14. ALLERGIC RHINITIS

Ray S. Davis

Allergic rhinitis, often referred to as hay fever, is a symptom complex characterized by sneezing, watery rhinorrhea, and nasal obstruction. Allergic rhinitis can be seasonal, occurring only several months each year, or perennial, occurring continuously throughout the year.

The incidence of allergic rhinitis in the general population is about 10%. The children of atopic parents—those with allergic rhinitis, asthma, or eczema—are 80 times more likely to develop allergic rhinitis. Conversely, approximately 80% of patients with allergic rhinitis have a strong family history of atopy. Although allergic rhinitis generally begins in late childhood, it can begin in adolescence.

Although the genetic tendency to develop allergic rhinitis is an important factor, a person must first become sensitized to one or more allergens. The symptoms occur during subsequent exposure of the person to these allergens.

Exposure to allergens such as pollens, house dust, animal danders, and molds can stimulate an atopic person's immune system to produce IgE. This IgE is produced by sensitized B-lymphocytes and is antigen specific. IgE produced in the serum becomes fixed to mast cells in tissues and basophils in the blood. Then, upon repeated exposure of the person to that particular antigen, the reaction of the antigen with the IgE molecules fixed to the mast cells in the nasal mucosa causes release of mast cell chemical mediators into the surrounding tissues. These mediators are responsible for the clinical symptoms in allergic rhinitis. The principle chemical mediator in mast cells is histamine, but there are other mediators that are known to participate in the production of the symptoms (e.g., leukotrienes, eosinophil chemotactic factors, and prostaglandins). These mediators cause dilatation of postcapillary venules, increased vascular permeability, mucosal edema, and goblet cell secretion. These physiologic alterations are manifested in the clinical symptoms of allergic rhinitis discussed in the next section.

Clinical Presentation

Seasonal allergic rhinitis is characterized by sneezing, watery rhinorrhea, and nasal obstruction. Other manifestations include itching of the nose, eyes, palate, and pharynx. Physical examination of a patient with allergic rhinitis often reveals many of the following signs: skin and facial pallor, dark circles underneath the eyes ("allergic shiners") caused by periorbital edema from venous obstruction, mouth breathing ("gaping habitus"), an accentuated horizontal line across the lower eyelids (Dennie's line), and a transverse nasal crease from the "allergic salute," an upward rubbing of the nose to relieve itching. Nasal mucosa will generally be pale and swollen, but may be inflamed. Rhinorrhea is usually thin, watery, and copious. Thirty to fifty percent of children with allergic rhinitis may have eustachian tube dysfunction that may be associated with chronic serous otitis media or sinusitis from chronic edema and obstruction of the antra of the sinuses.

Laboratory evaluation can be useful in the diagnosis of allergic rhinitis. Immediate hypersensitivity skin testing done by the puncture method (see Chap. 7) is often useful in confirming the clinical history, identifying the offending pollen in seasonal allergic rhinitis, and suggesting which environmental allergen is responsible for producing symptoms in perennial allergic rhinitis. Eosinophilia in nasal secretions is another helpful test in confirming allergic rhinitis, but it is not always present especially when symptoms are under control. Often patients with allergic rhinitis have elevated serum IgE levels, but this test is expensive and generally is not necessary to make the diagnosis.

Perennial allergic rhinitis is more difficult to diagnose than is seasonal allergic rhinitis. The clinical symptoms are the same; however, symptoms do not correspond to any particular pollen season. Although the symptoms are perennial, there may be exacerbations corresponding to seasons when the patient has pollen allergy in addition to allergy to environmental factors. Skin testing will generally show many immediate reactions to various pollens and household inhalants, such as house dust, animal danders, and molds. Cell types present in the nasal mucosa and serum IgE levels are similar to those seen in seasonal allergic rhinitis.

A "priming" effect occurs in patients with allergic rhinitis upon repeated antigen exposure. The concept of the priming effect states that a larger dose of antigen is required to produce symptoms when the nasal mucosa has been unchallenged, but that after a week or more of daily exposure, less antigen will be required to produce the same degree of symptoms. This explains why many patients continue to have severe symptoms at the end of a pollen season when the pollen counts are very low. Furthermore, the priming effect is a rational explanation why many patients with allergic rhinitis will be more sensitive to other nasal irritants (e.g., tobacco smoke and strong odors) during pollen season than during the off season.

Differential Diagnosis

The difficult diagnostic challenge is in differentiating perennial allergic rhinitis from nonallergic rhinitis with eosinophilia syndrome (NARES) and from vasomotor rhinitis. These entities are generally more difficult to treat than allergic rhinitis and, therefore, should be accurately differentiated from allergic rhinitis.

NARES is a pseudoallergic rhinitis that can be mistaken for perennial allergic rhinitis because of its similar clinical presentation and the presence of eosinophils in the nasal secretions. NARES generally begins in adulthood, in contrast to allergic rhinitis, which generally begins in late childhood. Its cause is unknown, but it does not appear to be an IgE-mediated disorder. Immediate hypersensitivity skin tests to pollens and household inhalants are negative and the serum IgE level is normal. A family history of atopy is uncommon and symptoms are predominantly those of nasal obstruction, with only occasional sneezing and rarely nasal or ocular itching. Physical examination is similar to perennial allergic rhinitis except that in NARES nasal polyps are present in approximately 30% of cases. Sinusitis is also more common in NARES.

Vasomotor rhinitis is a perennial condition of hyperreactivity of the nasal mucosa to a variety of stimuli including temperature and humidity changes, air conditioning, smoke, odors, and emotions. Like NARES, it does not appear to be IgE mediated, is generally not associated with nasal eosinophilia or elevated serum IgE levels, and is not associated with a family history of atopy. The mechanism most often proposed for vasomotor rhinitis is a neurogenic imbalance causing abnormal vascular control of blood flow leading to stasis within the sinusoids and, hence, nasal obstruction. Vasomotor rhinitis can begin in early childhood, but more commonly is seen in adolescence and adulthood. Patients are acutely aware of their nasal congestion and often complain disproportionately to the physical findings. The physical examination generally reveals inflamed nasal mucosa without edema. Polyps rarely occur.

Seasonal allergic rhinitis is not usually associated with any **complications,** however, patients with perennial allergic rhinitis frequently have serous otitis media probably caused by eustachian tube dysfunction. Other complications that have been noted in perennial allergic rhinitis include chronic sinusitis and orthodontic problems such as malocclusion from persistent mouth breathing.

Treatment

Once the diagnosis of allergic rhinitis is confirmed by history, physical examination, and appropriate laboratory data, a rational therapeutic regimen can be established. The therapeutic regimen should be based upon (1) avoidance of suspected allergens, (2) symptomatic medication, and (3) immunotherapy. Avoidance of suspected allergens, or environmental control, is discussed in detail in Chapter 23. Control over one's environment is paramount to any successful medical regimen in the treatment of allergic rhinitis, and is often the easiest, least expensive, and most beneficial of the three factors involved in a therapeutic regimen.

Symptomatic medication for allergic rhinitis is frequently combined with environmental control. These medications include oral antihistamines and decongestants, topical decongestants, cromolyn solutions, and steroids. Antihistamines are the most commonly prescribed drugs for allergic rhinitis (see Chap. 37). While the over-the-counter preparations may be effective (e.g., chlorpheniramine maleate, or Chlor-Trimeton, 2–4 mg b.i.d. to q.i.d.), sustained-release preparations by prescriptions are generally more potent. Oral decongestants such as phenylpropanolamine and phenylephrine are alpha-adrenergic agents. They seem to be effective in reducing nasal mucosal edema, either when used alone or in combination with antihistamines. Caution is necessary when these agents are used in patients with hypertension. Topical decongestants such as oxymetazoline hydrochloride and xylometazoline hydrochloride are also effective in shrinking swollen nasal mucosa, but should not be used more than twice daily for more than 5 consecutive days because a physiologic rebound phenomenon can occur. This phenomenon of rebound mucosal edema from abuse of "nasal sprays" is also known as rhinitis medicamentosa (see Chap. 15). Cromolyn solutions in 2 to 4% concentrations have shown mixed success in the treatment of allergic rhinitis and should be considered on an individual basis. A 4% cromolyn solution for nasal use is currently on the market under the trade name Nasalcrom. Topical nasal steroids such as beclomethasone and flunisolide have been shown to be very efficacious in the treatment of allergic rhinitis with minimal systemic absorption of the drug and thus minimal adrenal suppression. Although short courses of oral corticosteroids (i.e. prednisone) are occasionally necessary to control severe allergic rhinitis, adverse systemic side effects such as adrenal suppression occur frequently with these drugs and thus they should be avoided whenever possible.

Immunotherapy has been clearly established to be effective in controlling the symptoms of allergic rhinitis in many studies. Immunotherapy appears to be most effective in seasonal allergic rhinitis especially when the symptoms occur during a defined season and skin tests to the pollen(s) present in that season are positive. Graded doses of aqueous allergens are injected into the patient on a weekly basis until a maintenance level is achieved, and then the frequency of injections can be changed to every three to four weeks. (For details on consideration of patients for immunotherapy, general procedures for use, and proposed mechanisms of action of immunotherapy, see Chap. 38.)

Bierman, C. W., Pierson, W. E., and Donaldson, J. A.   Diseases of the Nose. In C. W. Bierman and D. S. Pearlman (Eds.), *Allergic Diseases of Infancy, Childhood, and Adolescence*. Philadelphia: Saunders, 1980. Pp. 511–525.
An article with an emphasis on management.
Buckley, J. M., and Pearlman, D. S.   Controlling the Environment. In C.W. Bierman and D. S. Pearlman (Eds.), *Allergic Diseases of Infancy, Childhood, and Adolescence*. Philadelphia: Saunders, 1980. Pp. 300–310.
This is one of the best reviews of environmental control.

Coffman, D. A.   A controlled trial of disodium cromoglycate in seasonal allergic rhinitis. *Br. J. Clin. Pract.* 25:403–406, 1971.
Double-blind prospective study that established good response to cromolyn.

Marsh, D. G., Meyers, D. A., and Bias, W. B.   The epidemiology and genetics of atopic allergy. *N. Engl. J. Med.* 305:1551–1559, 1981.
This is an excellent review of a complex subject.

Mullarkey, M. F.   A clinical approach to rhinitis. *Med. Clin. North Am.* 65:977–986, 1981.
Presents a very concise but complete review.

Mullarkey, M. F., Hill, J. S., and Webb, D. R.   Allergic and non-allergic rhinitis: Their characterization with the attention to the meaning of nasal eosinophilia. *J. Allergy Clin. Immunol.* 65:122–126, 1980.
A group of patients without evidence of immunologic nasal disease were identified. Forty percent had nasal eosinophilia and were classified as eosinophilic nonallergic rhinitis. These patients had a high prevalence of nasal polyps and were significantly more responsive to medical therapy than either nonallergic patients without eosinophilia or allergic patients.

Munch, E., et al.   An open comparison of dosage frequencies of beclomethasone diproprionate in seasonal allergic rhinitis. *Clin. Allergy* 11:303–309, 1981.
Comparative study that shows effectiveness of intranasal corticosteroids.

Mygind, N.   Clinical investigation of allergic rhinitis and allied conditions. *Allergy* 34:195–208, 1979.
This is a good discussion of history, physical, and laboratory approaches.

Mygind, N., and Weeke, B.   Allergic and Nonallergic Rhinitis. In E. Middleton, C. E. Reed, and E. F. Ellis (Eds.), *Allergy: Principles and Practice* (2nd ed.). St. Louis: Mosby, 1983. Pp. 1101–1118.
Complete review that includes differential diagnosis of other forms of rhinitis.

Norman, P. S.   Allergic Rhinitis. In L. M. Lichtenstein and A. S. Fauci (Eds.), *Current Therapy in Allergy and Immunology, 1983–84.* Ontario, B.C.: Decker, 1983. Pp. 1–13.
This is an authoritative and current review on the treatment of allergic rhinitis.

Norman, P. S.   Review of nasal therapy: Update. *J. Allergy Clin. Immunol.* 72:421–432, 1983.
The most recent review of the actions and side effects of nasal steroids and nasal cromolyn.

Rachelefsky, G. S., et al.   Sinus disease in children with respiratory allergy. *J. Allergy Clin. Immunol.* 61:310–314, 1978.
This study defines the prevalence of sinus disease in children with allergic disease (mostly asthma) and gives clinical and laboratory diagnostic criteria.

Settipane, G. A., and Chafee, F. H.   Nasal polyps in asthma and rhinitis. A review of 6,037 patients. *J. Allergy Clin. Immunol.* 59:17–21, 1977.
Good population study reviewing frequency of nasal polyps in various populations; details relationship between nasal polyps, allergy, aspirin intolerance, and so on.

Trzeciakowski, J. P., and Levi, R.   Antihistamines. In E. J. Middleton, C. E. Reed, and E. F. Ellis (Eds.), *Allergy: Principles and Practice* (2nd ed.). St. Louis: Mosby, 1983. Pp. 575–592.
Complete review of pharmacologic and therapeutic aspects of antihistamines.

Williams, H., and McNicol, K. N.   Prevalence, natural history and relationship of wheezy bronchitis and asthma in children. An epidemiologic study. *Br. Med. J.* 4:321–325, 1969.
A classic review; observations are still very true.

15. CHRONIC NONALLERGIC RHINITIS

Karl M. Altenburger

Chronic inflammation of the nasal mucosa (rhinitis, "sinus") is a common condition affecting a large portion of the population (estimates as high as 20%). It can be sufficiently debilitating to interfere with a person's daily activities and sleep, and it is a frequent reason for appointments with a physician. The person generally has a history of perennial nasal congestion of variable duration (a few months to many years) often associated with rhinorrhea and postnasal drip.

Table 8. Chronic nonallergic rhinitis

Known causes and associations
  Infections
  Anatomic dysfunction
    Congenital (e.g., choanal atresia)
    Traumatic (e.g., septal deformity)
    Adenoidal hypertrophy
    Foreign body
    Cerebrospinal fluid rhinorrhea
    Tumors, polyps
  Drug induced
    Topical (rhinitis medicamentosa)
    Systemic (reserpine, guanethidine, phentolamine, aspirin, alcohol, birth control pills)
  Hormonal (hypothyroidism, pregnancy, menstruation, menopause)
  Atrophic rhinitis
  Chronic irritant exposure (e.g., cigarettes)
  Miscellaneous
    Horner's syndrome, Kartagener's syndrome and other disorders of ciliary function,
    physical inactivity, Wegener's granulomatosis, cystic fibrosis
Etiology unknown
  Associated with nasal eosinophilia
  Associated with nasal mastocytosis
  Not associated with nasal eosinophilia

Occasionally the condition is truly allergic (IgE mediated) and this association has been discussed in detail in Chapter 14. Often no associated allergens can be identified and the symptom complex is then referred to as chronic nonallergic rhinitis.

The causes of chronic nonallergic rhinitis are variable and are outlined in Table 8. Persons with chronic nonallergic rhinitis are often incorrectly grouped together under the term *"vasomotor" rhinitis,* referring to a suspected instability of the nasal neurovascular unit. Vasomotor rhinitis should be distinguished from vasomotor instability. Vasomotor instability is also termed *nasal hyperreactivity, nasal hypersensitivity,* or *nasal dyspnea.* It can be best defined as an exaggerated or hyperresponsive cholinergic reactivity leading to exaggerated nasal turbinate swelling and hypersecretion. This vasomotor instability is characterized by alternating nostril congestion and symptoms in response to recumbency, alcohol intake, temperature and humidity changes, and other nonspecific irritants (inert dust, smoke, fumes, aerosols, powders, and strong odors). Such vasomotor instability may occur because of any inflammatory, noninflammatory, or structural cause of chronic rhinitis. Its presence is not diagnostic of a specific disorder, but rather indicates general nasal malfunctioning. Vasomotor instability should be seen as conceptually analogous to the relative bronchial instability observed in asthma of widely divergent etiology.

The diagnosis of intrinsic or primary vasomotor rhinitis should be entertained only after all the known causes for nasal disease have been excluded by extensive, thorough evaluation. Keeping the known causes and associations in mind, the evaluation is begun with a thorough history. The following questions are of special interest: What is the pattern of the illness from its onset and how has it affected the patient? Are there daily or seasonal exacerbations or remissions? What symptoms predominate (i.e., obstruction, discharge, anosmia)? What is the character of the nasal secretions? What precipitating factors have been identified and what has provided relief? The examination focuses on the nasal mucosa, but care must be used not to overlook important associated findings in the ears, eyes, mouth, and throat. All sinuses should also be thoroughly palpated. Adequate visualization, using a nasal speculum with adequate lighting, is essential, and the application of a topical vasoconstrictor is often necessary. An important laboratory aid involves scraping the nasal mucosa with a calcium alginate swab, which is then smeared and stained, eliciting the presence of eosinophils, neutrophils, and mast cells. Once all of this information has been gathered, further testing may be indicated (i.e., sinus x-ray, allergy skin tests, and so on).

If a cause can be identified the treatment is straightforward (e.g., antibiotics for bacterial infections, and so on). When an etiology cannot be found a number of general measures may be tried. These general measurers can also be useful in facilitating a response to a specific intervention, such as discontinuing the use of topical decongestants in rhinitis medicamentosa. Reducing exposure of the nasal mucosa to irritants—cigarette smoke, dust, and so on—is always important. Dust control measures are focused on the person's bedroom. The benefit of routine normal saline irrigations cannot be over emphasized. This is most easily accomplished by using a nasal spray bottle filled with salt water (⅛ teaspoon table salt plus ⅛ teaspoon baking soda plus 1 cup of water). Several sprays are generously applied in each nostril at least 3 times a day. Other techniques are nearly impossible to perform and compliance with these procedures is minimal. These procedures include using bulb syringes and nasal douches and sniffing salt water from cupped hands. Irrigations and nasal secretions are then blown gently from the nose; forceful blowing must be avoided. Exercise, and the resultant sympathetic nerve discharge, can be an important adjunct to therapy, especially in the young and middle-aged person.

The routine use of an antihistamine-decongestant combination is often beneficial. Most normotensive individuals tolerate these quite well. Although the soporific side effects of antihistamines can be troublesome, tolerance to these side effects usually develops within 3 weeks. A large variety of single agents, preferably from different classes of antihistamines, is generally sufficient. Sustained release agents, even for children (for whom capsules can be opened and divided), are preferred as they need to be used only twice daily.

Corticosteroids are often very useful in the treatment of these disorders. They seem especially effective in those persons with nasal eosinophilia, but are extremely useful in rhinitis medicamentous, which is not associated with eosinophilia. Generally the use of topical agents is sufficient although the occasional patient may require systemic steroids for 5 to 7 days. Both beclomethasone and flunisolide are currently approved for nasal use by the FDA. Beclomethasone is preferred by this author for adults and children older than age 12 because of its ease of administration, compact container, and decreased incidence of topical irritation (stinging). The initial dose is one spray in each nostril 3 times a day immediately following a normal saline irrigation (package insert directions should be carefully followed). Flunisolide has the advantage of being approved for use in children older than age 6. The recommended starting dose is two sprays in each nostril twice a day. Effects are usually apparent with either agent after 1 week. When the desired effect has been achieved the dose should be gradually tapered to the lowest tolerable dose. Rare side effects of these agents (e.g., intranasal candidal infection, epistaxis) have been mentioned after long-term use.

Close follow-up of any treatment plan is mandatory. The results are often rewarding although the disorder can occasionally be frustrating and difficult to treat. In either case an understanding and compassionate approach is required.

Chatterjee, S. S., Nassar, W. Y., Wilson, O., and Butler, A. G.   Intranasal beclomethasone dipropionate and intranasal sodium cromoglycate: A comparative trial. *Clin. Allergy* 4:343–348, 1974.
   Both therapies were well tolerated and effective without significant adverse reactions. Two therapies were not compared in the same patients.

Hendeles, L., Weinberger, M., and Wong. L.   Medical management of noninfectious rhinitis. *Am. J. Hosp. Pharm.* 37:1436–1454, 1980.
Good review of the pharmacologic management with an especially good review of the use of antihistamines.

Jacobs, R. L., Freedman, P. M., and Boswell, R. N.   Nonallergic rhinitis with eosinophilia (NARES syndrome). Clinical and immunologic presentation. *J. Allergy Clin. Immunol.* 67:253–262, 1981.
A review of this subgroup is presented.

Jalowayski, A. A., and Zeiger, R. S.   A Practical Guide for the Examination of Nasal Cytology in the Diagnosis of Nasal Disorders. Manual available by writing Rhinotechnics, P.O. Box 84058, San Diego, California 92138. 1980.
Detailed demonstration for obtaining, staining, and quantifying cell types identified and worth reading.

Knight, A., et al.   Immunologic parameters in perennial rhinitis. *Clin. Allergy* 9: 159–166, 1979.
What we know and what we do not know about this subject.

Mullarkey, M. F.   The classification of nasal disease: An opinion. *J. Allergy Clin. Immunol.* 67:251–252, 1981.
Presents a state-of-the-art opinion.

Mullarkey, M. F., Hill, J. S., and Webb, D. R.   Allergic and nonallergic rhinitis: Their characterization with attention to the meaning of nasal eosinophilia. *J. Allergy Clin. Immunol.* 65:122–126, 1980.
The presence of eosinophils is most valuable in predicting their response to therapy.

Mygind, N., and Weeke, B.   Allergic and Nonallergic Rhinitis. In E. Middleton, C. E. Reed, and E. F. Ellis (Eds.), *Allergy: Principles and Practice* (2nd ed.). St. Louis: Mosby, 1983. Pp. 1101–1118.
Complete review that includes differential diagnosis of other forms of rhinitis.

Siegel, C. J., and Dockhorn, R. J.   An evaluation of childhood rhinorrhea. *Ann. Allergy* 48:9–11, 1982.
Nasal cytology is useful in childhood rhinorrhea.

Spector, S. L., English, G., and Jones. L.   Clinical and nasal response to treatment of perennial rhinitis. *J. Allergy Clin. Immunol.* 66:129–137, 1980.
Clinical response to treatment associated with a loss of nasal eosinophils, and correlated with decreased inflammation on biopsy.

Tennenbaum, J. L.   Allergic Rhinitis. In R. Patterson (Ed.), *Allergic Diseases: Diagnosis and Management.* Philadelphia: Lippincott, 1980. Pp. 179–203.
A good general review of the subject.

Vilsvik, J. S., and Jenssen, A. O., and Walstad, R.   The effect of beclomethasone dipropionate aerosol on allergen induced nasal stenosis. *Clin. Allergy* 5:291–294, 1975.
Another article that reinforces the usefulness of this drug.

Zeiger, R. S., and Schatz, M.   Chronic rhinitis: A practical approach to diagnosis and treatment. *Immunol. Allerg. Pract.* 4:63–78, 108–118, 1982.
Excellent review with a very practiced approach to the problem.

16. SINUSITIS AND NASAL POLYPS
Allen D. Adinoff

One of the major target organs of allergic disease is the mucosa of the upper respiratory tract. Therefore, it is not surprising that disorders of the paranasal sinuses occur in many persons with allergic disease. Indeed, significant radiologic abnormalities are said to occur in up to 50% of persons with chronic rhinitis. Many of these sinuses are infected with aerobic and anaerobic bacteria and, occasionally, viruses. Treatment of persistent rhinorrhea or nasal obstruction may be frustrated if coexisting sinus disease goes unrecognized. Sinusitis may also complicate asthma. Many asthmatic symptoms may be more difficult to control if sinusitis is present. Treatment of sinus disease may make severe steroid-dependent asthma easier to control. Nasal polyps can also be found in a small percentage of persons with either chronic rhinitis or asthma.

Sinusitis

The paranasal sinuses develop from outpocketings of the nasal mucous membranes and include the maxillary, ethmoidal, frontal, and sphenoidal sinuses. The maxillary sinuses are present as slits at birth and may be infected in newborns. The ethmoidal sinuses are also present at birth. Frontal sinuses develop from the anterior ethmoids but do not pneumatize the frontal bone until 1 to 2 years of age. Often, one frontal sinus is absent. The sphenoidal sinus is not visible until approximately 3 years of age. The maxillary sinuses are the largest. The proximity of the maxillary sinuses to the upper teeth is important because dental pain can often be confused with sinusitis. The maxillary sinuses are roofed by the orbit and bordered medially by the nasal cavity. Drainage occurs posteriorly via the middle meatus. The ethmoidal sinuses are arranged in three pairs between the nasal cavity and medial orbit. A thin plate of bone, often incomplete, separates the ethmoidal sinuses from the orbit and is a common route for spreading infection. The anterior and middle ethmoidal sinuses drain anteriorly via the middle meatus, while drainage of the posterior ethmoidal sinuses occurs through the superior meatus. The frontal sinuses extend dorsally above the orbit and anteriorly to the cranial fossa. Because they are derived from the anterior ethmoidal sinuses, their drainage is via the anterior middle meatus. The sphenoidal sinuses are the most deeply placed. They are directly below the sella turcica and immediately anterior to the brain stem. The cavernous sinuses are located laterally and drainage occurs through the sphenoid-ethmoidal recess.

Radiographic examination of the paranasal sinuses involves three projections. The occipitomental (Water's) projection is used most commonly and maximizes visualization of the maxillary and frontal sinuses as well as the orbits and nasal septum. An occipitofrontal (Caldwell's) projection is best for viewing the ethmoidal air cells. A lateral projection allows visualization of the sphenoidal sinus and the posterior wall of the frontal sinus.

The physiologic functions of the sinuses are not fully known. Clearly they are poorly designed for bipeds as their lowest points are often below their respective drainage ostia. Olfaction, voice response, production of protective mucus, lessening of skill weight, and dampening of sudden pressure changes are some proposed functions.

Sinusitis is defined as an inflammation of the mucous membranes lining the paranasal sinuses. The process may be suppurative or nonsuppurative, acute, subacute, or chronic. Nearly 15 to 25% of asymptomatic persons have abnormal radiologic findings, suggesting that sinusitis is more common than was expected, or that radiologic changes may persist long after acute symptoms have subsided. Sinusitis usually accompanies conditions that predispose to obstruction of the sinus ostia, thereby preventing the normal clearance of mucus and bacteria. Other factors that need to be considered in sinusitis include cilia dysmotility syndromes and immune deficiency states (Table 9).

Acute suppurative sinusitis presents as a closed space infection. Fever, disproportionate malaise, and sinus pain are common. The pain may be either over the sinuses or referred. It often intensifies with bending or coughing and is usually worse in the evening. Nasal discharge is bloody or purulent. Soft tissue swelling is common in children and the sinuses are often tender. The nasal turbinates are red and swollen. Often purulent material can be seen at the sites of drainage and can identify the affected sinus. Transillumination may be helpful in adults, although considerable experience is needed for valid interpretation. Virtually 100% of opaque sinuses are infected whereas normal transilluminating sinuses nearly always yield no organisms. Radiologic examination is more sensitive than trans-

Table 9. Factors predisposing to sinusitis

Obstruction
  Anatomic
    Deviated nasal septum
    Polyps (especially in cystic fibrosis)
    Tumors
    Foreign bodies
    Adenoids
  Functional
    Upper respiratory tract infections
    Allergic and nonallergic rhinitis
    Rhinitis medicamentosa
Immune deficiency
  IgA deficiency
  Hypogammaglobulinemia
  Neutropenia: chemotactic defects
  Chronic granulomatous disease
  Secondary factors (e.g., chemotherapy, diabetes mellitus)
Abnormalities of cilia
  Kartagener's syndrome
  Other cilia dysmotility syndromes

illumination. Sinuses that show opacification or air-fluid levels almost always are infected. Mucous membrane thickening of 5 to 8 millimeters or greater is also highly correlated with sinus contamination. Computerized axial tomography has become extremely useful in delineating the extent of disease in certain patients. Frequently, retro-orbital extension from an infected maxillary sinus that is asymptomatic can be diagnosed before the disease is clinically apparent.

The only method for reliable identification of infecting organisms is direct aspiration of the sinuses, either by sinus puncture or surgery. Nasopharyngeal cultures have been routinely unreliable, showing poor correlation to predominant species of bacteria obtained directly from the sinuses. Recently, however, it has been suggested that the method of plating the cultures may account for the disparity between the cultures of aspirated fluid and the nasopharyngeal cultures. In a study comparing simultaneous cultures of the nasopharynx and middle ear exudates obtained by tympanocentesis, it was found that if the nasopharyngeal culture swab was plated directly onto appropriate solid agar rather than into trypticase soy broth, preferential growth of nonpathogens is reduced and greater yield of a single pathogen is obtained. Studies using this technique comparing direct sinus aspirates with nasopharyngeal cultures have not been done. The possibility of identifying pathogens without directly invading the sinuses is an exciting prospect.

The bacteriology of acute sinusitis has been well studied. *Streptococcus pneumoniae, Hemophilus influenzae* (nontypable) and *Branhamella catarrhalis* are most routinely found and are usually sensitive to ampicillin, amoxicillin, or trimethoprim and sulfamethoxazole. Other streptococcal species, gram-negative organisms, *Staphylococcus aureus,* anaerobes, and viruses are less commonly seen.

Medical treatment is aimed toward restoration of sinus drainage and eradication of infecting organisms. Ampicillin or amoxicillin in generous doses should be the primary antibiotic, although trimethoprim and sulfamethoxazole can be used in penicillin-sensitive patients. If an organism has been isolated, in vitro sensitivities can be used as a guide to therapy. Antibiotics should be supplemented with systemic decongestants as well as topical vasoconstricting agents (e.g., ephedrine or phenylephrine). Many patients require narcotic analgesics. Topical corticosteroids probably should not be used in bacterial sinusitis. Proper duration of treatment is uncertain although most sources recommend at least 10 to 14 days. Most treatment failures are caused by resistant organisms or the development of complications. Chronic sinusitis and osteomyelitis are not uncommon complications. Other complications may extend beyond the confines of the sinuses. Periorbital cellulitis and abscess or orbital abscesses can occur via a direct spread through the bony walls of the ethmoidal sinuses. Alveolar abscesses in the upper incisors via spread from the maxillary sinuses have been seen. Life-threatening complications such as subdural empyemas, brain abscesses, meningitis, and cavernous sinus thrombosis may also rarely occur.

While acute sinusitis appears to be a clear clinical entity, **chronic suppurative sinusitis** is less consistently defined. Many sources define chronic sinusitis as a sinus disease that fails to respond to medical management, while other authors define it in terms of mucosal changes—hypertrophy or fibrosis—seen on radiologic examination of the sinuses. Most would agree that sinus disease present for 2 to 3 months represents chronic sinusitis. The process appears to be common in that 15 to 25% of normal, asymptomatic subjects have radiographic abnormalities. Chronic sinusitis seems to be more common in patients with allergy or asthma or both, approaching an incidence of 50% of this patient population.

In contrast to acute sinusitis, symptoms of chronic sinusitis may be insidious or absent. Fever and sinus tenderness are unusual and headaches and malaise are very uncommon. Persistent rhinorrhea and nasal obstruction, chronic cough, postnasal drip, sore throat, and a fetid breath are symptoms that seem to correlate with radiographic abnormalities and contaminated sinus aspirates. However, clinical findings of chronic sinusitis may also be subtle and are often difficult to differentiate from chronic rhinitis alone. Edematous inflamed turbinates with purulent material are usually seen. Evidence of posterior pharyngeal irritation such as hypertrophy of posterior lymphoid follicles and anterior cervical adenopathy are also commonly observed. Radiographic confirmation is usually needed. Of all the sinus abnormalities seen on radiographic examination, opaque sinuses are most likely to be infected; air-fluid levels are rarely seen. As with acute sinusitis, mucous membrane thickening of 5 to 8 millimeters or greater correlates better with chronic signs and symptoms and positive aspirates than do the more minimal changes.

Organisms recovered from chronically inflamed sinuses yield a more diverse variety than those seen in acute sinusitis. Anaerobic bacteria are the only organisms recovered in 40 to 60% of positive bacterial aspirates, but they may also be mixed with aerobes. *Bacteroides* species, anaerobic gram-positive cocci, and *Fusobacterium* species are most commonly and consistently isolated and are sensitive to penicillin. The frequent involvement of anaerobes in chronic sinusitis is probably related to the poor drainage and increased intranasal pressure that develops during inflammation, reducing the oxygen tension by decreasing the mucosal blood flow. The lowering of the oxygen content and pH of the sinus cavities supports the growth of anaerobic organisms by providing them with an optimal oxidation-reduction potential. *Hemophilus influenzae,* hemolytic streptococci, and *Staphylococcus aureus* are the most common aerobic organisms. Viruses—adenovirus, rhinovirus, and influenza A—may also be recovered. The presence of unusual organisms should alert the clinician to the possibility of an underlying disease. Patients with cystic fibrosis or ciliary dysmotility syndromes may harbour *Pseudomonas aeruginosa* in their sinuses. Mucormycosis, aspergillosis, or candidiasis may be the primary cause of infections in patients with primary or secondary immune deficiency conditions. Granulomatous disease of the paranasal sinuses, including tuberculosis, syphilis, leprosy, and vascular granulomatous processes such as Wegener's, is uncommon. Parasitic infestation of the paranasal sinuses is extremely rare.

Treatment of chronic sinusitis is often frustrating, although the use of antimicrobials and methods to promote drainage (medical or surgical) still holds. The antibiotic used depends on the results of the sinus aspirate culture. Occasionally ampicillin or amoxicillin is given without culturing the sinus and the result followed clinically. Absence of a response to the primary antibiotic should be pursued by aspiration and culture so that the appropriate antibiotic can be selected. Medical drainage with systemic decongestants and topical vasoconstrictors should also be used. Treatment with topical corticosteroids may be useful, but is controversial in cases where sinuses are known to be infected. Treatment should continue for 3 to 4 weeks. Radiographic improvement correlates well with sterilization of the sinuses. Because the chronically inflamed sinus mucosa often has a poor blood supply with microabscesses within crypts, medical treatment may be unsuccessful. Surgical procedures, however, such as sinus aspiration and lavage or removal of hypertrophic mucosa with postoperative drainage are not uniformly successful. Vidian neurectomy has limited application.

Nasal Polyps

Nasal polyps have been described for more than 3000 years. Various treatment methods have been employed, many of which are used today with some modification. The incidence of nasal polyps is not known, although it appears to be higher in allergic populations. While most texts quote figures of 15 to 25%, a recent survey of more than 6000 adult patients with asthma and rhinitis found only a 4.2% incidence of nasal polyps. Polyps occur in less than 1% of allergic children. Polyps are more common in patients with asthma, especially if the patients are nonallergic, and their frequency increases with age. Fourteen percent of patients with polyps have aspirin intolerance (mostly bronchospasm). Approximately 6% of patients with cystic fibrosis have nasal polyps. Nasal mastocytosis also predisposes to polyps. Nasal polyps are also common in patients with the well-established triad of reversible obstructive airways disease, chronic sinusitis, and aspirin idiosyncracy.

The pathogenesis of polyps is not known. Chronic inflammation of the nasal mucosa, abnormal vasomotor responses, and mechanical problems from increased interstitial fluid pressure and edema are believed to play a role. Histologic and biochemical studies have not resolved the enigma of the causes of polyps. Grossly, polyps may have a papillary, glandular, or cystic appearance. Microscopically, the epithelium may range from normal-appearing ciliated columnar epithelium to squamous metaplasia. The stroma consists of a highly edematous, fine reticular network with infiltrates of eosinophils and plasma cells. IgA and IgE are found in concentrations greater than is expected from passive filtration. Histamine, serotonin, norepinephrine, leukotrienes C and D (formerly known as slow-reacting substance of anaphylaxis, or SRS-A), and eosinophilic chemotactic factor of anaphylaxis (ECF-A) have been found with polyps.

The most common clinical features of nasal polyps are nasal airway obstruction and rhinorrhea; anosmia is a frequent complaint. The nasal discharge varies from clear, watery secretions to tenacious, purulent material. Nasal examination is most effective when the normal mucosa is shrunken by a topical vasoconstrictor (1% cocaine or 1% ephedrine). Nasopharyngeal examination is usually unnecessary to identify most polyps because they are most common in the upper part of the lateral nasal wall, around the middle turbinate. Polyps are rounded or pear-shaped, usually soft and gelatinous, and have a "peeled grape" appearance. They are usually mobile and insensitive to manipulation, and will pit with palpation. Radiologic examination will reveal the presence of soft tissue masses within the nasal chambers. Findings consistent with chronic sinusitis are almost always present. Several tumors and neoplasms have the clinical appearance of nasal polyps. Unilateral polyps in particular should alert the clinician to the possibility of another disease process. Meningoceles, nasal dermoids, juvenile nasopharyngeal angiofibromas, and squamous cell carcinomas are the most important entities to consider.

The treatment of nasal polyps, whether medical or surgical, is often frustrated by their recurrence within several weeks to months. Medical treatment should include systemic decongestants and topical vasoconstrictors. Antibiotics are useful if chronic sinusitis is found. Aspirin avoidance should be maintained if idiosyncracy is recognized. Steroids may be administered by aerosol, local injection, or systemically. Local injection of steroids, usually triamcinolone acetonide (Kenalog-40) 0.5 to 1.0 ml at various sites with a 27-gauge needle, will often cause regression of the polyps. Systemic corticosteroids (e.g., prednisone 40 mg per day for 5–7 days) will often produce dramatic improvement in nasal airway obstruction. Patients may require steroid maintenance with alternate-day prednisone or an aerosolized steroid with low absorption (e.g., beclomethasone) to prevent recurrence. Surgical treatment should be considered in those patients who do not respond to medical treatment or those with complications. Intranasal polypectomy may be performed with local anesthesia as an outpatient procedure. Because the origin of tissue is often located within the sinus, however, recurrence is common. Most polyps arise from the ethmoidal sinus; therefore, external ethmoidectomy with removal of diseased sinus tissue is considered to be the most definitive procedure.

Sinusitis and Polyps: Relationship to Asthma

It has long been recognized that sinusitis and asthma are related, although the nature of the association is unclear. Chronic sinusitis is found in approximately 50% of patients with asthma. Although no control studies have been done, the cumulative experience has been that steroid-dependent asthmatic patients with sinusitis frequently will have significant improvement in their pulmonary status if associated sinusitis is treated aggressively. Very often steroid dosages can be dramatically reduced or discontinued. The author's approach to such patients is as follows: (1) Asthmatic patients in whom symptoms and radiologic examination suggest sinusitis should be treated medically with antibiotics (ampicillin), decongestants (topical for 3–4 days and systemic), and topical steroids for 3 to 4 weeks. (2) If no improvement in symptoms or sinus roentgenograms is seen and the asthma is severe, antral puncture and lavage should be performed. (3) If the organism recovered is resistant to the initial antibiotic used, the appropriate antimicrobial should be employed. (4) If sinus disease continues, aggressive sinus surgery should be considered. It should be remembered that these guidelines apply only to severe, usually steroid-dependent asthmatic patients as sinus surgery is not always successful and is not without its complications.

There are many possible mechanisms by which sinus disease could aggravate underlying asthma. (1) Nasal obstruction could lead to mouth breathing of relatively cold, unhumidified air causing bronchoconstriction. (2) Postnasal drip could aggravate cough and produce bronchospasm. (3) Direct aspiration of purulent nasal discharge could produce airways obstruction. Radiolabelled material placed in the nasopharynx can be found in the lungs; a reflex mediator pathway via the afferent trigeminal nerve from the sinus to the dorsal vagal nucleus in brain stem reticular formation and then to broncial smooth muscle fibers via the efferent vagus nerve has been proposed to explain this occurrence. (4) Enhancement of beta-adrenergic blockade could exist.

The relationship of nasal polyps to asthma has also long been recognized. The earlier literature suggested that asthmatic patients often tended to develop more severe, often intractable asthma after polypectomy; however, recent studies do not support this relationship.

Summary and Conclusions

Sinusitis accompanies any process in the upper respiratory tract that predisposes to obstruction or impediment of normal sinus drainage. Persons with nasal allergy and asthma are a highly susceptible group. Acute sinusitis presents as a closed space infection and is treated by antibiotics with medical or surgical drainage. Early recognition is important as complications can be life-threatening. In the vast majority of cases organisms are sensitive to ampicillin. Chronic sinusitis is a more indolent process with more subtle signs and symptoms. It may aggravate asthmatic symptoms, and aggressive treatment of the sinusitis may be accompanied by improvement in pulmonary status. Causative organisms are predominantly anaerobic bacteria that are sensitive to penicillins. The presence of an unusual organism should alert the clinician to the possibility of an underlying disease. Treatment of chronic sinusitis, whether medical or surgical, should be aggressive although both methods are often unsuccessful.

Nasal polyps are found in approximately 4% of adults with asthma and rhinitis. Unilateral polyps should alert the clinician to the possibility of a tumor or neoplasm.

Brook, I.   Chronic sinusitis in children. *J.A.M.A.* 246:967–969, 1981.
Aspiration of chronically inflamed sinuses yielded primarily anaerobes often mixed with aerobic bacteria.
Downing, E., Braman, S., and Settipane, G.   Bronchial reactivity in patients with nasal polyps before and after polypectomy (abstr.) *J. Allergy Clin. Immunol.* 69:102, 1982.
Bronchial hyperreactivity in asthmatic and nonasthmatic persons before and after polypectomy is discussed.
English, G. M.   Nasal Polyps and Sinusitis. In E. Middleton, Jr., C. F. Reed, and E. F. Ellis (Eds.), *Allergy: Principles and Practice* (2nd ed.). St. Louis Mosby, 1983. Pp. 1215–1248.
Evans, F. O., et al.   Sinusitis of the maxillary antrum. *N. Engl. J. Med.* 293:735–739, 1975.
The bacteriology of acute maxillary sinusitis obtained by needle aspirates is discussed.
Freda, A. J., Jacobs, R. L., and Culver, W. G.   Primary nasal polyposis (abstr.) *J. Allergy Clin. Immunol.* 69:148, 1982.
Methacholine bronchial provocation in patients with primary polyposis is discussed. These patients may represent an incomplete example of aspirin-triad asthma.
Gottlieb, M. J.   Relationship of intranasal disease in the production of asthma. *J.A.M.A.* 85:105–108, 1925.
An early study concerning the relationship of sinusitis in bronchial asthma; mechanisms of pathogenesis are discussed.
Hamory, B. H., et al.   Etiology and antimocrobial therapy of acute maxillary sinusitis. *J. Infect. Dis.* 139:197–210, 1979.
A classic and often referenced study of needle aspirates of adults with acute sinusitis.
Miles-Lawrence, R., Kaplan, M., and Chang, K.   Methacholine sensitivity in nasal polyposis and the effects of polypectomy (abstr.) *J. Allergy Clin. Immunol.* 69:102, 1982.
Nasal polypectomy does not significantly increase bronchial hyperreactivity.
Rachelefsky, G. S., et al.   Sinus disease in children with respiratory allergy. *J. Allergy Clin. Immunol.* 61:310–314, 1978.
The association of sinus disease with respiratory allergy is discussed. Clinical signs and symptoms show correlation with positive X-rays.
Sampter, M., and Lederer, F. L.   Nasal polyps: Their relationship to allergy, particularly to bronchial asthma. *Med. Clin. North Am.* 42:175–179, 1958.
Patients with asthma who seemed to worsen after polypectomy were more likely to have aspirin idiosyncracy.
Scramm, V., Jr., and Effron, M.   Nasal polyps in children. *Laryngoscope* 90:1488–1493, 1980.

Antral-choanal polyp was the most frequently observed nasal mass found in patients. Surgical procedure for nasal polyposis in children is discussed.

Schwartz, R., et al.   The nasopharyngeal culture in acute otitis media. *J.A.M.A.* 241:12170–1273, 1979.
Using solid agar plating techniques, cultures of the nasopharynx correlated well with those obtained by direct tympanocentesis.

Settipane, G. A., and Chafee, F. H.   Nasal polyps in asthma and rhinitis. A review of 6037 patients. *J. Allergy Clin. Immunol.* 59:17–21, 1977.
The incidence of nasal polyps in adult patients with asthma and rhinitis was 4.2%. The association of polyps with other categories of allergic diseases is discussed.

Slavin, R. G., et al.   Sinusitis and bronchial asthma. *J. Allergy Clin. Immunol.* 66:250–257, 1980.
Treatment of sinusitis in many patients with severe asthma resulted in improvement of pulmonary status.

Wald, E. R., et al.   Acute maxillary sinusitis in children. *N. Engl. J. Med.* 304:749–754, 1981.
The bacteriology of acute maxillary sinusitis in children obtained by direct needle aspirates is discussed.

Wald, E. R., Pang, D., Milmore, G. J., and Schramm, V. L., Jr.   Sinusitis and its complications in the pediatric patient. *Pediatr. Clin. North Am.* 28:777–798, 1981.
Presents an excellent review with extensive reference lists.

17. OTITIS MEDIA AND ALLERGIES
Don A. Bukstein and Kathleen C. Davis

Otitis media, or middle ear effusion, is a collection of fluid in the middle ear resulting in decreased mobility of the tympanic membrane. This inflammation of the middle ear may or may not be infectious. Acute, or suppurative, otitis media is most often the result of infection, either bacterial or viral. Chronic, or serous, otitis media has many forms, including mucoid and nonsuppurative otitis media. Infection (or more accurately growth of bacterial organisms) is reported in 25 to 40% of cases of serous otitis media. It is difficult to determine whether the associated infection is the cause of the effusion; infection could be the result of secondary bacterial growth in the effusion, which is an excellent culture media.

The prevalence of otitis media in infants and children is 15 to 20% with a peak occurence between 6 and 36 months of age. The incidence of otitis media in groups of allergic children is slightly higher than the incidence in nonatopic children. Bluestone (1978) described a seasonal variation in episodes of secretory otitis media, with an increased incidence in early spring and winter and a decreased incidence in summer. Otitis media occurs with increased frequency in males, in members of lower socioeconomic groups, in Eskimos and American Indians, in children with abundant nasopharyngeal lymphoid tissue, in infants fed cow's milk in the supine position, and in children with cleft palate. The extent to which host infection and environmental factors interact to influence the prevalence and incidence of otitis media has not been established.

Most authors agree that abnormal function of the eustachian tube is involved in the pathogenesis of the effusion in otitis media. The eustachian tube connects the ear and nasopharynx allowing it to carry out three physiologic functions: (1) ventilation of the middle ear, (2) clearance of secretions produced in the middle ear, and (3) protection of the middle ear from nasopharyngeal secretions. Several mechanisms have been proposed for the dysfunction of the eustachian tube in production of the effusion in otitis media: (1) Functional obstruction from persistent collapse can be caused by increased compliance of the tube or an abnormally active opening mechanism. This obstruction is common in otherwise normal infants and younger children in whom the cartilage supporting the eustachian tube is not fully developed, and is routinely seen in infants with unrepaired cleft palate and in many children with repaired cleft palates. (2) Intrinsic mechanical obstruction can be caused by inflammation from an inadequately treated infection or possibly by allergy. (3) Extrinsic obstruction can be secondary to a tumor or possibly an adenoidal mass. (4) Abnormal patency, where the tube has a low resistance and opens easily, allowing easy access of nasopharyngeal secretions to the middle ear, may be a fourth cause for eustachian tube dysfunction.

Whether or not otitis media is a manifestation of allergic disease per se is still a matter of debate. A reduction of eustachian tube permeability after a reagin-induced nasal crisis in atopic subjects has been described. However, in other studies where antigen was instilled intranasally middle ear effusion was not demonstrated. Analyses of IgE and eosinophils in middle ear effusion have also yielded conflicting reports. Some studies show that the effusion is a transudate of serum, while other studies have found an increase of IgE and eosinophils in the effusion when compared with plasma. Friedman and colleagues (1983) conducted provocative nasal challenges in a group of patients with IgE-mediated allergic rhinitis. Their results conclusively demonstrated that eustachian tube obstruction can be induced by nasal antigen challenge.

Bluestone's study (1978) demonstrated that when a patient with nasal obstruction swallows the nasopharyngeal pressure is first positive and then negative. Positive nasopharyngeal pressure and nasal obstruction caused secretions from the nasopharynx to be insufflated into the middle ear. Subsequent negative nasopharyngeal pressures were shown to cause obstruction of the eustachian tube. It is speculated that this may be the mechanism for the development of effusion in the middle ears of patients with allergic rhinitis.

At this point it seems that the theory of mechanical obstruction as outlined in Bluestone's study is the most likely explanation to account for the effusion in patients with allergic rhinitis. A prospective study of eustachian function in allergic patients is underway to establish whether pollen inhalation during allergy season can produce changes in eustachian tube function. The model of allergy-induced eustachian tube obstruction defined by Friedman and colleagues (1983) should be useful in the study of middle ear disease in allergic individuals.

Clinically, patients with secretory otitis media may present in a variety of ways. Older children may complain of itching, popping, or stuffed-up ears. Some complain of hearing loss or a sensation of fullness in the ear. Young children often do not complain of symptoms but may present with delayed language development because of impaired hearing.

Diagnosis is made by combining a physical examination with audiometry and tympanometry, when indicated. Examination with a pneumatic otoscope may reveal decreased mobility of the tympanic membrane. The tympanic membrane usually appears dull and retracted with air-fluid levels or bubbles. On the other hand, the tympanic membrane may look relatively normal. It is in these cases that tympanometry, which measures the compliance of the tympanic membrane, and audiometry, which may show a conductive hearing loss, are indicated. These techniques are also a useful way to follow the resolution of chronic otitis media. Evaluation of chronic middle ear effusion should include a thorough search for an underlying cause (e.g., paranasal sinusitis, upper respiratory tract allergy, submucous cleft palate, or a nasopharyngeal tumor).

Treatment of patients with secretory otitis media is varied and none has been shown to be effective in acceptable clinical trials. However, of all the medical treatments that have been advocated, a trial of an antimicrobial agent appears to be the most appropriate in persons who have not received an antibiotic in the recent past. Most authors recommend decongestants and antihistamines, however, these are also of unproved efficacy. In fact, a study by Olson and colleagues (1978) suggests that the use of decongestants may even be associated with an increased incidence of serous otitis. In this study, patients with history of allergy were treated with either decongestants or placebo during episodes of acute otitis media. Fifty-six percent of the patients treated with decongestants developed secretory otitis media whereas only 29% of the placebo-treated group developed the problem.

Topical decongestant nose sprays are also recommended for use during acute allergic exacerbations; their use should be strictly limited to 3 or 4 days to prevent development of rhinitis medicamentosa. Adrenocorticosteroids, in the form of intranasal beclomethasone, are of unproved benefit in the treatment of chronic otitis media. Although no controlled studies are available, hyposensitization may benefit those difficult patients with chronic middle ear effusion and a concomitant nasal allergy that has been unresponsive to vigorous drug therapy. Adenoidectomy is not generally thought to be beneficial for the majority of children with an atopic history and middle ear effusion. Patients with refractory effusions are often treated with myringectomy and placement of a ventilation tube.

Complications of middle ear effusion include conductive hearing loss, suppurative otitis media, and cholesteatoma. Impairment of cognitive, linguistic, and speech development has been reported in children with persistent or episodic conductive hearing loss. The degree and duration of the hearing loss required to produce such defects have not been defined. Adequate diagnosis and early intervention should prevent these complications.

Bluestone, C. D. Otitis media in children: To treat or not to treat? *N. Engl. J. Med.* 306:1399–1404, 1982.
Reviews the most reasonable approach to the treatment of otitis media.
Bluestone, C. D. Eustachian tube function and allergy in otitis media. *Pediatrics* 61:753–760, 1978.
A good review of the topic with helpful diagrams illustrating the pathogenesis of otitis media.
Bluestone, C. D., Bernstein, J. M., and Douglas, G. S. Otitis Media. In E. Middleton, C. E. Reed, and E. F. Ellis (Eds.), *Allergy: Principles and Practice* (2nd ed.). St. Louis: Mosby, 1983. Pp. 1275–1296.
Presents a thorough discussion of the subject.
Crifo, S., Cittadini, S., DeSeta, E., and Andriana, G. Eustachian tube permeability during the nasal provocation test. *Rhinology* 15:81–85, 1977.
Decreased eustachian tube permeability was demonstrated after experimentally induced nasal allergy.
Dockhorn, R. J. Otolaryngologic allergy in children. *Otolaryngol. Clin. North Am.* 10:103–112, 1977.
Symposium that includes a discussion of allergic rhinitis and serous otitis media.
Fernandes, D., Gupta, S., Sly, R. M., and Frazer, M. Tympanometry in children with allergic respiratory disease. *Ann. Allergy* 40:181–184, 1978.
Evaluation of tympanometry as an adjunct to treatment of allergic children.
Friedman, R. A., et al. Immunologic-mediated eustachian tube obstruction: A double-blind crossover study. *J. Allergy Clin. Immunol.* 71:442–447, 1983.
The findings of this study suggest an allergic basis for eustachian tube obstruction and possibility for the development of otitis media with effusion.
Henderson, F. W., et al. A longitudinal study of respiratory viruses and bacteria in the etiology of acute otitis media with effusion. *N. Engl. J. Med.* 306:1377–1383, 1982.
An excellent study demonstrating the importance of respiratory tract virus infection as an antecedent to otitis media with effusion.
Kjellman, N. I. M., Harder, H., Hansson, L.-O., and Linwall, L. Allergy, otitis media and serum immunoglobulins after adenoidectomy. *Acta Paediatr. Scand.* 67:717–723, 1978.
A study of otitis media before and after adenoidectomy.

Miller, D. L., and Friday, G. A.   Allergic diseases of the nose and middle ear in children. *Ear Nose Throat J.* 57:100–115, 1978.
Thorough discussion of the allergic aspects of otitis media.

Olson, A. L., et al.   Prevention and therapy of otitis media by oral decongestant: A double-blind study in pediatric practice. *Pediatrics* 61:679–684, 1978.
Demonstrated no difference in prevention or treatment with or without use of decongestants.

Paradise, J. L.   Otitis media during early life: How hazardous to development? A critical review of the evidence. *Pediatrics* 68:869–879, 1981.
Critical examination of the question whether otitis media with effusion in early life results in hearing loss leading to developmental delay.

Sade, J., and Weissman, Z.   Middle ear mucosa and secretory otitis media. *Arch. Otorhinolaryngol.* 215:195–205, 1977.
Discussion of histology of mucosa and mucus in middle ear.

ASTHMA

18. ASTHMA: GENERAL EVALUATION AND ASSESSMENT
Karl M. Altenburger

The general evaluation and assessment of a patient with suspected or proved reactive airways disease depends almost totally on eliciting a detailed history and on the performance of a thorough physical examination. Except in the case of the infant or young child where the differential diagnosis of asthma is extensive, the diagnosis of asthma is generally straightforward and can be made from this history and physical examination, as well as from a characteristic chest roentgenogram that does not suggest other disease. The purpose of the patient evaluation involves much more than establishing a diagnosis: it should serve to define how this disease process interacts with and controls the patient's environment. The object of therapy should be to return control to the patient.

The approach to the patient's history requires obtaining a large amount of information. For the sake of completeness it is best to follow an outline (Table 10). The history begins with defining the nature of the patient's symptoms (the usual reason for the visit). While relief from these symptoms is desired, the goals of the patient need to be defined. The pattern of the patient's symptoms is of particular importance, especially in the more severe asthmatic patient where the character and response to treatment of acute attacks can often be predicted by reviewing the course of previous episodes. Precipitating factors for the patient's symptoms should be identified so that the patient can be counseled to avoid situations that might aggravate symptoms, or taught to use a preventive form of therapy when faced with unavoidable situations. The past history from onset and diagnosis (often discordant) and the clinical course provide useful clues of the impact of this disease on the patient. The family history may occasionally suggest a cause for chronic pulmonary disease other than asthma, such as cystic fibrosis. The general medical history should emphasize acute or chronic neurologic (e.g., seizures, headaches), cardiovascular (e.g., arrhythmias), gastrointestinal tract (e.g., "sensitive stomach," gastroesophageal reflux, vomiting, diarrhea), and dermatologic (e.g., eczema, urticaria, contact sensitivities) problems. Finally the psychological and financial impact of this chronic illness needs to be fully appreciated. In the process of obtaining a complete history, the attitudes of the patient and the family toward the diagnosis and treatment of asthma should become apparent. This information is especially critical to the design and acceptance of the treatment plan.

The physical examination focuses on the upper and lower respiratory tract, however, important details of other systems should not be overlooked (Table 11). The presence of a pulsus paradoxus should be sought, especially if the patient is symptomatic. It is also important to ask the patient how he or she is breathing. Signs of airway obstruction in a patient who denies disability provide an important clue about the patient's perception of his or her disease. During auscultation of the chest, one should listen carefully for wheezing throughout expiration, during both normal quiet respirations and with forced expiration. Even small children can easily perform this maneuver (e.g., "blow out the birthday candles").

Laboratory aids (Table 12) that assist in the diagnosis and management of asthma abound. The performance of spirometry (FVC, FEV_1, FEF_{25-75})* before and after inhaled bronchodilators is mandatory. Correlating the obtained values with impressions gained during the history and physical examination will influence the patient's management. An initial chest x-ray film (posteroanterior and lateral) is useful if a normal x-ray film has not been obtained since the onset

FVC = forced vital capacity; FEV_1 = forced expiratory volume in 1 second; FEF25–75% = forced xpiratory flow rate between 25 and 75% of vital capacity.

Table 10. Information to be obtained from patient's history

Relative prominence of wheezing, dyspnea, cough, sputum production, chest pain, fatigue
  History of cyanosis, syncope, seizures, respiratory arrest
  Presence and relative prominence of upper respiratory tract symptoms
Pattern of symptoms
  Perennial, seasonal, or perennial with seasonal flare
  Continuous, paroxysmal, or continuous with paroxysms
  Frequency (e.g., days or months of symptoms)
  Diurnal variation
  Geographic variation
Precipitating or aggravating factors
  Allergens (pollens, mold, dust, animal danders, rarely food)
  Nonspecific irritants
  Weather changes
  Exercise
  Infections
  Emotional stress
  Aspirin or other drugs
  Sinusitis
  Noncompliance with medical regimen
  Other
Profile of typical attack
  Prodromal signs and symptoms
  Tempo of progression
  How handled
  Usual outcome
Impact of disease
  Impact on patient
    Number of hospitalizations and emergency visits
    Number of school or work days missed
    Limitation of activity
    Effect on growth, development, behavior
  Impact on family
    Disruption of family routines or restriction of activities
    Conflicts among family members
Development of disease
  Age of onset; age of diagnosis
  Trend of severity
  Major changes in course
  Previous workup and therapy
  Present management
  History of steroid use
Family history
General medical history (with emphasis on chronic neurologic, cardiovascular, gastro-intestinal tract, and dermatologic problems; adverse reactions to foods, drugs, insect stings)
Environmental survey
  Physical environment (including description of work and home)
  Typical daily routine
Assessment of the family
  Intactness of family
  Responsibility for care
  Knowledge about and attitudes toward asthma
  Adequacy to manage asthma (interest, intelligence, maturity, psychologic, and economic resources)

Source: Adapted from F. Leffert, *J. Pediatr.* 97:876–885, 1980.

Table 11. Physical examination: important signs in evaluation of a patient with asthma

Vital signs: Pulsus paradoxus, height, weight (with percentiles), and so on.
General appearance: Ill, healthy
Skin: Cyanosis, dry, eczema
Eyes: Inflammation, cataracts
Ears: Tympanic membrane motility and appearance
Nose: Inflammation, secretions, polyps
Sinuses: Tenderness, transillumination
Mouth/throat: Adenopathy, postnasal discharge, thyroid
Chest: Symmetry, anteroposterior diameter, excursion, aeration, wheezing (tidal volume, forced expiration), prolonged expiratory phase, rales
Heart: Rhythm, murmurs
Abdomen: Apparent hepatosplenomegaly from a depressed diaphragm, bowel sounds
Genitalia: Development
Extremities: Clubbing, cyanosis
Neurologic: Mentation

Table 12. Laboratory tests useful for diagnosing asthma

Essential
  Spirometry
Often useful
  Chest roentgenogram
  Sinus roentgenograms
  Allergy skin testing
  Complete blood count and eosinophil count
  Cortisol level if patient is taking steroids
Other
  As indicated by history and physical examination

of symptoms. Allergy skin testing is often useful. Using properly applied and controlled skin tests, the role of IgE-mediated factors in the disease can be evaluated (see Chap. 7). Depending on the patient's history and examination, other tests may be indicated, however, a number of tests are commonly employed that are of little or no value to the physician or patient and only serve to increase the cost of medical care unnecessarily. Physicians working in this area should be aware of the American Academy of Allergy's Position Paper governing such procedures (see also Chap. 56).

It is essential to obtain a complete portrait of the asthmatic patient in order to design a rational, acceptable treatment plan, which improves the chances of compliance. Such a plan develops over months after many physician-patient interviews. The considerable time involved should be stressed during the initial visits so that the patient can develop appropriate expectations. The patient should also understand that asthma cannot be cured; its course can only be modified. Successful treatment allows the patient to be more in control of his or her environment and ensures normal participation in educational, social, physical, and work-related activities.

Aaronson, D. W. Asthma: General Concepts. In R. Patterson (Ed.), *Allergic Diseases, Diagnosis and Management* (2nd ed.). Philadelphia: Lippincott, 1980. Pp. 231–278. *Differential diagnosis and general approach are clearly explained.*

Brooks, S. M.   The evaluation of occupational airways disease in the laboratory and work place. *J. Allergy Clin. Immunol.* 70:56–66, 1982.
This is a useful guide centered on occupational immunologic lung disease and is worth reading.
Cherniack, R. M.   *Pulmonary Function Testing.* Philadelphia: Saunders, 1980.
Everything you ever wanted to know about pulmonary function testing.
Green, L. W., Goldstein, R. A., and Parker, S. R.   Workshop on self-management of child-hood asthma. *J. Allergy Clin. Immunol.* 72:519–626, 1983.
This is the report of an excellent workshop.
Leffert, F.   Management of chronic asthma. *J. Pediatr.* 97:875–885, 1980.
Mandatory reading on the assessment of chronic asthma management in children.
Leffert, F.   Asthma: A modern perspective. *Pediatrics* 62:1061–1069, 1978.
Good review of the evolution of our thinking about this chronic illness and the current approach.
Lichtenstein, L. M., and Austin, K. F. (Eds.).   *Asthma: Physiology, Immunopharmacology, and Treatment. Second International Conference on Asthma.* New York: Academic, 1977.
The discussions are especially worthwhile. The third symposium was held in Spring 1983.
McFadden, E. R., and Ingram, R. H.   Asthma: Perspectives, Definition and Classifications. In A. P. Fishman (Ed.), *Pulmonary Diseases and Disorders.* New York: McGraw-Hill, 1980. Pp. 562–566.
A historical perspective on asthma.
Middleton, G., Reed, C. E., and Ellis, E. F. (Eds.).   *Allergy: Principles and Practice* (2nd ed.). St. Louis: Mosby, 1983.
Several good chapters are included on approach to asthma in children and adults.
Panel on Asthma.   Asthma and other allergic diseases. *NIAID Task Force Report.* NIH Publication No. 79–387, May 1979. Pp. 111–189.
The impact of asthma on our population. Committee recommendations are of special interest.
Scoggin, C. H., and Petty, T. L.   *Clinical Strategies in Adult Asthma.* Philadelphia: Lea & Febiger, 1982.
Assessment in adults.
Weiss, E. B., and Segal, M. S. (Eds.).   *Bronchial Asthma: Mechanisms and Therapeutics.* Boston: Little Brown, 1976.
A good, Encyclopedic reference although most of the information here is at least 10 years old.

19. DIFFERENTIAL DIAGNOSIS OF THE WHEEZING INFANT
Nick George Anas

Normal breathing is inaudible without the use of a stethoscope because the velocity of air flow in the tracheobronchial tree is too low to produce adequate sound. Airway narrowing results in increased air velocity, thus creating turbulent flow and noisy breathing. Diseases characterized by obstruction of intrathoracic airways cause wheezing that tends to be most prominent during the expiratory phase of respiration, whereas extrathoracic tracheal obstruction results in inspiratory stridor. This differentiation is often difficult to make in an infant.

The signs and symptoms of airways obstruction in older children and adults are most often obvious and include progressive dyspnea, wheezing (often both expiratory and inspiratory), prolongation of expiration, and coarse and fine rales. In contrast, infants frequently show only nonspecific signs of respiratory distress such as retractions, tachypnea, and noisy breathing—often making the diagnosis of a particular entity by history and physical alone very difficult. Additional problems can come from the incorrect description of a variety of adventitious sounds associated with respiration such as rhonchi, stertor, and stridor as "wheezing." The sounds caused by obstruction in varying sites of the airways are not always wheezing in the strict sense. A precise diagnosis of the disease process responsible for abnormal sounds in the chest in infancy often requires knowledge of the large number of other diseases that can cause partial tracheobronchial obstruction. A failure to make an accurate diagnosis can result in needless prolongation of illness or even death.

Differential Diagnosis and Evaluation

The causes of intrathoracic airways obstruction in the wheezing infant can be divided into intraluminal and extraluminal processes. Intraluminal obstruction can be caused by bronchoconstriction, excessive mucus production, edema of the walls of the airway, and foreign material lodged in the airway. The extraluminal causes are primarily congenital malformations that result in compression of a portion of the tracheobronchial tree. A complete differential diagnosis is listed in Table 13 and serves as the format for the remaining discussion.

The sudden onset of wheezing and respiratory distress in an infant who has previously been well is due most commonly to **foreign body aspiration.** The circumstances preceding the onset of respiratory compromise should be learned,

Table 13. Differential diagnosis: The wheezing infant

Anatomic and mechanical
  Foreign body
  Vascular anomalies
  Developmental anomalies
    Sequestration
    Lobar emphysema
    Congenital cysts
  Tracheobronchomalacia
  Adenopathy
Infections
  Bronchiolitis
  Pneumonia
Pulmonary parenchymal disease
  Asthma (reactive airways disease)
  Cystic fibrosis
  Bronchopulmonary dysplasia
  Alpha$_1$-antitrypsin deficiency
  Shock lung (adult respiratory distress syndrome)
Cardiac: congestive heart failure with pulmonary edema
  Congenital defects
  Acquired diseases
Gastrointestinal
  Gastroesophageal reflux
  Congenital malformations of the esophagus
  Swallowing
Toxicologic
  Beta-adrenergic blocking agents
  Histamine releasers
  Anticholinesterase inhibitors
Others
  Allergic bronchopulmonary aspergillosis
  Hypersensitivity pneumonitis
  Collagen vascular diseases
  Immune complex diseases
  Metabolic acidosis
  Neurogenic pulmonary edema

with emphasis placed on a history of coughing or choking and evidence of food or toy parts found near the child. Keep in mind that symptoms present acutely after foreign body aspiration can resolve spontaneously and can be followed by a symptom-free interval ranging from weeks to years before chronic symptoms caused by the foreign body start. The location of the foreign body in the tracheobronchial tree will affect both the physical findings and the degree of respiratory distress. Objects lodged within the larynx, trachea, or main stem bronchi result in severe air hunger and constitute a medical emergency, whereas those located in peripheral airways may be a cause of recurrent pneumonia and wheezing. Partial obstruction of the airway may cause a ball-valve effect with localized wheezing, air trapping, and hyperresonance. A foreign body that is chronically imbedded often completely obstructs a lobe or segment, and diminished air entry and dullness to percussion will be found by physical examination. Roentgenograms of the upper airway and larynx should be obtained when inspiratory stridor is present. Comparison of chest roentgenograms taken during inspiration and expiration may demonstrate unilateral hyperinflation or a shift of the mediastinum at end expiration. Fluoroscopy of the chest may show decreased diaphragmatic movement on the side of the aspirated foreign body (most often the right side). Rigid bronchoscopy must be performed to confirm the diagnosis and to remove the foreign body.

Intrinsic abnormalities of the respiratory tract or the cardiovascular system are important causes of chronic, recurrent wheezing in the infant. Vascular anomalies such as double aortic arch compress both the esophagus and the trachea, resulting in dysphagia as well as respiratory signs and symptoms. A barium esophagram often demonstrates posterior indentation of the respiratory tract, and angiography of the great vessels will outline the abnormal anatomy. Surgical correction ameliorates all problems in most cases. Congenital lobar emphysema should be a diagnostic consideration in the infant who develops respiratory distress in the first few weeks to months of life. Localized wheezing in the upper lobes and roentgenographic findings of unilateral hyperinflation compressing the mediastinum are indicators. Resection of the abnormal lung is the recommended treatment. Pulmonary sequestrations and congenital cysts are less common causes of wheezing. Surgical intervention is indicated when there is respiratory compromise or recurrent infection.

Infectious agents are responsible for the majority of cases of wheezing in infants. Bronchiolitis is an acute viral infection of the small airways characterized by tachypnea, wheezing, and hyperaeration. Roentgenograms of the chest demonstrate hyperinflation without prominent infiltrates. The wheezing associated with bronchiolitis is not usually altered by the administration of bronchodilators, thus differentiating it from asthma. Criteria for hospital admission include apnea, a resting respiratory rate greater than 60 per minute, the presence of intercostal retractions or nasal flaring, or significant arterial blood gas abnormalities ($PaO_2 \leq 60$ mm Hg; $PaCO_2 \geq 45$ mm Hg). Inpatient therapy includes the use of humidified oxygen to maintain a PaO_2 of 50 to 80 mm Hg, intravenous fluid support, and chest physiotherapy. Mechanical ventilation is indicated when the $PaCO_2$ exceeds 60 to 65 mm Hg. A trial of bronchodilators is recommended for hospitalized infants with moderate or severe expiratory wheezing. Antibiotics are not helpful in acute viral bronchiolitis, and steroids have never been proved efficacious. Antiviral agents such as ribavirin are presently being investigated.

Pneumonias in infancy are caused by a variety of agents: viruses (respiratory syncytial, parainfluenza, influenza, adenoviruses), bacteria (*Streptococcus pneumoniae, Hemophilus influenzae, Staphylococcus aureus*), and atypical organisms (*Chlamydia trachomatis,* cytomegalovirus, and *Pneumocystis carinii*). Respiratory signs include cough, labored breathing, crackles, and wheezes. Roentgenographic patterns vary from platelike atelectasis to generalized infiltrates with hyperinflation. Treatment consists of the respiratory support outlined in the preceding paragraph. Antibiotics are indicated if a bacterial etiology is confirmed.

Asthma is a common cause of recurrent and reversible wheezing and cough, and is discussed in detail elsewhere in this book. Asthma may occur in infants as young as 2 or 3 months, but more often is seen at 8 to 10 months of age. Since the IgE type I mechanism can function in early infancy, many physicians feel that allergy to inhalants or foods may play a role even in asthma that starts in infancy. Viral respiratory tract infections, however, are probably the most important causative factor of wheezing episodes in this age group. Although signs and symptoms of asthma may appear in the first two years of life, confirmation of this diagnosis is often not possible because a beneficial response to subcutaneous or inhaled beta-adrenergic agents is difficult to document. This response to beta-adrenergic agents should be documented on several occasions before a definitive diagnosis of reactive airway disease can be made.

Cystic fibrosis (CF), the most common cause of chronic suppurative lung disease in children, is an inherited disorder of the exocrine secretory glands. In the majority of cases, wheezing occurs when viscid mucus obstructs airflow in both central and peripheral airways. The diagnosis should be suspected in any infant whose wheezing is associated with chronic cough, digital clubbing, cyanosis, diffuse infiltrates and hyperaeration on the chest roentgenogram, or sputum containing *Pseudomonas aeruginosa, Staphylococcus aureus,* or *Aspergillus fumigatus.* Patients with CF may also have a bronchospastic component to their wheezing that will often respond at least partially to bronchodilators. However, it is important to note that in the young child asthma cannot always be distinguished from CF because the signs other than wheezing and chronic cough may not have had time to develop. The diagnosis is confirmed by demonstrating a sweat chloride level greater than 60 mg/L using the quantitative pilocarpine iontophoresis technique. Any infant suspected of having CF should be referred to the regional Cystic Fibrosis Center for diagnosis and long-term therapy.

Bronchopulmonary dysplasia is the sequela of hyaline membrane disease of prematurity that has required treatment with prolonged mechanical ventilation and a high concentration of inspired oxygen. Pathologically, there is damage to ciliated epithelial cells, interstitial fibrosis, alveolar destruction, pulmonary vascular smooth muscle hypertrophy, and lymphatic engorgement. Wheezing results from obstruction of the airways by mucus, bronchiolar compression by enlarged lymphatics, or pulmonary edema. Treatment should include oxygen, postural drainage, and diuretics. Up to 50% of the children who have had severe bronchopulmonary dysplasia in infancy develop a clinical course in the second or third years of life that is difficult to distinguish from asthma with wheezing that responds to use of standard bronchodilators. The approach to these children is similar to the approach to the child with asthma who did not have problems in infancy.

Congestive heart failure ("cardiac asthma") is a cause of wheezing in infants resulting from compression of small airways by fluid, engorged pulmonary veins, or enlargement of the left atrium. The most common causes of congestive heart failure with pulmonary edema in the infant are endocardial fibroelastosis, viral myocarditis, ventricular septal defect with a large left-to-right shunt, severe aortic stenosis, and paroxysmal atrial tachycardia. Treatment aimed at improving cardiac output includes the use of inotropic agents, diuretics, and, when possible, surgical correction of the cardiac lesion.

Gastroesophageal reflux (GER) secondary to an incompetent lower esophageal sphincter has been associated with recurrent cough and wheezing in infancy. Chronic aspiration is the most likely cause of the pulmonary disease associated with GER, although there is some evidence that autonomic reflex stimulated by reflux of gastric contents into the lower esophagus may cause bronchospasm.

GER may be diagnosed with varying sensitivity by barium studies of the upper GI tract, esophageal pH monitoring, esophageal manometry, esophagoscopy, and lung scans after a radioactive technetium meal. Medical management includes maintaining the infant in an upright position after feeding, thickening of the formula with cereals, and bedtime antacids. Fundoplication may be necessary.

Congenital malformations of the esophagus have an incidence of about 1 in 4000 live births. Approximately 90% of these infants have a proximal esophageal atresia and a distal tracheoesophageal fistula (TEF). The diagnosis should be suspected in any newborn with excessive oral secretions and respiratory distress, and is confirmed by inability to pass a nasogastric tube. Less commonly, TEF (H-type fistula) without atresia results in chronic cough, wheezing, and choking during feedings. Diagnosis of the later condition may be made with a barium swallow, but often requires simultaneous esophagoscopy and bronchoscopy to document the connection by the passage of dye.

Swallowing dysfunction may be associated with recurrent pulmonary disease. Swallowing is an important function of the pharynx. Any disease process that interferes with either the structure or the function of the pharynx may result in aspiration, and associated chronic wheezing. These types of problems are seen in infants with cleft palate, cranial nerve palsies, neuromuscular diseases, severe asphyxial brain damage, and familial dysautonomia (Riley-Day syndrome).

Pharmacologic agents that cause bronchospasm include beta-adrenergic blocking agents (e.g., propranolol) and histamine releasers (e.g., morphine, curare); however, they are clinically important only in individuals with underlying reactive airways disease. The accidental ingestion of organophosphates such as parathion and methylparathion (the constituents of many insecticides) can cause wheezing, cough, dyspnea, and an increase in bronchopharyngeal secretions from the inhibition of serum anticholinesterase. Treatment includes the administration of atropine and pralidoxine chloride.

Allergic bronchopulmonary aspergillosis (associated with cystic fibrosis or asthma), hypersensitivity pneumonitis, pulmonary involvement by collagen vascular diseases, Goodpasture's syndrome, and the immune complex diseases rarely occur in infancy, but are well-described causes of wheezing and respiratory distress in older children and adults. Kussmaul respiration (increased depth and rate of tidal breathing) is seen in infants with diabetic ketoacidosis or after the accidental ingestion of toxic amounts of salicylates. This abnormal breathing pattern, which may result in high airflow rates causing wheezing, can be mistaken for intrinsic pulmonary disease.

Abdulmajid, O. A., Ebeid, A. M., Motaweh, M. M., and Kleibo, I. S. Aspirated foreign bodies in the tracheobronchial tree: Report of 250 cases. *Thorax* 31:635–640, 1976.
  Outlines the clinical presentation of children with foreign body aspiration.
Berquist, W. E., et al. Gastroesophageal reflux–associated recurrent pneumonia and chronic asthma in children. *Pediatrics* 68:29–35, 1981.
  Interesting and thought-provoking study of the relationship between gastroesophageal reflux, asthma, and chronic pneumonitis in young children.
Brasher, G. W. Clinical aspects of infantile asthma. *Ann. Allergy* 35:216–220, 1975.
  A brief but good presentation of the clinical aspects of infantile asthma.
Dunsky, E. Bronchiolitis: Differentiation from infantile asthma. Pediatr Ann. 6:45, 47–51, 55–56, 1977.
  Simple review that highlights the similarities as well as the differences between bronchiolitis and infantile asthma.
Euler, A. R. Use of bethanechol for the treatment of gastroesophageal reflux. *J. Pediatr.* 96:321–324, 1980.
  Most believable assessment to date on the role of medical therapy in the treatment of gastroesophageal reflux.

Fulginiti, V. A., and Clyde, W. A.   Workshop on bronchiolitis. Bethesda, Md.: U.S. Department of Health, Education and Welfare, DHEW Pub. No. (NIH) 77–1242, 1977.
  The world's experts gather their experience on bronchiolitis.
Glezen, W. P., and Denney, F. W.   Epidemiology of acute lower respiratory disease in children. *N. Engl. J. Med.* 288:498–505, 1973.
  A classic study highlighting Mycoplasma as well as the common respiratory viruses in the etiology of acute lower respiratory tract disease.
Law, D., and Kosloske, A. M.   Management of tracheobronchial foreign bodies in children: A reevaluation of postural drainage and bronchoscopy. *Pediatrics* 58:362–367, 1976.
  Presents reasonable suggestions on the management of tracheobronchial foreign bodies.
Lenney, W., and Milne, A. D.   At what age do bronchodilator drugs work? *Arch. Dis. Child.* 53:532–535, 1978.
  One of the few studies aimed at this controversial issue.
McIntosh, K., et al.   The association of viral and bacterial respiratory infections with exacerbations of wheezing in young asthmatic children. *J. Pediatr.* 82:578–590, 1973.
  This study supports viral (not bacterial) infections as the primary precipitant of exacerbations of wheezing.
Milner, A., and Henry, R. L.   Acute airway obstruction in children under 5. *Thorax* 37:641–645, 1982.
  Excellent review of the natural history, prognosis and treatment of acute airways obstruction in children under the age of 5 years.
Murray, J. F.   *The Normal Lung: The Basis for Diagnosis and Treatment of Pulmonary Disease.* Philadelphia: Saunders, 1976.
  An easy-to-understand book on pulmonary physiology.
Rudolph, A. M.   *Pediatrics* (16th ed.). New York: Appleton-Century-Crofts, 1977.
  Presents a physiologic approach to pediatric diseases.
Simpson, W., Hacking, P. M., and Court, S. D.   Radiologic findings in RSV infection in children. The radiological findings in respiratory syncytial virus infection in children. II. The correlation of radiological categories with clinical virological findings. *Pediatr. Radiol.* 2:155–160, 1974.
  Radiographic differentiation of respiratory syncytial virus infections from other viral lower inspiratory infections in children.
Tal, A., et al.   Dexamethasone and salbutamol in the treatment of acute wheezing in infants. *Pediatrics* 71:13–18, 1983.
  Combination of the two drugs resulted in the best rate of clinical improvement in acutely wheezing infants.
Williams, H. E., and Phelan, P. D.   *Respiratory Illness in Children.* Oxford: Blackwell, 1975.
  This book is the most complete compendium of childhood lung diseases.
Wohl, E. and Chernick, V.   State of the art—bronchiolitis. *Am. Rev. Respir. Dis.* 118:759–781, 1978.
  Excellent review that stresses the pathophysiology of bronchiolitis.

20. OUTPATIENT TREATMENT OF ASTHMA
Ray S. Davis

Clinicians frequently encounter patients with complaints of intermittent dyspnea, chronic coughing, and wheezing, which are suggestive of asthma. The first step in the management of these patients is to establish a firm diagnosis of asthma. A thorough history must be taken and a physical examination performed. Laboratory tests, including a chest roentgenogram, a sweat test, serum immunoglobulins, pulmonary function testing before and after inhaled bronchodilators, and allergy skin tests, are also useful, especially in considering causes of wheezing other than asthma.

The diagnosis of asthma—reversible obstructive airways disease–can be made in several ways: (1) by demonstrating an increased forced expiratory volume at 1 second (FEV_1) by 20% or more after inhalation of a bronchodilator; (2) by demonstrating a decreased FEV_1 by 20% or more following a standard methacholine or histamine challenge; or (3) by demonstrating a decreased FEV_1 by 20% or forced expiratory flow between 25 and 75% of forced vital capacity (FEF25–75%) of 35% or more following a standard exercise challenge. Although other methods exist, these three are the most practical and meet the American Thoracic Society's criteria for the diagnosis of asthma. Once the diagnosis of asthma is made, the clinician must provide the patient with a treatment regimen based on the patient's disease severity.

A thorough treatment regimen should include (1) avoidance of precipitants of the asthma whenever possible, (2) pharmacologic management, and (3) consideration of immunotherapy. Avoidance of suspected or confirmed precipitants is most preferable, but since asthma is a multifactorial disease, complete avoidance of all precipitants is not always possible. Both avoidance of possible precipitants and immunotherapy are thoroughly reviewed in chapters 23 and 38. This chapter is concerned only with the pharmacologic management of asthma once the diagnosis has been established.

Bronchodilator therapy in the 1980s provides the clinician with a multitude of theophylline and beta$_2$-sympathomimetic preparations from which to chose. Various factors such as disease severity, tolerance to side effects and the availability of serum theophylline levels are major determinants as to the individualization of drug regimens. The clinician must also remember that patient compliance is inversely proportional to the number of medications prescribed. The following discussion attempts to provide a rationale for the choice of medication for mild, moderate, and severe asthmatics. No attempt is made to suggest dosages for medications, since the *Physician's Desk Reference* and many standard textbooks can be consulted.

Mild Asthma

Mild asthma, for the purposes of this discussion, is defined as asthma associated with not more than three prolonged wheezing attacks per year. These patients often have mild wheezing with exercise or during intense exposure to irritants, but those episodes are almost always transient and easily controlled. Often, mild asthmatic patients have significant morbidity from these episodes, keeping them from school or work, requiring acute treatment in an emergency room, or even requiring occasional hospital admission for more intensive therapy. The general principle in the approach to these patients is to treat wheezing episodes promptly and not to let a more prolonged attack, which might need intensive therapy, develop. Many authorities prefer the use of an inhaled beta$_2$-sympathomimetic agent in these patients when the first signs of coughing or wheezing occur. The major benefit of inhaled beta$_2$ sympathomimetics is that they have almost immediate bronchodilatory effects with minimal side effects. Metaproterenol and albuterol generally afford relief of clinical bronchospasm for 4 to 6 hours. Although metaproterenol and albuterol metered-dose inhalers* are approved for use only in patients aged 12 years and older, many physicians use these drugs in children after obtaining parental approval if other preparations have proved to be less effective.

During their infrequent attacks of asthma, many patients need theophylline or

---

*The stigma of rising asthmatic patient deaths in England in the 1960s that was linked to the increased use of metered-dose aerosols led many physicians to refrain from their use. However, close scrutiny of this issue has shown the aforementioned link to be falsely associated, since a rise in asthmatic patient deaths in the United States and Australia did not occur during the 1960s with a similar rise in the use of metered-dose inhalers.

an oral beta$_2$ sympathomimetic in addition to the inhaled bronchodilators to provide more continuous bronchodilation. An indication for the use of an oral preparation is the need for an inhaled bronchodilator more than four times in a 24-hour period. Both classes of oral bronchodilators are equally effective, but both take much longer to provide adequate bronchodilatation when compared with metered-dose aerosols, and both are frequently associated with undesirable side effects. One example is the gastrointestinal side effects seen in some children with ingestion of even extremely low amounts of theophylline. Some patients who can not tolerate theophylline because of these side effects can tolerate an oral beta$_2$-sympathomimetic agent. Conversely, patients who have been treated with a beta$_2$-sympathomimetic agent alone and experienced extreme skeletal muscle tremors, may tolerate a theophylline preparation. Whatever drug regimen is selected for treatment of the intermittent attacks must be continued for at least a week following clearing of clinical symptoms, because significant airways obstruction can persist even after the physical examination has become normal, and clinical symptoms may recur if bronchodilators are discontinued prematurely.

Although many mildly asthmatic patients remain completely asymptomatic between their occasional episodes of clinical bronchospasm, some mildly asthmatic patients continue to have occasional episodes of cough or mild wheezing between the more significant attacks. These episodes often become evident after exercise or during the night. The clinician should closely monitor any patients who have persistent evidence of mild bronchospasm in between occasional episodes of acute asthma. In these patients, pulmonary functions in the office or mini-peak flowmeters used at home may objectively establish the presence of significant bronchoconstriction that is not appreciated by the patient or even by careful physical examination. It is well established that asthmatic patients can have abnormal pulmonary functions even while they are completely asymptomatic. Although the abnormal pulmonary functions may not be sufficient to induce symptoms at rest, they may cause enough airflow obstruction so that minimal exercise or a mild viral infection may lead to a severe asthma attack. Therefore, in mild asthmatics who are not entirely well between acute episodes close monitoring of their pulmonary functions is necessary. Frequent reevaluation in these patients may ultimately lead to a reclassification of the patient into the moderately severe category. These patients generally require continuous medication to improve their pulmonary functions and symptoms.

Moderate Asthma

Moderate asthma, for the purposes of this discussion, is defined as asthma associated with attacks that occur on a regular basis, at least once a month, whether the symptoms are perennial or just seasonal. Although this discussion is directed toward the moderately severe perennial asthmatic patient, most of this discussion applies also to the moderately severe seasonal asthmatic patient.

Patients who experience exacerbations of their asthma with a frequency of at least once a month, are frequently absent from school or work and are often limited in their recreational activities. Generally, a medical regimen sufficient for the mild asthmatic patient is not sufficient for the moderately severe asthmatic patient, and chronic daily therapy is necessary.

The use of **metered-dose aerosol** three or four times daily may provide adequate bronchodilatation of sufficient duration to obviate the need for oral medication and, if successful, can have significant advantages for the patient. However, when a metered-dose aerosol alone is not adequate, the addition of an **oral beta$_2$ sympathomimetic** in low doses three to four times daily can potentiate the bronchodilatory effects of the inhaled drugs. Use of the inhaled form of the drug with the low-dose oral drug can minimize the frequent side effects that are seen when higher doses of oral beta$_2$ sympathomimetics are taken alone.

Many allergists and pulmonologists use sustained-release oral **theophylline** preparations as the drug of choice in the treatment of moderately severe asthmatic patients who require daily medication. Sustained-release theophylline preparations taken twice daily can often maintain the patient's serum theophylline level close to the therapeutic range (10–20 µg/ml), and alone may provide adequate bronchodilatation. Patients should be carefully monitored for early signs of toxicity, such as nausea and irritability. With the increased use of sustained-release preparations and serum theophylline levels, clinicians have become aware of how complex the use of this drug can be and how difficult it can be to avoid toxicity. This is especially true when attempts are made to maintain serum theophylline levels in the upper portion of the therapeutic range (see Chap. 30 for details).

When theophylline alone on a daily basis is not sufficient to provide adequate relief of dyspnea, coughing, and wheezing, and after compliance has been demonstrated by adequate theophylline levels, the addition of a beta$_2$ sympathomimetic to the medical regimen may be useful. Many times, the addition of a beta$_2$ sympathomimetic, either by inhalation or orally, three to four times daily provides adequate relief of symptoms. When relief of symptoms is not sufficient after the addition of a beta$_2$ sympathomimetic by either the inhaled or oral routes, the addition of both might provide the desired relief of symptoms. There is good evidence that relatively low doses of both theophylline and beta$_2$ sympathomimetic can provide the same degree and duration of bronchodilatation with fewer side effects than either drug alone in higher doses.

Cromolyn sodium is useful only when inhaled. It can be inhaled as a powder with a spinhaler or as a liquid with standard nebulization equipment. It appears to be at least as useful as theophylline as a primary drug for maintenance therapy in the patient with moderately severe asthma. It is effective in blocking allergen-induced bronchospasm, and may be especially useful in moderately severe asthmatics who have identifiable allergic precipitants. It is also an excellent drug in the prevention of exercise-induced bronchospasm. Cromolyn is more widely prescribed in Europe than is theophylline.

The major benefit of cromolyn is that it has virtually no side effects in comparison with theophylline and beta$_2$ sympathomimetics. On the other hand, its usefulness is limited because (1) it is relatively expensive, (2) compliance may be difficult for some patients as it may have to be used four times daily, and (3) it is not a bronchodilator. Inhalation of the powder can be irritating and thus produce cough that can exacerbate asthma. However, this side effect can generally be avoided by use of the spinhaler after an inhaled beta$_2$-sympathomimetic agent. The use of the liquid form by nebulization obviates the irritant response and will allow the continued use of cromolyn even during an acute exacerbation of asthma.

Exacerbations of asthma can occur intermittently in an otherwise well-controlled moderately severe asthmatic patient. When compliance of the drugs used for ongoing therapy has been ensured (e.g., by measuring adequate theophylline levels) and the patient does not achieve adequate bronchodilatation by increasing the use of a routinely inhaled beta$_2$-sympathomimetic agent, short courses of high-dose **corticosteroids** are indicated. Generally, prednisone is the drug of choice because the half-life of the drug is short and it is associated with a minimum of adrenal gland suppression. Prednisone is also inexpensive. Most other preparations, such as dexamethasone and prednisolone, offer no advantages over prednisone in the effectiveness of asthma control.

For acute exacerbations, prednisone, 2 mg/kg/day, is given for 2 to 3 days, either once in the morning or divided into two or three daily doses. In the majority of cases the maximum amount of drug needed, even in adults or heavier children, is 60 mg per day. Most physicians then gradually taper the daily dose by about 10 mg per day over the succeeding week, while others stop the prednisone course after 3 to 4 days without tapering the dose. There is probably no risk of adrenal crisis and shock from discontinuing the prednisone abruptly after only several days of therapy, as short courses of prednisone in the doses above do not appear to cause significant adrenal suppression.

The parenteral injection of aqueous allergens over time as a treatment for asthma is still controversial (see Chap. 38). The development of polymerized antigens for **immunotherapy** promises to provide a better preparation with higher immunogenicity (immune system blocking ability) and lower allergenicity (adverse effects). FDA approval of polymerized allergen extracts is pending. Many physicians feel that a trial of immunotherapy is indicated in atopic patients with moderately severe seasonal asthma in the hope of improving symptoms and minimizing other chronic medication, especially corticosteroids.

The physician who is treating a moderately or severely asthmatic patient must constantly reevaluate the patient both subjectively and objectively toward the goal of minimizing the amount of medication in the patient's regimen, especially since patient compliance is inversely proportional to the number of drugs in the regimen. Subjective evaluation can take the form of daily home symptom diaries, which the patient is asked to fill out and bring to the routine office visits. Objective evaluation usually includes periodic pulmonary function tests and often the use of small plastic devices (mini-peak flowmeters) for measuring the patient's peak flows at home. Chest auscultation alone is not a substitute for pulmonary functions.

Severe Asthma

Severe asthma, for the purposes of this discussion, is defined as asthma that occurs at least once a week. Most severely asthmatic patients are by definition perennial asthmatic patients, but their condition may be even worse during seasonal exacerbations.

Pharmacologic management is difficult with severely asthmatic patients as they usually require the chronic daily use of oral theophylline, oral or inhaled beta$_2$ sympathomimetics, and cromolyn, as well as corticosteroids. Even after maximizing therapy, "break-through wheezing" can occur in these patients on an intermittent basis and may lead to hospitalization for more intensive therapy (see Chaps. 3 and 4).

The need for frequent short courses of high-dose **prednisone** (twice a month or more) in a patient with asthma generally necessitates placing that patient on alternate-day prednisone (i.e., 1 day on prednisone, given early in the morning, and the next day off all prednisone). Alternate-day prednisone minimizes the adrenal suppression that invariably occurs with daily prednisone. However, there are some patients whose asthma can be controlled only by daily prednisone. Because of the high incidence of serious side effects from the chronic use of corticosteroids (e.g., cataracts, hypertension, obesity and adrenal crises), the physician should attempt to use the lowest possible dose that affords adequate control of clinical wheezing and normalizes daily activity as much as possible. **Inhaled corticosteroids** (e.g., beclomethasone) are available as a powder in pressurized metered-dose inhalers. These inhaled corticosteroids appear to act locally on the lung tissue with minimal systemic absorption, thus reducing the serious side effects that are seen with oral corticosteroids. Many authorities use inhaled beclomethasone to help lower the daily required dose of oral prednisone in the hope of minimizing the systemic side effects of chronic prednisone usage.

Atropine sulfate has definite bronchodilatory effects when solubilized and inhaled by nebulization either alone or in combination with a beta$_2$-

sympathomimetic agent. Several studies attest to its clinical utility, but to date it has not been approved by the FDA for use in the treatment of asthma. When mixed with a beta$_2$-sympathomimetic agent for inhalation use, atropine seems to be able to potentiate the bronchodilatory effects of the beta$_2$ agent for up to several hours. Certainly, consideration of the use of atropine must be given in a severely asthmatic patient after other FDA approved drugs have failed.

Troleandomycin (TAO) is a macrolide antibiotic in the erythromycin group that has been used in several research studies of severe asthmatics who appeared to be refractory to all other combinations of approved drugs. TAO appears to have a "steroid-sparing" effect in that severely asthmatic patients who require daily corticosteroids are able to tolerate significantly lower doses of corticosteroids while taking TAO. TAO does prolong corticosteroid half-life, but appears to have other effects as well: most of the patients tolerate lower doses of corticosteroids and they lose their cushingoid appearances. TAO, although approved for use as an antibiotic, is not approved for use in asthma therapy and should be reserved as a drug of last choice, to be used only by physicians experienced in its use (see Chap. 36).

Bundgaard, A., et al.   Short-term physical training in bronchial asthma. Brit. *J. Dis. Chest* 77:147–152, 1983.
  The authors found that short-term physical therapy is well tolerated by adult patients with asthma and that exercise can improve maximum O$_2$ consumption, while decreasing the need for aerosol bronchodilator therapy.
Ellis, E. F.   Asthma in childhood. *J. Allergy Clin. Immunol.* 72:526–539, 1983.
  This article is an excellent overview.
Hendeles, L., Weinberger, M., and Wyatt, R.   Guide to oral theophylline therapy for the treatment of chronic asthma. *Am. J. Dis. Child.* 132:876–880, 1978.
  This article is the basic "how to" of theophylline therapy.
Hill, D. J., Landau, L. I., McNicol, K. N., and Phelan, P. D.   Asthma—The physiological and clinical spectrum in childhood. Respiratory function studies in its assessment. *Arch. Dis. Child.* 47:874–881, 1972.
  The authors present a thorough review of pulmonary pathophysiology and pulmonary function abnormalities in asthma.
Jenne, J. W.   A critique of dosing strategies for beta-2 adrenergic agents and theophylline. *Lung* 159:295–314, 1981.
  Fantastic review article documenting research studies that show the benefits of various combination regimens of bronchodilators.
Konig, P.   Conflicting viewpoints about treatment of asthma with cromolyn: a review of the literature. *Ann. Allergy* 43:293–306, 1979.
  Everything you always wanted to know about cromolyn, but were afraid to ask.
Landan, L. I.   Outpatient evaluation and management of asthma. *Pediatr. Clin. North Am.* 26:581–601, 1979.
  This article is an excellent summary of the subject.
Leffert, F.   Asthma: A modern perspective. *Pediatrics* 62:1061–1069, 1978.
  Presents a nice, concise review of the various theories of the pathophysiology of asthma.
McFadden, E. R., Kise, R., and deGroot, W. J.   Acute bronchial asthma. Relations between clinical and physiologic measurements. *N. Engl. J. Med.* 288:221–225, 1973.
  Classic study that showed how important objective pulmonary functions are in demonstrating airways obstruction in patients who are asymptomatic.
Pak, C. C. F., Kradjan, W. A., Lakshminarayan, S., and Marini, J. J.   Inhaled atropine sulfate. Dose-response characteristics in adult patients with chronic airflow obstruction. *Am. Rev. Respir. Dis.* 125:331–334, 1982.
  This study reviews other studies of inhaled atropine. They recommended a dose of inhaled atropine sulfate of 0.025 mg/kg to a maximum of 0.05 mg/kg.
Rachelefsky, G. S., Katz, R. M., and Siegel, S. C.   Albuterol syrup in the treatment of the young asthmatic child. *Ann. Allergy* 47:143–146, 1981.
  A study that shows oral administration of albuterol (salbutamol) was very effective and safe in children as young as 5 years.

Swarts, C. L., and Hyde, J. S.   Long-term efficacy and safety of nebulized metaproterenol solution in bronchial asthma. *Chest* 70:617–620, 1976.
  This study showed that nebulized metaproterenol was better than nebulized isoproterenol.
Tattersfield, A. E., and McNicol, M. W.   Salbutamol and isoproterenol. A double-blind trial to compare bronchodilators and cardiovascular activity. *N. Engl. J. Med.* 281:1323, 1969.
  One of the earliest and best studies comparing the two drugs by double-blind trial. Salbutamol had a longer duration of action with fewer cardiovascular side effects.
Weber, R. W., Petty, W. E., and Nelson, H. S.   Aerosolized terbutaline in asthmatics. Comparison of dosage strength, schedule, and method of administration. *J. Allergy Clin. Immunol.* 63:116–121, 1979.
  Presents a study of the dose response characteristics of inhaled terbutaline.
Wyatt, R. W., Waschek, J., Weinberger, M., and Sherman, B.   Effects of inhaled beclomethasone dipropionate and alternate-day prednisone on pituitary-adrenal function in children with chronic asthma. *N. Engl. J. Med.* 299:1387–1392, 1978.
  Classic article comparing inhaled steroids to alternate-day steroids. Both caused some adrenal suppression and the combination had an additive effect.

21. EXERCISE-INDUCED ASTHMA
Shmuel Kivity

Exercise-induced asthma (EIA) can be defined as acute reversible airway obstruction that is induced by exercise in asthmatic patients. EIA is very common in young, active asthmatic patients, reaching an incidence of 90% in some reports.

Typically, strenuous exercise induces bronchoconstriction during the first 10 minutes following the exercise. The brochospasm increases over the next 5 to 10 minutes, with gradual spontaneous resolution. Without treatment symptoms of severe bronchoconstriction may not subside for an hour or longer.

In a susceptible patient the severity of EIA is proportional to the severity and duration of exercise. Brief exercise, even if strenuous, does not usually cause symptoms. Intermittent exercise is often well tolerated by the asthmatic patient. The worst type of exercise is that which usually lasts for longer periods, such as middle distance running or certain gymnastics. Paradoxically, even longer and more strenuous exercise such as cross-country running is well tolerated by some, and the patients find they are able to "run through" their asthma. Among the various strenuous exercises, swimming is the least likely to trigger asthma and is the most recommended form of exercise.

A careful history often reveals symptoms characteristic of EIA. The signs and symptoms of EIA do not differ from those of other forms of asthma except that they are usually of short duration, are self-limiting, and are totally reversible. There is no sure way to predict the severity of EIA in a given patient without proper testing. An exercise challenge permits quantitative assessment of the degree of EIA. It also evaluates the ability of various medications to inhibit EIA. Exercise testing in the office or pulmonary function laboratory is an important part of the diagnosis and treatment of EIA.

Exercise testing should be carried out while the effects of theophylline preparations and beta$_2$ agonists are minimal (the last dose of each drug will be dependent on the duration of action). The best exercise stimulus, established through numerous investigations, consists of continuous running for 6 to 8 minutes, sufficient to produce a heart rate close to 85% of the patient's maximal heart rate (177–180 beats per minute). The type of running can take many forms, such as free running in a corridor or running up and down stairs.

Pulmonary function equipment such as the Wright peak flowmeter or a simple spirometer measuring forced expiratory volume in 1 second (FEV_1) can be used to give a quantitative assessment of the degree of bronchoconstriction. A drop of 20% from baseline of either peak expiratory flow rate or FEV_1 is diagnostic of EIA. When more precise testing is needed, the degree of EIA can be assessed by using a treadmill or cycle ergometer. This equipment allows quantitation of the amount of exercise performed and makes electrocardiographic monitoring practical. Complete pulmonary functions, including measurements of lung volumes, are done prior to and 7 to 10 minutes following exercise. An occasional patient with clinically significant EIA can have changes in lung volumes alone without apparent alterations in flow rates.

Exercise tests should not be performed in asthmatic patients who are short of breath prior to testing or in patients with cardiac or other severe systemic disease. Since exercise can occasionally induce severe wheezing, measures such as oxygen, aerosol bronchodilators, and epinephrine should be available to treat these symptoms.

Even after 30 years of extensive research in this field, the physiologic mechanisms responsible for EIA are not fully understood. Clearly, the initial event in the induction of EIA is directly related to the degree of heat loss that occurs during exercise; the amount of heat loss is dependent on the level of minute ventilation at which the asthmatic patient is breathing, as well as on the temperature and humidity of the inspired air. Voluntary isocapnic hyperpnea or exercise in cool dry air will induce significant EIA, which can be blocked by breathing warm (37° C) humid air (100%).

Efforts should be made to encourage free exercise activity and participation in school, recreational, and competitive sports. At the same time the asthmatic child should be encouraged to participate in those activities that are least likely to cause symptoms, such as swimming and other intermittent activities.

Four groups of drugs are important in the pharmacologic prevention of EIA: (1) aerosolized beta$_2$ agonists, (2) cromolyn sodium, (3) theophylline-containing preparations, and (4) aerosolized atropine. Aerosolized beta$_2$ agonists are the most effective and can be used by inhaling one or two whiffs 5 to 10 minutes prior to a planned activity. Albuterol and metaproterenol are more effective than isoetharine and isoproterenol because they provide longer protection (4–6 hours). These drugs also can be used in relieving postexertional bronchoconstriction. Inhaled cromolyn sodium powder (aerosolized cromolyn sodium solution for small children), is also very effective when used just before exercise, but it does not relieve bronchoconstriction that has occurred. Theophylline-containing and newer calcium channel blocker drugs prevent EIA to a lesser degree than beta$_2$ agonists and cromolyn sodium.

Anderson, S., Seale, J. P., Ferris, L., Schoeffel, R., and Lindsay, D. A.   An evaluation of pharmacotherapy for exercise-induced asthma. *J. Allergy Clin. Immunol.* 64:612–624, 1974.
This is an excellent review of the subject.
Anderson, S. D., Silverman, M., Konig, P., and Godfrey, S.   Exercise-induced asthma. *Br. J. Dis. Chest* 69:1–39, 1975.
A review article that discusses the clinical pattern, physiologic response, possible mechanisms, and treatment of EIA.
Katz, R. M.   Asthma and sports. *Ann. Allergy* 51:153–160, 1983.
This review discusses the medical and physical problems associated with asthma and exercise.
Kivity, S., and Souhrada, J. F.   Hyperpnea: The common stimulus for bronchospasm in asthma during exercise and voluntary isocapnic hyperpnea. *Respiration* 40:169–177, 1980.
Emphasizes the fact that the degree of bronchoconstriction is dependent primarily on the amount of hyperpnea achieved during exercise and not the type of exercise.

McFadden, E. R., and Ingram, R. H.   Exercise-induced asthma. *N. Engl. J. Med.* 301:763–769, 1979.
  Presents a discussion of the new heat loss theory.
Patel, K. R.   Calcium antagonists in EIA. *Brit. Med. J.* 282:932–933, 1981.
  This is an editorial on the use of these drugs on EIA.
Tinkelman, D. G., Cavanaugh, M. J., and Cooper, D. M.   Inhibition of exercise-induced bronchospasm by atropine. *Am. Rev. Respir. Dis.* 114:87–91, 1976.
  Demonstrated the ability of inhaled atropine sulfate to block EIA in 17 of 18 patients studied.

22. OCCUPATIONAL ASTHMA
Don A. Bukstein

Occupational asthma is a reversible airways obstruction that results from an occupational exposure to organic and inorganic dusts, gases, vapors, or fumes. The diagnosis of occupational asthma is important in treatment. When persons with occupational asthma are identified, their coworkers must be evaluated so that serious medical consequences can be avoided before symptoms appear. Good epidemiologic data on the prevalence of occupational asthma are difficult to obtain because it is not a reportable disease. The overall prevalence has been estimated to be 2% of adult patients with asthma; however, the incidence varies widely with the geographic location, age, sex, and exposure to different industrial agents.

Pathophysiology
Several different mechanisms acting alone or in combination may cause occupational asthma (Table 14). This type of asthma may result from a single irritant mechanism or from several distinct mechanisms (see Table 14) producing similar effects by way of a common final pathway. The bronchospastic response pattern may be immediate—within minutes—or late—within a few hours after exposure. The pathogenesis is defined by the physicochemical properties of the offending substance. Some substances, such as toluene diisocyanate, trigger attacks in trace amounts, whereas others, such as grain dusts, require large amounts. Host factors are probably important but are currently not identified precisely. The atopic worker may be more likely to develop an allergic type of occupational asthma, such as that in platinum sensitivity. However, in most forms of occupational asthma that produce a late form of bronchoconstriction, atopy is not a predisposing factor.

The complex pathophysiology involved in occupational asthma is exemplified by the multiple pathogenic mechanisms involved in workers exposed to trimellitic anhydride. These workers may develop any of the following syndromes:

1. Pulmonary disease-anemia syndrome consisting of dyspnea, a restrictive respiratory defect, hypoxemia, and anemia. Workers with this syndrome have high levels of IgG antibodies against trimellitic proteins and trimellitic-coated erythrocytes.
2. Late respiratory systemic syndrome occurring 4 to 8 hours after trimellitic anhydride exposure, characterized by cough, wheezing, dyspnea, malaise, fever, and arthralgias. This syndrome is associated with high levels of IgG and IgA antibodies against trimellitic proteins.
3. Immediate type rhinitis and asthma syndrome associated with IgE antibodies against trimellitic proteins.

Table 14. A partial listing of etiologic agents

Type of agent	Representative occupation or industry
Specific immediate hypersensitivity	
Animal proteins	Breeders, drug research workers
Enzymes (animal)	Drug
Enzymes (plant)	Food
Plant proteins	Granary workers, bakers, cottonseed oil producers, farmers, food processors, green coffee and castor bean workers
Vegetable gums	Food, printing
Anhydrides	Plastics, drugs, epoxy resins
Platinum salts	Refining
Dyes	Cloth dyeing
Antibiotics	Pharmaceutical
Metallic salts	Metal plating, tanning, cement
Other chemicals	Hairdressers, plastics, rubber
Fluxes	Aluminum, soldering, electronics
Irritant (nonspecific)	
Nonparticulates	
Sulfur dioxide	Refrigeration
Fluorocarbon propellants	Beauticians
Inert particulates	
Lactose and talc	Pharmaceutical
Pharmacologic (nonimmunologic)	
Cotton, flax, jute	Textile
Toluene diisocyanate	Polyurethane foam, manufacturers
Hexamethylene diisocyanate	Auto, plastics, paint
Organophosphates	Pesticide workers, farmers, fumigators
Solder flux	Electronics industry

4. Irritant response syndrome that may occur after significant exposure to trimellitic anhydride powder.

Clinical assessment plus a determination of the type of antibodies to trimellitic proteins may clarify whether or not clinical symptoms following exposure to trimellitic anhydride are due to immunologic respiratory disease.

A large number of occupational agents cause asthma through a known or suspected **immediate hypersensitivity** (allergenic) **reaction.** "Allergic" occupational asthma occurs in the person who has IgE antibodies to an occupational allergen. Although this usually occurs in an atopic person with a history of hay fever, asthma, or eczema, isolated allergenic sensitivity to an occupational allergen without a concomitant personal or family history is not uncommon.

Large molecular weight proteins from either animals or plants are potent occupational allergens. Small-molecular-weight inorganic and organic chemicals can combine with a somatic protein carrier and acquire allergenic properties. Examples of the latter mechanism include antibiotics (dry powders and vapors), platinum salts, heavy metals, dyes, and anhydride chemical derivatives.

Byssinosis, bronchospasm induced by cotton dust, is attributed to a histamine-releasing agent isolated by heat distillation from aqueous extracts of cotton bract. There is no evidence of allergenic sensitivity to components of cotton bracts or fiber. Similar mechanisms might also be responsible for asthma occurring in people working with toluene diisocyanate, western red cedar, pine resin, and solder flux. Several studies have demonstrated that extracts of some of the materials responsible for occupational asthma can cause direct in vitro activation of the complement system. Whether or not these findings are related to the production of the clinical syndromes is unknown.

Increased bronchial reactivity is a feature of all types of asthma. Occupational exposure to **inert particles** and to **irritant gases,** such as sulfur dioxide and fluorocarbons, may produce reflex bronchospasm by direct stimulation of irritant receptors localized in the submucosa of the bronchial wall. Late-onset bronchoconstriction may be caused by a chemical inflammatory response resulting from toxic concentrations of sulfur dioxide, nitrogen dioxide, ozone, ammonia, halogen gases, strong acid fumes, and organic solvents. Soluble vapors usually cause upper airway bronchitis. Insoluble vapors that can penetrate to the smaller airways may produce an alveolitis and pulmonary edema.

Evaluation and Diagnosis

As Osler has suggested, "Listen to the patient, he is telling you the diagnosis." A detailed description of the history and symptoms (Table 15) should be obtained. History is of prime importance because the physical examination is usually unrewarding.

Table 15. Important aspects of patient history in occupational asthma

Occupation
  Duties
  Nature of exposure in workplace
    Present duration (hours/day, days/week)
    Type of exposure (gas, dust)
    Nature of precautionary measures
    Adherence to these measures
    Duration of exposure (months or years)
Symptoms
  Ocular
  Nasal
  Chest
  Skin (urticaria, angioedema)
  Other
Onset of symptoms
  In relation to exposure (immediate or delayed)
  In relation to duration of occupational exposure (time after initial work exposure, weekends)
  Pattern of attack (immediate, late, recurrent, nocturnal)
Severity of symptoms
  Conscious of exposure (mild irritation)
  Significant acute or chronic symptoms in terms of discomfort or disability
  Hospitalization, work loss
Duration of symptoms (after exposure ended)
  Persistence (overnight, weekends)
Previous work experience (occupational exposure)
History of related or unrelated symptoms (current or remote)
  Rhinitis
  Asthma
  Eczema
  Smoking history (cough and sputum production)
  Animal exposure
Comments and opinions of exposed subjects

Evaluation of suspected occupational asthma may include investigation of possible allergic etiology. The atopic potential of the patient can be determined by skin testing with routine allergens and examination of blood, sputum, and nasal secretions for eosinophils. Skin or radioallergosorbent testing (RAST) with materials from the workplace is rarely helpful because of the chemical properties of the suspected agents.

Pulmonary function studies are extremely useful for establishing the diagnosis. Routine spirograms away from work may be normal; however, evaluations before, during, and after work may be diagnostic. Patterns of deterioration and improvement in serial peak expiratory flow rates at home and at work may be able to document the association between airways obstruction and the patient's work area. In general, measurements that allegedly measure small airway function and distribution of inspired air (frequency dependence of dynamic lung compliance, single breath nitrogen test with determination of the alveolar plateau and closing volume, and comparison of maximal expiratory flow curves during exhalation of helium and air) may show abnormalities before the forced expiratory volume in 1 second (FEV_1) is abnormal. However, the clinical importance and predictive value of these tests will have to await additional studies in patients with occupational asthma. Most patients with occupational asthma show bronchial hyperreactivity to histamine or methacholine, but it is not known if the hyperreactivity is a cause or a result of the occupational disorder. The advantage of this test is that it may be positive in a person whose baseline studies are normal.

A bronchial provocation test is the single most diagnostic test. For this test, the patients perform their exact work with actual industrial materials under careful supervision in a controlled laboratory setting; measurements of pulmonary function are serially recorded. Inhalation challenges can also be performed with aerosolized material or in an environmental chamber. Bronchial provocation tests with inert substances (e.g., lactose) and with different types of dusts found in the work environment can help identify the inciting factor and exclude nonspecific bronchial hyperreactivity. Extreme care must be used in selecting the doses of inhaled materials, and observation of the patient should be extended to cover late reactions. In patients with late or complex reactions and for substances for which there is no satisfactory skin test or antigen for the radiosorbent assay, bronchial provocation may be the only way of making the diagnosis (e.g., toluene diisocyanate sensitivity) with certainty.

Treatment and Prevention

As with nonoccupationally induced asthma, treatment should be individualized to suit the needs of the patient. Alteration of the working conditions to minimize or avoid contact with offending agents should be attempted earnestly before the institution of drug therapy. Some workers have asthma of such severity that they must give up their job or be reassigned to other work; other workers can continue to work at a lower level of exposure or with devices such as masks and ventilatory hoods that decrease exposure.

The indications for pharmacologic therapy are similar for all types of asthma. Cromolyn may be especially effective. Corticosteroids, both inhaled and oral, are also efficacious in blocking the late reactions often seen in occupational asthma. Immunotherapy is potentially useful in only a small number of occupational allergens, such as animal dander. Immunotherapy is costly, time consuming, and may not give complete protection.

The decision to send a patient back to work with medical management involves the ethical dilemma of whether individuals shown to develop asthma on inhalation of particular occupational materials should continue to work with medication. Thus, a patient who is aware of the potential risks involved in continuing his or her present occupation should be given protective measures to minimize exposure. This patient should also have periodic pulmonary function testing, chest roentgenograms, and immunologic testing to aid in the early detection of increasing airway obstruction or parenchymal lung disease. Also uncertain are the long-term effects on respiratory function of those patients who have ceased exposure to the causative agent.

The prevention of occupational asthma could be aided by strict screening of atopic patients at high risk for sensitization and by avoiding exposure to potential pulmonary irritants or allergens in high-risk industries. Better monitoring of airborne chemicals and dust as well as a strong program of education and of pulmonary and immunologic testing with high-risk industries will also aid in the reduction of occupational asthma.

It is difficult to generalize about the long-term effects of work-related asthma. The prognosis is excellent if a responsible allergen can be avoided and if other factors contributing to the patient's asthma are minimal. Some types of work-related asthma are associated with generalized bronchial hyperirritability that may persist even under non-work-related conditions. There may also be a cross reactivity on exposure to antigenically similar substances. Occupational asthma probably does not predispose the patient to other unrelated allergic conditions or to other forms of chronic pulmonary disability.

Andrasch, R. A., Bardana, E. J. Jr., Koster, F., and Pirofsky, B.   Clinical and bronchial provocation studies in patients with meat wrapper's asthma. *J. Allergy Clin. Immunol.* 58:291–298, 1976.
Presents the best description of meat wrapper's asthma.

Bernstein, I. L.   Occupational asthma. *Clin. Chest Med.* 2:255–272, 1981.
A current review of the literature focusing on pathophysiology, etiology, diagnosis, treatment, and prevention of occupational asthma.

Chan-Yeung, M.   Fate of occupational asthma: A followup study of patients with occupational asthma due to western red cedar (Rhuja plicata). *Am. Rev. Respir. Dis.* 116:1023–1029, 1977.
A demonstration that nonspecific bronchial hyperreactivity persisted in patients who left exposure.

Dally, M. B., et al.   Hyperreactivity to platinum salts: A population study (abstr.). *Am. Rev. Respir. Dis.* 121(Suppl.):230, 1980.
This is a discussion of occupational asthma secondary to platinum sensitivity.

Gross, N. J.   Allergy to laboratory animals: epidemiologic, clinical and physiologic aspects, and a trial of cromolyn in its management. *J. Allergy Clin. Immunol.* 66:158–165, 1980.
The use of cromolyn in the management of preventing the clinical manifestations of hypersensitivity to laboratory animals is nicely outlined.

Karr, R. M. N., et al.   Occupational asthma. Allergy grand rounds. *J. Allergy Clin. Immunol.* 61:54–65, 1978.
A thorough description of the proper evaluation and treatment of patients with occupational asthma to toluene diisocyanate.

Lam, S., Wong, R., and Yeung, M.   Nonspecific bronchial reactivity in occupational asthma. *J. Allergy Clin. Immunol.* 63:28–34, 1979.
Attempt to establish methacholine inhalation test as a simple, safe, and useful procedure in initial assessment of patients suspected to have occupational asthma by demonstrating that a negative methacholine challenge in the presence of a positive history of occupational asthma could exclude that diagnosis.

Mason, R. J.   Occupational Pulmonary Disease. In J. B. Wyngaarden and L. H. Smith (Eds.), *Cecil Textbook of Medicine.* Philadelphia: Saunders, 1982, Pp. 395–404.
An excellent concise review of occupational pulmonary medicine.

Pepys, J.   Inhalation challenge tests in asthma. *N. Engl. J. Med.* 293:758–759, 1975.
This article is a description of the usefulness in doing inhalation challenge tests in asthma.

Pepys, J., and Hutchcroft, B. J.   Bronchial provocational tests in the etiologic diagnosis and analysis of asthma. *Am. Rev. Respir. Dis.* 112:829–859, 1975.

Detailed descriptions of examples where bronchial provocational testing established the diagnosis of occupational asthma.

Sale, S. R., Roach, D. E., Zeiss, C. R., and Patterson, R.   Clinical and immunologic correlations in trimellitic anhydride airway syndromes. *J. Allergy Clin. Immunol.* 68:188–193, 1981.

In previous studies these authors correlated symptoms caused by trimellitic anhyride inhalation with antibody activity. This study suggests that clinical assessment plus total antibody determination may aid in diagnosis of immunologic respiratory disease caused by trimellitic anhydride powder.

Thiel, H., and Ulmer, W. T.   Baker's asthma: Development and possibility for treatment. *Chest* 78 (2 Suppl.):400–405, 1978.

A general discussion of the diagnosis and treatment in baker's asthma.

23. ALLERGIC AND IRRITANT TRIGGERS OF ASTHMA
Mark Holbreich

Asthma is a disease characterized by a heightened responsiveness of the bronchial tree to a diversity of stimuli. Exposure to these stimuli will produce bronchospasm in most asthmatic patients. A few persons respond only to a single stimulus. Exercise and infection are two of the most commonly implicated triggers. Emotional upset, certain drugs, gastroeosphageal reflux, and sinus disease are other factors thought to play a role in asthma. Allergen and irritant exposure, including pollution and climatic changes, are also important precipitants of asthma.

Allergy
The most commonly recognized triggers of allergic asthma include pollens, house dust, mold spores, and animal danders. Pollen grains of seed plants are carried by the wind. A number of trees, grasses, and weeds produce abundant quantities of allergenic pollen. In most areas of the country trees and grasses pollinate in the spring, while weeds are fall pollinators. Not all pollens are implicated in allergic disease. Most flowering and fragrant plants are insect-pollinated and present little problem. Pollen production for a particular region may vary significantly from year to year based on a variety of climatic conditions. Numerous guides exist detailing seasonal pollen counts and predominant allergenic plants in each geographic area. When pollen-induced asthma is suspected the relationship must be confirmed by comparing skin-test data, local pollen counts, and seasonal flares of asthmatic symptoms for each person.

House dust is an important inhalant allergen. It is made up of a variety of allergenic components, including textile fiber, human and animal skin and hair, plant fibers, pollen grains, mold spores, and household insects such as cockroaches, moths, and mites. The mite Dermatophagoides pteronyssimus is one of the major allergenic components of house dust. The mite content of house dust specimens varies greatly, depending on the geographic area and source material. They predominate in humid environments and are most numerous in samples from mattresses and carpeted areas around beds. Skin-test sensitivity is frequently noted in asthmatic patients, and direct challenge of the bronchial tree by mite antigen can result in bronchospasm in a large number of patients with large, positive epicutaneous skin tests. Symptomatic sensitivity is often suggested by increased symptoms during the winter months when the home is poorly ventilated and central heating is used, although mites actively breed in the warm, humid summer months and symptoms during this period may pre-dominate.

Airborne mold spores are encountered universally in nonpolar areas. They grow under most climatic conditions. Although a damp, warm environment is ideal for many molds, each mold has conditions that are the most favorable for its growth. Unlike allergens such as pollens and animal dander, which come from obvious sources, airborne molds originate from inapparent microscopic growth. *Alternaria* and *Claudosporium* (*Hormodendrum*) are the most commonly en-countered outdoor molds. They predominate during the growing season and are found largely in plant soil and vegetable matter. During the winter months indoor sources of mold (infrequently cleaned and overly used humidifiers, house-plants, crawl spaces, damp basements and bathrooms) are predominant. *Penicil-lium, Aspergillus,* and *Fusarium* are the most commonly encountered indoor mold spores during these months. The exact clinical impact of mold exposure on respiratory allergic disease, particularly asthma, is largely unknown. It is gener-ally believed to play a significant role.

Hypersensitivity to animal dander is well recognized. Dander is made up of epidermal scales of an animal's skin and all animals shed dander (albeit some more than others and some appear to be more allergenic than others, but none are nonallergenic). Animal saliva and hair are also allergenic. Individuals with cat and dog dander sensitivity will usually react similarly on exposure to all breeds of cats and dogs, although occasionally an individual will become sensitized to a single breed. Domestic animals produce large quantities of dander regardless of hair length or breed. Other common household pets that can be highly allergenic are guinea pigs, rabbits, hamsters, and gerbils. Often a patient will state that their animal bothered them when they first acquired it but not now. It is unlikely that they have become "hyposensitized." It is more likely that, instead of obvious acute symptoms with exposure, the patients are having constant low-grade symp-toms (a poor situation medically because they are always in a more reactive state). This may be confirmed by the history of recurring acute symptoms for a short period of time when the patients return home after having been away from the animal for 2 to 3 weeks.

A wide variety of less commonly encountered animal allergens have also been implicated in respiratory allergy. These include animals such as horses and cat-tle. Furthermore, rodent hair, urine, and saliva are potent sensitizers, and respi-ratory symptoms secondary to exposure to these have been well documented in laboratory workers. Plant fibers including jute, kapok, cottonseed, flaxseed, orris-root and pyrethrum are also potentially allergenic.

Certain food sensitivities have been noted as precipitants of asthma. In the vast majority of well-documented cases of asthma caused by foods, ingestion of the food was also associated with either cutaneous or gastrointestinal signs and symp-toms. Asthma precipitated by foods is more common in the pediatric age group than among adults. Before a restricted or elimination diet is introduced, the correlation between ingestion of a particular food and symptoms must be estab-lished. This is done through a careful history, skin testing, elimination diets, and food challenge (see Chap. 41).

Environmental Aspects of Asthma

Air pollution in major industrial areas is rich in sulfur dioxide, sulfuric acid, carbon monoxide, and particulate matter, including dust and soot. In regions with large numbers of cars and sunny days, pollution is also characterized by carbon dioxide, carbon monoxide, and ozone, produced through a photochemical reaction. Industrial pollution and automobile pollution may exist separately or together.

Retrospective studies of major air pollution catastrophes show a marked in-crease in morbidity and mortality among asthmatic patients. Prospective studies on asthma and air pollution have found a positive correlation between the concentration of various air pollutants and the aggravation of asthmatic symptoms. However, an accurate evaluation of the complex role that air pollution plays in airways disease is difficult. Not only are there numerous pollutants, but pollen and mold counts and meteorologic conditions also vary during the periods of study. Nevertheless, the following recommendations can be made for asthmatic patients during air pollution alerts: (1) They should remain indoors as much as possible. (2) They should use an air conditioner. (3) They should minimize their exposure to other irritants (e.g., dust, smoke, sprays). (4) They should institute regular bronchodilator therapy or add rapid-acting bronchodilators to their regimen. (5) They should wear a mask with carbon filters for necesary, transitory periods outdoors.

Climatic conditions include temperature (irritant effect, especially cold), barometric pressure (ion effect), wind velocity (irritant effect), and humidity. Like air pollution, meteorologic conditions affect bronchial reactivity in certain persons. Bronchospasm induced by cold air is an example of a direct influence of the weather on asthma. This bronchospasm probably results from irritation of the parasympathetic receptors in the upper airway producing vagal stimulation and reflex bronchospasm. One example of a possible indirect climatic effect is the increased mold and dust mite proliferation in damp environments. Relocation of the family is often suggested as a means of avoiding harsh climatic conditions. Reports of improvement with a change in climate are anecdotal only and there is no way to predict whether a given individual will benefit from a change.

Numerous **nonspecific irritants** adversely affect many asthmatic patients. These include any strong odors such as paint or perfume, any type of particulate matter such as chalk dust, or anything that produces cough on inhalation. The cough is a protective mechanism and is self-limiting in normal persons. In asthmatic patients however, the cough can trigger reflex bronchospasm as well. Tobacco smoke is one of the best known irritants. Smoking tobacco has long been known to be a major factor in the morbidity and mortality of lung disease and is clearly contraindicated in asthmatic patients. More recently, increased interest has centered around passive exposure to cigarette smoke: exposure to sidestream cigarette smoke causes significant airways obstruction in asthmatic patients. Passive exposure to cigarette smoke in childhood asthma may increase the risk of chronic lung disease in later life. Some investigators have noted an improvement in the asthma of children whose parents give up smoking. Physicians should encourage elimination of cigarette smoking, especially for parents who smoke around their children.

Asthmatic patients frequently report sensitivity to a variety of other nonspecific irritants in addition to cigarette smoke. Household sprays, paint, varnish, and nailpolish remover are often mentioned. Exposure to these products should therefore be limited.

Environmental Control in Allergy

A careful and complete **environmental survey** (Table 16) is central to the allergy evaluation. It details the presence of potential allergens and irritants in the home, school, or workplace. Occasionally a home visit is required (Table 17).

A physician recommending changes in the patient's environment must base the recommendations on proved or highly suspected precipitating factors. The broader the change, the more evidence a physician needs. A physician must consider the possible financial burden of the recommendations.

Because **house dust** can be both an allergen and an irritant, it is reasonable to control house dust exposure if the history is suggestive, regardless of the skin-test results. Efforts to control house dust exposure should be concentrated in the

Table 16. Environmental Survey

Where do you live (city or rural) _____
Number of indoor plants _____ Age of house (years) _____ House construction
(brick, wood, etc.) _____ Are any rooms damp or musty? _____ Do you have a(n)
Air cleaner _____ Air humidifier _____ Dehumidifier _____ Air conditioner _____
Type of carpet (wool, synthetic, jute) Bedrooms _____ Living room _____
    Den _____ Dining room _____
And pad (rubber, ozite, hair) Bedrooms _____ Living room _____
    Den _____ Dining room _____
How old is your Pillow _____ Mattress _____
Do you have any Stuffed furniture _____ Feather comforters _____
Is your pillow _____ Feather _____ Foam rubber _____ Dacron _____ Other _____
Encased in plastic
Is your mattress _____ Foam rubber _____ Cotton _____ Innerspring & cotton _____
Waterbed _____ Encased in plastic _____ Other
What kinds of grasses, shrubs, and trees are in the immediate vicinity of your house?

Do you have pets? List number and kind (dog, cat, birds, horses, etc,)

Do your pets spend time indoors? _____ Yes _____ No
What type of work do you do? _____
Are you exposed to anything at work or school that might aggravate your condition?
Which things? _____

Have you missed any time from work or school because of your allergies? How much time?

Do you have any other exposures from hobbies, recreational activities, and so on?

---

bedroom but other rooms, especially those frequented by the patient, should be
included.
    The following steps should be taken to maintain a dust-free room:

1. Dust-collecting objects (toys, books, pillows, and so on) should be kept to a
   minimum.
2. Carpeting should be vacuumed weekly (or more often if indicated) and sham-
   pooed occasionally.
3. The room should be dusted daily with a damp rag.
4. Curtains should be kept dust free (tumble in dryer on "air only" or "fluff").
5. Closets in the patient's bedroom should not be used for storage and only the
   current season's clothes should be kept there; closet floors should be kept clean
   and the closet door kept closed.
6. Hot-air vents in homes with forced-air heat should be closed and sealed with
   tape. Alternately, five or six layers of cheesecloth can be placed behind the
   heating vent cover to filter the warm air. Furnace filters should be replaced or
   cleaned each month during the winter season.
7. The mattress and box spring should be encased in a mite-proof, airtight cover
   for persons with significant sensitivity to house dust mites.
8. More extensive modification of the environment (carpet and curtain removal,
   air filtration, cleaning heating ducts, and so on) should be considered only
   when more simple measures fail to produce improvement in the patient's
   condition.

Table 17. Home Visit Information

Name _____ Date _____

OUTSIDE ENVIRONMENT
Location _____ How long in location? _____
Type of planting within one block of house: Trees _____ Grass _____
  Shrubs _____ Other _____
Are there any animals kept in the immediate neighborhood? List number and kind.
_____

Type of planting in patient's yard: Grass _____ Shrubs _____Trees _____
  Dirt yard _____

HOUSE
House construction _____
Age of house _____ Size _____
Number living in home Adults _____Children _____
Type of air conditioning _____ Filter _____
Type of heating _____ Filter _____
Central humidifier _____ Electronic filter _____
Carpet type _____ Age _____ Carpet pads _____
Type of window coverings _____ Age _____
  Washable _____
Furnishings _____
Cleaning _____ Dust control _____ Odors _____
  Sprays _____
Unusual hobbies or occupations _____
Indoors _____ Outdoors _____

PATIENT'S BEDROOM
No. sleeping in room _____ No. of beds _____ Type of mattress _____
  Springs _____ Pillows _____ Blankets, quilts, spreads _____
Carpet/pads _____
Window coverings _____ Washable _____
Stuffed toys _____ Furniture _____
Where are toys stored? _____ Dust catchers _____
Sleep with windows: Open _____ Closed _____
Sleep with closet: Open _____ Closed _____

COMMENTS:

RECOMMENDATIONS:

Molds are found primarily outdoors. Indoor mold growth is usually a reflection of what has been outdoors, but the indoor growth can be encouraged by humidity and moisture. Humid coastal areas present a better environment for both indoor and outdoor mold growth than do more arid regions. Areas prone to mold growth include damp or musty basements and crawl spaces; rubber, jute, horsehair, and other organic underpads for carpets; bathroom shower stalls; feather and foam rubber pillows and mattresses; refrigerator drip trays; home humidifiers and vaporizers; and evaporator-type air conditioning units. Houseplants apparently are not a problem as long as they are healthy.

The following steps should be taken to reduce indoor mold growth:

1. Replace damp or musty carpet and carpet pads.
2. Seal off damp crawl spaces.
3. Decrease humidity in a damp basement by using a dehumidifier.
4. Regularly clean shower stalls, bathtubs, and shower curtains (at least monthly) with liquid bleach (e.g., Clorox) or a disinfectant (e.g., Lysol). If mold growth is significant, bathroom walls and floors should be washed four times a year with 1:750 solution of 17% benzalkonium chloride (Zephiran Chloride; 1 fluid ounce in 1 gallon of tap water). Zephiran Chloride is available without prescription from most pharmacies.
5. Replace foam rubber pillows and mattresses with polyester.
6. Clean portable humidifiers and vaporizers with liquid bleach (Clorox) weekly. A capful of Clorox may be added to each refill of large portable humidification units. Central humidifiers can be a major source of mold if the reservoir is not cleaned regularly. Humidifiers without a reservoir may be best. Air conditioning units especially swampcoolers can also be a source of mold. Portable units may be sprayed with Lysol periodically to remove mold growth.
7. Do not use paraformaldehyde crystals—once recommended for indoor mold control—because of their potential carcinogenic effect.

Elimination of the family pet is often a difficult task. If the patient has minimal sensitivity, a significant decrease in **dander** exposure may be accomplished by keeping the animal outdoors or out of the bedroom both day and night. When significant dander sensitivity exists, total elimination of the animal is necessary. Dander in heating ducts and carpets may be a continuing source of exposure for 4 to 6 months after the animal is gone; therefore, professional cleaning of the carpet and ductwork is suggested after the animal is removed from the home. Animal dander may be the principal allergic constituent of house dust in areas where animals are present.

Pollens from trees and weeds travel many miles; therefore, removal of trees within the yard is not particularly effective unless a given plant is right outside a bedroom window or in the direct path of the wind currents to the bedroom window. In contrast, grass pollen travels much shorter distances, and attempts to reduce pollination in the patient's yard, such as frequent mowing, may be useful. Someone in the family other than the grass-sensitive person should be responsible for the upkeep of the yard.

A few simple, general recommendations will significantly decrease pollen exposure during the pollen season. (1) Bedroom windows and doors should be kept closed as much as possible. (2) After playing or working outside, the pollen-sensitive person should shower and put on fresh clothing. (3) Room or central air conditioners will significantly decrease indoor pollen counts if they recirculate indoor air instead of drawing in pollen from the outside air. Windows and doors must be kept closed. Attic fans will obviously only aggravate the problem by pulling air through the patient's bedroom and through the house.

Central and portable electrostatic air filtration systems will remove most pollen as well as mold spores and animal dander. Cigarette smoke and other gaseous materials (pollution and so on) are best removed by adding, in front of the regular filter, a carbon or "activated charcoal" filter to the unit. Poorly designed portable electrostatic units may produce ozone, an irritant to asthmatic patients. Central units remove airborne particulate matter as the air circulates through a central heating or cooling system. Air must be continually moving for these units to be effective, so the fan usually has to operate constantly. High efficiency particulate air (HEPA) filters are the most efficient, removing virtually all airborne particles. They are expensive ($350–500) and at present are available only as portable units. They can usually be rented for a month or more, providing an adequate trial period to assess their benefit before purchase.

Buckley, J. M., and Pearlman, D. S.   Controlling the Environment. In C. W. Bierman and D. S. Pearlman (Eds.), *Allergic Diseases of Infancy Childhood and Adolescence.* Philadelphia: Saunders, 1980. Pp. 300–310.
Contains practical points on environmental control.

Girsh, L. S., Shubin, E., Dick, C., and Schulaner, F. A.   A study on the epidemiology of asthma in children in Philadelphia. The relation of weather and air pollution to peak incidence of asthmatic attacks. *J. Allergy Clin. Immunol.* 39:347–357, 1967.
Definite relationship between these factors was observed in this study.

Holbreich, M., and Strunk, R. C.   Precipitating factors in childhood asthma. *Respir. Ther.* 11:74–78, 1981.
Presents a systematic review of precipitating factors in childhood asthma and a detailed bibliography.

Khan, A. U.   The role of air pollution and weather changes in childhood asthma. *Ann. Allergy* 39:397–400, 1977.
Prospective study demonstrating relationship between asthmatic attacks and high levels of ozone and carbon monoxide. However, all factors played only a minor overall role.

Lopez, M., and Salvaggio, J. E.   Climate-Weather-Air Pollution. In E. Middleton, E. Reed, and E. F. Ellis (Eds.), *Allergy: Principles and Practice* (2nd ed.). St. Louis: Mosby, 1983. Pp. 1203–1214.
Presents a complete review of irritant precipitants.

Mathews, K. P.   Other Common Inhallant Allergens. In C. W. Bierman and D. S. Pearlman (Eds.), *Allergic Diseases of Infancy, Childhood and Adolescence.* Philadelphia: Saunders, 1980. Pp. 248–259.
Details house dust and dander allergens.

Solomon, W. R.   Common pollen and fungus allergens. In C. W. Bierman and D. S. Pearlman (Eds.), *Allergic Diseases of Infancy, Childhood and Adolescence,* Philadelphia: Saunders, 1980. Pp. 219–247.
This book is very complete, including regional pollen guides.

Weiss, S. T., Tager, I. B., Speizer, F. E. and Rosner, B.   Persistent wheeze. Its relation to respiratory illness, cigarette smoking, and level of pulmonary function in a population sample of children. *Am. Rev. Respir. Dis.* 122:697–707, 1980.
Contains more information about effects of passive smoking on asthma.

Zweiman, B., et al.   Effect of air pollution on asthma: A Review. *J. Allergy Clin. Immunol.* 50:305, 1972.
Presents a good overview of the subject.

Resource Information
Pollen Guides
Statistical Report of the Pollen and Mold Committee of the American Academy of Allergy, 1981. American Academy of Allergy, 611 East Wells Street, Milwaukee, WI 53202.
Pollen Guide for Allergy. Hollister-Stier, P.O. Box 3145, T.A., Spokane, WA 99220.

Companies supplying air filters and other equipment for environmental control
Air Techniques Inc. 1801 Whitehead Road, Baltimore, MD 21207. (301-944-6037) makes a Cleanaire HEPA filter.
Allergen-Proof Encasings, Inc. 1450 E. 363rd St. East Lake, OH (800-321-1096) makes mattress and pillow encasings.

Bio-tech Systems, P.O. Box 25380, Chicago, IL (800-621-5545) makes inexpensive furnace filters.

Mason Engineering, 242 W.Devon Ave. Bensenville, IL 60106 (312-595-5700) makes Cloud-9 HEPA FILTER.

Research Products Corp., Madison, WI (800-356-9652) makes humidifiers and air cleaners.

Vitaere Corp., 8113 Broadway, Elmhurst, NY 11373 (212-335-8589) makes HEPA Filter.

24. INFECTION AND ALLERGIC DISEASE
Fernan Caballero and Don A. Bukstein

Both epidemiologic and clinical studies have linked viral infections with the exacerbation of asthmatic symptoms. Viruses are especially important precipitants of bronchospasm in asthmatic children, but they can precede and precipitate bronchospasm in both children and adults. There is also some evidence that viral infections may initiate the development of allergic sensitization in infants predisposed genetically to the development of allergy.

Respiratory syncytial virus (RSV) infection has been found to trigger more than 50% of asthmatic attacks in children up to 5 years of age. Other commonly implicated viruses are parainfluenza and rhinovirus; rarely, influenza A, A2, and B, enterovirus, and adenovirus have caused attacks. Rhinovirus has been associated with exacerbation of asthma at all ages, while influenza A and B have been associated with exacerbation of asthmatic symptoms primarily in adults.

Several investigators have postulated that viral infections induce bronchospasm by producing an abnormality in autonomic regulation, specifically by decreasing beta$_2$-adrenergic responsiveness in cells. In vitro studies demonstrate that culturing lymphocytes from asthmatic patients with live influenza virus vaccine or rhinovirus in vitro reduces the increase in cyclic adenosine monophosphate (cAMP) seen in the lymphocytes after incubation with isoproterenol and other beta$_2$ agonists. Viral infections may also induce impaired beta-adrenergic responsiveness to the beta$_2$ agonists in airway smooth muscle, thereby producing the bronchospasm that occurs during those infections. This altered beta-adrenergic responsiveness may also result in increased release of leukocyte lysosomal enzymes, which produce inflammation. This process may accentuate the viral-induced inflammatory response, increasing the severity and duration of the viral infection in the patient with asthma. The reason(s) that viral infection decreases beta$_2$ adrenergic activity in asthmatic patients but not normal subjects is not known.

Viral infections are also known to induce transient increases in nonspecific airway smooth muscle reactivity in persons without asthma or other underlying lung disease. This effect can persist for up to 6 weeks. Long-term persistence of nonspecific airway reactivity in these otherwise normal subjects is not documented, though the condition may exist. One example may be children who have had a history of spasmodic croup and continue for several years to have an increased response to inhaled histamine, a finding characteristic of increased airways reactivity. The reason for this increase in nonspecific airways reactivity may be one of the following: (1) inflammation in small airways induced by viral infection; (2) sensitization of rapidly adapting airway receptors of the vagal nervous system; (3) blunting of the bronchial smooth muscle response to beta-adrenergic stimulation; (4) augmentation of histamine release; or (5) increased synthesis of bronchospastic leukotrienes.

Current data suggest that damage induced to the rapidly adapting vagal receptors in the lung may be primarily responsible for increased bronchial sensitivity to histamine in normal subjects after viral infections. This epithelial damage is not necessarily, however, the only factor; many viruses that severely damage epithelium in the airways do not necessarily provoke an asthmatic response, and viruses that produce increased reactivity, such as RSV and rhinovirus, do not severely damage airway mucosa.

Asthmatic patients appear to be at a higher risk for the development of viral infections than normal subjects. Several epidemiologic studies demonstrate that asthmatic patients have more viral infections than nonasthmatic members of the same household. Allergic infants seem to be more susceptible to the development of viral bronchiolitis, and the bronchiolitis that they have is more severe. In older children and adults with asthma, many respiratory viruses cause an exaggeration of the already increased airways reactivity characteristic of asthma and this exaggeration seems to persist much longer than in normal subjects. The reason for the increased susceptibility of asthmatic patients to viral infection is not known. Attempts to describe a pattern of immunodeficiency in these patients have not been successful. Asthma may interfere with mucociliary defense mechanisms in a subtle way and thereby enhance the viral infections, however, no such abnormalities have been described. The role of IgE in the pathogenesis of wheezing has also been the subject of recent investigation. The presence of virus-specific IgE was found more frequently and in higher titers in RSV-infected patients with wheezing than in RSV-infected patients without wheezing. The RSV-infected patients with wheezing also had higher histamine levels in their secretions. Again, the basis for such differences is not known.

Several studies have shown that exacerbation of asthmatic symptoms is not related to the presence of bacterial infection. The findings in the epidemiologic studies predicted the finding in subsequent studies that neither routine use of antibiotics in children with uncomplicated asthmatic attacks nor the use of bacterial vaccine in the treatment of asthma was of value.

Boushey, H. A., Holtzman, M. J., Sheller, J. R., and Nadel, J. A.   State of the art: Bronchial hyperreactivity. *Am. Rev. Respir. Dis.* 121:389–413, 1980.
Complete review of the methods of assessment, mechanisms of hyperreactivity, and their relation to asthma.
Busse, W. W., Anderson, C. L., Dick, E. C., and Warshaurer, D.   Reduced granulocyte response to isoproterenol, histamine, and prostaglandin E_1 after in vitro incubation with rhinovirus 16. *Am. Rev. Respir. Dis.* 122:641–646, 1980.
This study showed a blunted B-adrenergic response after in vitro virus challenge.
Empey, D. W., Laitinen, L. A., Jacobs, L., Gold, W. M., and Nadel, J. A.   Mechanisms of bronchial hyperreactivity in normal subjects after upper respiratory tract infection. *Am. Rev. Respir. Dis.* 113:131–139, 1976.
Airway epithelial damage with sensitization of receptors postulated as a possible mechanism for wheezing.
Frick, O. L., German, D. F., and Mills, J.   Development of allergy in children. I. Association with virus infections. *J. Allergy Clin. Immunol.* 63:228–241, 1979.
Eleven children with two allergic parents were followed prospectively. Immunologic evidence of allergic sensitization occurred in all 11 children 1 to 2 months following viral upper respiratory tract infections.
Ida, S., Hooks, J. J., Siraganian, R. P., and Notkins, A. L.   Enhancement of IgE-mediated histamine release from human basophils by viruses: Role of interferon. *J. Exp. Med.* 145:892–906, 1977.
IgE and interferon involvement on histamine release in leukocytes and atopics.
McIntosh, K., et al. The association of viral and bacterial respiratory infections with exacerbations of wheezing in young asthmatic children. *J. Pediatr.* 82:578–590, 1973.
Prospective study on an inpatient population in two consecutive seasons. No relation with bacterial infection was found.

Minor, T. E., et al.   Viruses as precipitants of asthmatic attacks in children. *J.A.M.A.* 227:292–298, 1974.
   Epidemiologic study of viruses involved in asthmatic attacks in children.

Mitchell, I., Inglis, H., and Simpson, H.   Viral infection in wheezy bronchitis and asthma in children. *Arch. Dis. Child.* 51:707–711, 1976.
   The authors present a prospective study with a large number of patients.

Perelmutter, L., Potvin, L., and Phipps, P.   Immunoglobulin E response during viral infections. *J. Allergy Clin. Immunol.* 64:127–130, 1979.
   Changes in IgE levels during viral infections in a large atopic and nonatopic population.

Reinherz, E. L., O'Brien, C., Rosenthal, P., and Schlossman, S. F.   The cellular basis for viral-induced immunodeficiency: Analysis by monoclonal antibodies. *J. Immunol.* 125:1269–1274, 1980.
   Variations of suppressor-helper cell ratio during the acute and convalescent phase of Epstein-Barr virus infection.

Rooney, J. C., and Williams, H. E.   The relationship between proved viral bronchiolitis and subsequent wheezing. *J. Pediatr.* 79:744–747, 1971.
   Retrospective and noncontrolled study with a high incidence of atopic children in whom a high incidence of persistent wheezing was found.

Shapiro, G. G., et al.   Double-blind study of the effectiveness of a broad spectrum antibiotic in status asthmaticus. *Pediatrics* 53:867–872, 1974.
   Prospective, double-blind study of 44 children and adolescents without evidence of bacterial infections in whom the treatment with broad-spectrum antibiotic did not modify the course of an asthmatic attack.

Sherter, C. B., and Polnitsky, C. A.   The relationship of viral infections to subsequent asthma. *Clin. Chest Med.* 2:67–78, 1981.
   Review of the available data on the relationship of viral infections to subsequent asthma, as well as the pathogens involved, with mention of possible mechanisms.

Stempel, D. A., and Boucher, R. C.   Respiratory infection and airway reactivity. *Med. Clin. North Am.* 65:1045–1053, 1981.
   Concise summary of mechanisms involved in virus-enhanced airway reactivity, with a brief reference to clinical background.

Twiggs, J. T., Larson, L. A., O'Connell, E. J., and Ilstrup, D. M.   Respiratory syncytial virus infection: Ten-year follow-up. *Clin. Pediatr.* 20:187–190, 1981.
   The longest follow-up study of children with RSV disease. No evidence of persistence of asthma was found.

Welliver, R. C.   Upper respiratory infections in asthma. *J. Allergy Clin. Immunol.* 72:341–346, 1983.
   This is an excellent review.

25. RELATIONSHIP BETWEEN GASTROESOPHAGEAL REFLUX AND ASTHMA

Michael E. Martin

Gastroesophageal reflux (GER) has been documented to occur in association with a variety of pulmonary disorders including recurrent pneumonia, recurrent "obstructive" bronchitis, pulmonary fibrosis, neonatal apnea, and asthma. An etiologic role for GER in causing the respiratory symptoms has been suggested by studies reporting amelioration of symptoms following antireflux medical therapy or antireflux surgery. Furthermore, some patients have convincing histories relating the onset of respiratory symptoms to the occurrence of gastrointestinal symptoms of GER. Evidence to support such a sequence of events has been reported recently in studies using continuous monitoring of distal esophageal pH. Using an intraluminal esophageal pH probe, we, as well as others, have documented that the onset of respiratory symptoms (e.g., cough, wheezing or apnea) is closely associated with the spontaneous reflux of gastric acid into the esophagus. The relationship of GER to asthma has many complexities, however.

Basic Aspects of Gastroesophageal Reflux

GER is the retrograde flow of gastric contents into the esophagus across an incompetent gastroesophageal (GE) junction. Normally a positive-pressure gradient exists from the abdominal cavity to the thoracic cavity, and antireflux mechanisms at the GE junction prevent the backward flow of gastric contents. Several physical factors may be involved in producing an effective GE junction but the most important mechanism appears to be the lower esophageal sphincter (LES). The LES is a 2- to 5-cm-long area of increased pressure at the GE junction that helps to prevent reflux of gastric contents. Prevention of reflux esophagitis probably depends on several factors including a competent LES, effective esophageal clearance by peristaltic mechanisms, and possibly local mucosal factors. Gastrointestinal symptoms of GER include vomiting, regurgitation (bitter taste), substernal and epigastric pain, and, late in the disease course, dysphagia.

The laboratory diagnosis of GER has been the subject of several recent comprehensive reviews. The two diagnostic procedures that correlate best with a history of GER in adults are esophageal acid perfusion (Bernstein test) and intraesophageal pH monitoring to detect acid reflux (Tuttle test).

The Bernstein test can diagnose esophagitis and evaluate the effect of acid infusion on pulmonary function. This test is preferred in adults and children who can perform pulmonary function tests and are reliable enough to report the subjective symptoms that occur during acid infusion. The Tuttle test can be used in children too young for the Bernstein test. If the facilities and expertise are available, overnight pH recording can be used to quantitate the severity of GER, and to observe for a sequence of reflux followed by wheezing.

Other less reliable tests include barium esophagram, esophageal manometrics to measure LES pressure, and scintigraphic monitoring. Although the esophagram by itself is not a reliable method of diagnosing GER, it should be done to define anatomic abnormalities such as a significant hiatal hernia, which might alter the therapeutic approach. More recently, the use of prolonged esophageal pH monitoring has been reported to be a very accurate test for the diagnosis of GER.

Relationship Between Gastroesophageal Reflux and Asthma

GER has been reported to occur in a high percentage of asthmatic children and adults. In previous studies, the incidence of reflux in asthmatic patients has ranged from 46 to 63%. The principle mechanism accounting for the high incidence of reflux has not been defined, but two causes have been suggested. The first is the effect of drugs commonly used to control asthma on LES pressure. Theophylline decreases LES pressure in animals and humans and could thereby predispose many asthmatic patients to reflux of gastric contents. The second cause is the abnormal pulmonary physiology associated with asthma. As previously stated, intrathoracic pressure is normally lower than intraabdominal pressure, resulting in a pressure gradient across the GE junction. Any changes that would increase the pressure gradient could result in more frequent reflux. Patients with asthma may have decreases in forced expiratory flow rates as well as hyperinflation. Breathing at higher lung volumes requires generation of greater negative intrathoracic pressures, and this would increase the pressure gradient across the LES and further predispose to GER.

GER may precipitate asthma directly by aspiration of gastric contents into the tracheobronchial tree or indirectly via a reflex arc begun by stimulating the lower esophagus. If aspiration of refluxed gastric contents occurs, there may be a history of recurrent pneumonia with pulmonary infiltrates on chest x-ray film. However, aspiration of extremely small amounts of refluxed acid material into the tracheobronchial tree may induce bronchoconstriction in asthmatic patients and not be associated with recurrent pneumonia. Aspiration can be documented in some asthmatic patients by using a lung scan after instillation of radioactive technetium in the stomach. The findings of Mansfield and Stein (1978) supported the involvement of a neurogenic reflex. Fifteen patients with asthma and GER had mild but significant bronchoconstriction following infusion of 0.1 N hydrochloric acid into the distal esophagus. Aspiration was very unlikely to have occurred during this procedure. In further studies using dogs with a chemically induced esophagitis, Mansfield and co-workers (1980) reported similar pulmonary responses of increased airways resistance following acid infusion into the distal esophagus. A very interesting finding was that the bronchoconstrictive response could be abolished by vagotomy.

It remains to be determined if GER has a significant clinical role in causing or exacerbating respiratory symptoms; however, there is direct and indirect evidence available that it may. While there are several reports in the surgical literature of the resolution or improvement of asthma symptoms after an antireflux surgical procedure, there are no well controlled surgical studies, and objective evidence of improvement in pulmonary function, symptoms, and reduced medication requirements is scant. In a recent double-blind crossover study of cimetidine versus placebo in asthmatic patients with GER, there was significant improvement in nocturnal wheezing scores in patients on the cimetidine antireflux medical regimen. This demonstration gives further support to the possibility that reflux may cause wheezing in some patients with reactive airways.

Importance of Gastroesophageal Reflux in Nocturnal Asthma
Nocturnal and early morning wheezing is a particularly significant and perplexing problem for many asthmatic patients, and the reasons for these exacerbations in any individual patient are far from clear. Many investigators have attempted to determine the basis for this phenomenon and many possible factors have been noted. These include elevated plasma histamine levels in the early morning hours and an increased airways reactivity to histamine and specific antigens during the nighttime hours when compared with the daytime hours. In general, nighttime asthma is almost always more prominent when the asthma is not well controlled during the day; however, some patients have asthma only at night. It has also been postulated that the occurrence of GER when the patient is recumbent may be responsible for some of the episodes of nocturnal cough and wheezing. Using overnight esophageal pH recordings to quantitate the severity of GER, we have documented a high incidence of GER (64%) in 25 severely asthmatic children. Furthermore, a highly significant statistical correlation ($r = 0.66, p = 0.001$) was found between the frequency of nighttime wheezing and the severity of GER as determined by the esophageal pH monitoring.

In summary, mounting evidence is being reported that supports a clinically important association between wheezing and GER in some patients with asthma. The role GER has in causing respiratory symptoms requires further investigation, but there is now data to suggest that in some patients, GER may cause exacerbations of asthma.

Diagnosis and Treatment
At present, confirmation of an association between GER and exacerbations of asthma is difficult and requires careful clinical observation. If an association between asthma and GER is suspected in a patient, the following approach is suggested:

1. Take a careful, thorough history and be especially alert to the following: (a)

unexplained nocturnal wheezing, (b) onset of respiratory symptoms during or after gastrointestinal symptoms of GER, and (c) history of aspiration or recurrent pneumonia or pulmonary infiltrates.

2. Review the therapeutic regimen for asthma and evaluate compliance to ensure optimal medical therapy, especially with medicine taken near bedtime.

3. Confirm the presence of GER with the following tests: (a) Berstein test, (b) Tuttle test, and (c) esophagram. These tests should be performed only if nocturnal symptoms are not controlled by good management of asthma in general.

4. If esophagitis or significant reflux is diagnosed, a medical antireflux regimen that includes the following should be tried for 4 to 6 weeks: (a) elevating the head of the bed at least 6 inches; (b) eliminating after-dinner snacks; (c) antacids: 15-30 ml p.c. and h.s.; and (d) cimetidine: 400 mg h.s.

5. Specific indications for surgical intervention are not well defined at present. The severity of the GER, the response to medical therapy, and the severity of the associated respiratory symptoms will need to be considered for the risk-benefit analysis. Until the etiologic role of GER in asthma is established, and until the results of controlled studies of therapy are available, a very conservative approach towards surgical intervention seems appropriate. In general, indications for surgery should be based primarily on gastrointestinal indications (e.g., hiatal hernia, prevention of esophageal stricture, recurrent bleeding) and not on asthma alone.

Arasu, T. S., et al. Gastroesophageal reflux in infants and children—comparative accuracy of diagnostic methods. *J. Pediatr.* 96:798–803, 1980.
Esophageal pH measurement is the most reliable test; esophagram is insensitive but highly specific.

Behar, J., Biancani, P., and Sheahan, D. G. Evaluation of esophageal tests in the diagnosis of reflux esophagitis. *Gastroenterology* 71:9–15, 1976.
Acid infusion test and esophageal pH study are the most accurate tests for GER.

Berquist, W. E., et al. Effect of theophylline on gastroesophageal reflux in normal adults. *J. Allergy Clin. Immunol.* 67:407–411, 1981.
Theophylline decreases lower esophageal sphincter pressure and induces GER in a high percentage of normal subjects and asthmatic patients.

Christie, D. L., O'Grady, L. R., and Mack, D. V. Incompetent lower esophageal sphincter and gastroesophageal reflux in recurrent acute pulmonary disease of infancy and childhood. *J. Pediatr.* 93:23–27, 1978.
GER is a factor in some patients with recurrent acute pulmonary disease.

Danus, O., Casar, C., Larrain, A., and Pope, C. E. Esophageal reflux—an unrecognized cause of recurrent obstructive bronchitis in children. *J. Pediatr.* 89:220–224, 1976.
The association between GER and asthmalike symptoms is documented.

Davis, R. S., Larsen, G. L., and Grunstein, M. M. Respiratory response to intraesophageal acid infusion in asthmatic children during sleep. *J. Allergy Clin. Immunol.* 72:383–397, 1983.
The authors concluded that during sleep the presence of acid in the lower esophagus can trigger bronchoconstriction in asthmatic children with a positive Bernstein test and that these children appear to be more susceptible to the bronchoconstrictive effects of intraesophageal acid at 4 to 5 a.m. than at midnight.

Euler, A. R., et al. Recurrent pulmonary disease in children: A complication of gastroesophageal reflux. *Pediatrics* 63:47–51, 1979.
Thirty patients with chronic asthma (27) or recurrent pneumonia (3) were studied; 63% had GER by esophageal pH measurement and other tests.

Fisher, R. S., and Cohen, S. Gastroesophageal reflux. *Med. Clin. North Am.* 62:3–20, 1976.
Presents a comprehensive review of the gastrointestinal aspects of GER.

Fonkalsrud, E. W., Ament, M. E., Byrne, W. J., and Rachelefsky, G. S. Gastroesophageal fundoplication for the management of reflux in infants and children. *J. Thorac. Cardiovasc. Surg.* 76:655–664, 1978.

Favorable pulmonary response to surgery for five patients with asthma. The author suggests cautious interpretation of studies regarding indications for surgery.

Goodall, R. J. R., et al. Relationship between asthma and gastro-esophageal reflux. *Thorax* 36:116–121, 1981.

Reports significant improvement in nocturnal wheezing scores in patients on cimetidine antireflux regimen. A double-blind crossover study design was used.

Herbst, J. J., Minton, S. D., and Book, L. S. Gastroesophageal reflux causing respiratory distress and apnea in newborn infants. *J. Pediatr.* 95:763–768, 1979.

The title is self-explanatory.

Johnson, L. F., and Demeester, T. R. Twenty-four hour pH monitoring of the distal esophagus. A qualitative measure of gastroesophageal reflux. *Am. J. Gastroenterol.* 62:325–332, 1974.

Accuracy and usefulness of prolonged esophageal pH monitoring in children and adults is assessed. The method for calculating reflux score is best described in paper by Jolley and colleagues.

Jolley, S. G., et al. An assessment of gastroesophageal reflux in children by extended pH monitoring of the distal esophagus. *Surgery* 84:16–24, 1978.

Accuracy and usefulness of prolonged esophageal pH monitoring in children and adults is assessed.

Mansfield, L. E., et al. Canine bronchoconstriction provoked by esophageal acid infusion (abstr). *J. Allergy Clin. Immunol.* 65:209, 1980.

Bronchoconstriction induced in dogs with esophagitis by acid perfusion of esophagus. The response was abolished by vagotomy.

Mansfield, L. E., and Stein, M. R. Gastroesophageal reflux and asthma: A possible reflex mechanism. *Ann. Allergy* 41:224–226, 1978.

Bronchoconstriction induced by acid perfusion of the distal esophagus in 15 asthmatic patients with confirmed GER.

Martin, M. E., Grunstein, M. M., and Larsen, G. L. Relationship of gastroesophageal reflux to nocturnal asthma. *Ann. Allergy* 49:318–322, 1982.

Sixty-four percent of 25 asthmatic children had abnormal GER during overnight esophageal pH study. There was a strong correlation between severity of GER and frequency of nocturnal wheezing symptoms.

Mays, E. E. Intrinsic asthma in adults—association with gastroesophageal reflux. *J.A.M.A.* 236:2626–2628, 1976.

Forty-six percent of 28 adults with severe asthma had GER diagnosed by esophagram, versus 5% incidence of abnormal esophagram in 468 control subjects.

Mays, E. E., Dubois, J. J., and Hamilton, G. B. Pulmonary fibrosis associated with tracheobronchial aspiration. A study of the frequency of hiatal hernia and gastroesophageal reflux in interstitial pulmonary fibrosis of obscure etiology. *Chest* 69:512–515, 1976.

Persistent GER and aspiration can cause pulmonary fibrosis.

Overholt, R. H., and Voorhees, R. J. Esophageal reflux as a trigger for asthma. *Dis. Chest* 49:464–466, 1966.

Fourteen of eighteen selected asthmatic patients with GER had moderate to dramatic improvement in their asthma after antireflux surgery.

Pope, C. E. Pathophysiology and diagnosis of reflux esophagitis. *Gastroenterology* 70:445–454, 1976.

Good discussion of neural and humoral mechanisms for control of reflux, including the role of cyclic AMP.

Shapiro, G. G., and Christie, D. L. Gastroesophageal reflux in steroid-dependent youths. *Pediatrics* 63:207–212, 1979.

Forty-seven percent incidence of GER by Tuttle test in 19 asthmatic patients who were taking therapeutic doses of theophylline.

Spaulding, H. S., et al. Further investigation of the association between gastroesophageal reflux and bronchoconstriction. *J. Allergy Clin. Immunol.* 69:516–521, 1982.

Decreased pulmonary function was observed after intraesophageal acid infusion in asthmatic patients with positive challenge. The response was the greatest in asthmatic subjects who associated reflux symptoms with attacks of asthma.

Stein, M. R., et al. The effect of theophylline on the lower esophageal sphincter pressure. *Ann. Allergy* 45:238–241, 1980.

Another study demonstrating that theophylline decreases lower esophageal sphincter pressure and induces GER in a high percentage of normal subjects and asthmatic patients.

Strobel, C. T., Byrne, W. J., Ament, M. E., and Euler, A. R.   Correlation of esophageal lengths in children with height: Application to the Tuttle test without prior esophageal manometry. *J. Pediatr.* 94:81–84, 1979.
Formula for accurate pH probe placement for esophageal pH study.

26. LATE ASTHMATIC RESPONSES
B. Lyn Behrens

The pulmonary response to an inhaled allergen in asthmatic patients sensitive to that allergen has characteristically been considered to occur immediately following the exposure. However, the use of allergen inhalation tests in asthmatic patients identified three patterns of response. The immediate asthmatic response (IAR) occurs within minutes after the exposure, peaks in intensity by 15 to 30 minutes, and resolves over 1 to 2 hours. A second pattern of response, termed the *late asthmatic response* (LAR), has a delayed onset after exposure of 2 to 4 hours, peaks by 6 to 12 hours, and resolves usually within 24 hours. An IAR followed by a LAR is termed a *dual asthmatic response* (DAR) and represents the third pattern. Similar timing of response patterns have been noted in the skin, following allergen skin tests, and in the nose in allergic rhinitis patients after nasal provocation testing.

More than a century ago, Blackley reported a prolonged asthmatic episode following a brief accidental pollen exposure and is credited with the first description of an LAR. In 1934, Stevens noted severe LAR after bronchial provocation tests and abandoned this form of testing because of the severity of asthmatic attacks precipitated. In 1952, Herxheimer suggested that LARs would increase the difficulty of identifying a precipitating agent, thereby increasing the probability of prolonged and excessive exposure and more severe clinical consequences. Further work by Pepys has demonstrated the relevance of these reaction patterns to occupational asthma. In the last decade, there has been increased interest in this phenomenon especially as it relates to the pathogenesis of severe asthma and therapeutic modalities for prevention and treatment.

Clinical Overview
Using bronchial challenge testing with various antigens, in extrinsic asthmatic patients, researchers have demonstrated all three response patterns in both children and adults (Table 18). Allergens that have been used in these studies include house dust, mite, animal dander, molds, ragweed, and grass pollens. The incidence of each pattern of responsiveness varies among studies, ranging from 20% IAR and 80% DAR in Warner's study of severe perennial asthmatic children to 53% IAR and 47% DAR in Booij-Nord's study of perennial asthmatic adults. Isolated LARs were identified in only four of the eight studies, varying from 7% in Robertson's study to 46% in Van Lookeran Champaigne's report. Preliminary reports indicate that exercise and foods may also be precipitins of the various patterns of response.

The pattern of response for each patient with the same antigen has been shown to be reproducible. The pulmonary response pattern is probably antigen specific, for studies in limited numbers of subjects have shown that different antigens can produce different patterns in the same person. Price and colleagues compared the pulmonary response pattern to the response pattern for the same allergen in the

Table 18. Response patterns of children and adults to various antigens

	Antigens and incidences of responses			Bronchial provocation test		
Source	Age	Agent	Number of patients	Immediate (patients/%)	Dual (patients/%)	Late (patients/%)
Van Lookeran Champaigme (1969)	Children	House dust	54	29/54		25/46
Booij-Nord (1972)	Adults	House dust	55	29/53	26/46	
Robertson (1974)	Adults	Ragweed	15	6/40	8/53	1/7
Warner (1976)	Children	Mite	60	10/20	50/80	
Gaultier (1979)	Children	House dust	61	26/43	13/21	22/36
Gross (1980)	Adults	Animals	12	6/50	6/50	
Hill (1981)	Children	Mites	13	2/15	6/46	
		Rye grass	13	2/15	11/86	5/38
Price (1982)	Children (18 total)	Mite	14	1/7	13/93	
		Cat dander	8	2/25	6/75	
		Timothy grass	15	4/27	11/73	

Table 19. Pulmonary bronchial reactivity

	Immediate response	Late response
Timing		
Onset	10 min	2–4 hr
Peak	10–15 min	5–12 hr
Duration	1–2 hr	24 hr to several days
Clinical		
Course	Rapid	Slow, progressive, severe
Symptoms and signs	Clinically evident, subjectively and objectively	Insidious until fully developed
Treatment		
Prophylaxis		
Cromolyn	+	+
Steroids, inhalation	−	+
Steroids, oral	Insignificant	+
Antihistamine	Insignificant	Insignificant
Atropine	Partial	Partial
Reversal		
Adrenergics	Rapid	Poorly responsive
Aminophylline	Responsive	Poorly responsive

skin, nose, and lungs; only 4 of 21 children studied showed the same response pattern to an allergen for the three target organs.

As noted already, the three patterns of asthmatic responses are differentiated from each other primarily by their time courses after bronchoprovocation testing. The three patterns can also be distinguished by their clinical course and the therapeutic agents that are useful for their prophylaxis and treatment. All these characteristics are summarized in Table 19.

Clinically immediate responses begin rapidly, with clearly identified evidence of bronchospasm both subjectively and objectively. A careful history can often identify the precipitants. By contrast, the LAR begins more gradually and insidiously. Often the pulmonary function tests deteriorate to a much greater extent than in the IAR before the changes are apparent to either the patient or the observer and, as would be expected, identification of exposure-symptom relationship is much more difficult than in the IAR.

The IAR and LAR respond differently to various medications. This is of interest both for therapeutic intervention and as an aid to understanding the underlying pathophysiologic differences between each response. Both cromolyn and steroids can be used to block the LAR, but only cromolyn blocks the IAR. Adrenergic agents and theophylline derivatives are effective medications for management of IAR, but are poorly effective for LAR. Steroids are the most effective drugs for reversing an LAR.

Clinical Relevance

LARs pose a major diagnostic dilemma in the identification of precipitants. This applies to both typical aeroallergens and occupational exposures. Robertson (1974), in reporting LAR with ragweed pollen allergy, compared the diurnal variation in pollen counts and the asthmatic symptoms. The highest pollen counts were present through the morning while LAR symptoms were most prominent in the evening. Delayed responses to occupational exposures may not be obvious because the asthmatic symptoms occur only in the evening, long after the patient has left work. Absence of the evening symptoms when the patient has not

Table 20. Steps in establishing the diagnosis of late asthmatic response

HISTORY
Delayed but consistent relationship to event or activity
Nocturnal asthma with pattern related to season or activity
Severe asthma
Effective cromolyn prophylaxis
Steroid dependency

SKIN TEST
Correlation with LCR and LAR not absolute

BRONCHOPROVOCATION TESTING
Occupational or event exposure—PEFR profile
Bronchial provocation testing with pulmonary function testing should be performed only
  by specialized laboratories

been at work during the day, such as on weekends or vacations, should provide the clue to the relationship. Thus, an LAR should be suspected when there is a consistent relationship between symptoms and an event, activity, or antigen exposure. Symptoms that consistently occur in the evening or at night may indicate the presence of an LAR.

In reviewing the clinical studies of patients with LAR, it can be noted that the majority of patients selected had severe asthma. This may be because patients with LAR have a more severe clinical course than asthmatic patients with only an IAR pattern. Warner and colleagues (1978) study of mite sensitivity in perennial asthmatic children supports this hypothesis. They showed a correlation between the presence of an LAR and the frequency of asthmatic attacks. Thirty of thirty-six children with an LAR in bronchoprovocation testing had two or more attacks per month, whereas 10 of 13 children with IAR only had no more than one attack per month.

Induction of an LAR in bronchoprovocation testing is associated with an increase in nonspecific responsiveness of the airways to substances such as methacholine. The increased nonspecific responsiveness following LAR lasted days to weeks in some subjects, long after all pulmonary function tests had returned to normal. This may be important clinically, providing a mechanism for a prolonged increase in symptoms after a limited antigen exposure.

A careful history and appropriate skin and bronchoprovocation tests are necessary to establish a diagnosis (Table 20). The first step is to elicit a careful history concentrating on the relationships between exposure of precipitins and the onset of symptoms, the severity of the asthma, and its response to therapy. On the basis of these historical criteria, a subpopulation of asthmatic patients at risk for LAR can be identified.

The second step involves the use of skin testing. Controversy exists about the value of a late cutaneous response in predicting an LAR. Boulet and colleagues (1983) suggested that the occurence of LAR from inhaled antigen could be suggested either by a wheal of 5 mm or less in the immediate response that proceeds to a later cutaneous response or by the occurence of a later cutaneous response from low concentrations of allergens. By contrast, Price and co-workers (1982) showed no direct correlation between skin and pulmonary responses for any antigens studied.

The third and currently only definitive diagnostic tool is bronchoprovocation testing to the suspected allergen, followed by periodic measurement of pulmonary function parameters over the ensuing 24 hours. The simplest methodology is allowing an intense natural exposure to the suspected precipitin, following the response with a mini-peak flowmeter to determine the pattern of change in peak expiratory flow rates (PEFR). PEFRs should be recorded before encountering the agent as a baseline and to ensure reproducibility of the measurement. For safety, baseline PEFRs should be at least 80% of the best previous values for the subject before the study is started. The subsequent measurement of PEFRs should continue through the time period when symptoms normally begin.

Using occupational exposure as an example of the application of this methodology, the test would be done after an absence of some days from work when baseline PEFRs are at their best. The subject would establish the baseline levels, encounter their usual work exposure for a defined time (30 minutes to 1 hour) early in the morning and do PEFRs over the subsequent 24 hours. Hourly recordings should be made until bedtime and continued through the night only if the patient is symptomatic. A final measurement is made 24 hours after the challenge. A decrease in the PEFR of 25% from baseline is considered significant. For comparison the PEFR profile should be obtained over the same time period without the exposure, with the subject on an identical therapeutic regimen. More definitive testing can be done by bronchoprovocation testing using repetitive challenges of measured concentrations of the antigen. This, however, requires more sophisticated testing equipment and personal experience in the testing procedure. If the latter is desired, the subject should be referred to a center where it can be safely performed.

As with all extrinsic asthma, avoidance of the precipitating agent is the best form of therapy. This can have great relevance in the management of subjects with occupational asthma.

For those allergens that cannot be avoided (e.g., pollens) therapeutic agents effective in blocking LAR should be used before exposure if the exposure is episodic, or continuously if the exposure cannot be predicted or occurs frequently. Cromolyn is the safest medication to use and should be instituted first. Steroids are also useful and may need to be considered. Obviously the risk-benefit ratio of steroid therapy should be carefully assessed for each patient before institution of these drugs in a therapeutic regimen. Since bronchial reactivity is increased after LAR, anticholinergic agents may prove helpful, but this has not been adequately evaluated. As noted previously, adrenergic agents and theophylline are not effective in either treatment or prevention of LARs. As the pathogenesis of the late asthmatic response is better understood, other therapeutic agents will probably become available.

Immunotherapy may be useful in patients with LAR. Mite-sensitive children who improve clinically following immunotherapy with mite antigen had a loss of the LAR in spite of persistence of IAR upon repeat bronchial challenge with mites. Studies with a small number of mold-sensitive subjects have also confirmed this finding. However, further studies need to be done to expand these observations before firm recommendations can be given.

Immunopathology and Pathophysiology

There have been three main thrusts in the research of the LAR. First, the late cutaneous response (LCR) has been studied in an attempt to understand the basic mechanism of delayed responses to antigens. In humans these reactions are initiated by IgE antibody to the allergen and are associated with mixed inflammatory cell infiltrate, which becomes predominantly mononuclear by 24 hours after antigen challenge. The LCR has also been shown to be altered by medication in a similar fashion to the LAR indicating mechanisms of the two reactions are probably similar (see Gleich, 1982, for more details).

Neutrophil chemotactic factor of anaphylaxis (NCF-A) is released by mast cells along with other mediators in immediate type hypersensitivity (see Kay and Lee,

1982). Following antigenic challenge in subjects with DAR, NCF-A has been shown to rise in the immediate phase, return toward baseline within 30 minutes, and then subsequently increase. The second rise in NCF-A precedes the pulmonary function changes of the LAR by up to 3 hours, indicating probable continued involvement of mast cells in the reaction.

Lastly an animal model has been developed to study the late asthmatic responses (see Shampain and colleagues, 1982). Using this model it has been shown that LAR occurs only when IgE-antigen-specific antibodies are present and that the reaction is blunted by the presence of IgG-antigen-specific antibodies. In addition, preliminary observations indicate that the LAR in the rabbit responds in the same manner to cromolyn and steroid pretreatment as noted in human LAR.

It is apparent that further studies will be necessary before the immunopathology and pathophysiology are delineated for the LAR. Clarification of the underlying pathophysiologic mechanisms is of more than theoretical interest for it may explain the basis of severe asthma and provide direction for usage of other therapeutic modalities both prophylactically and in reversal of the episodes.

Bernstein, I. L.   Cromolyn sodium in the treatment of asthma: Changing concepts. *J. Allergy Clin. Immunol.* 68:247–253, 1981.
Reviews the clinical usage of cromolyn sodium.

Booij-Nord, H., DeVries, K., Sluiter, H. J., and Orie, N. G. M.   Late bronchial obstructive reaction to experimental inhalation of house dust extract. *Clin. Allergy* 2:43–61, 1972.
Report of a study on house dust allergy in adults.

Booij-Nord, H., Orie, N. G. M., and DeVries, K.   Immediate and late bronchial obstructive reactions to inhalation of house dust and the protective effects of disodium cromoglycate and prednisolone. *J. Allergy Clin. Immunol.* 48:344–354, 1971.
Report on a study of asthmatic responses and the effects of medication.

Boulet, L. P., Hargreave, F. E., and Dolovich, J.   Prediction of late asthmatic responses to inhaled allergens (Abstr.). *J. Allergy Clin. Immunol.* 71:107, 1983.
Study report of the prediction of late asthmatic responses to inhaled allergens.

Cartier, A., et al.   Allergen-induced increase in bronchial responsiveness to histamine: Relationship to the late asthmatic response and change in airway caliber. *J. Allergy Clin. Immunol.* 70(3):170–177, 1982.
Study report on relationship of bronchial reactivity to late asthmatic responses.

Dahl, R.   Disodium cromoglycate and food allergy. *Allergy* 33:120–124, 1978.
Case report of dual asthmatic response evoked by food allergy.

Gaultier, C., et al.   Immediate and late bronchial reaction to house dust in children. *Bull. Eur. Physiopathol. Respir.* 15:1091–1102, 1979.
Report of a study on house dust allergy in children.

Gleich, G. J.   The late phase of immunoglobulin E-mediated reaction: A link between anaphylaxis and common allergic diseases? *J. Allergy Clin. Immunol.* 70:160–169, 1982.
Reviews the pathogenesis of late allergic responses.

Gross, N. J.   Allergy to laboratory animals. Epidemiologic, clinical and physiological aspects and a trial of cromolyn in its management. *J. Allergy Clin. Immunol.* 66:158–165, 1980.
Report of a study on allergy to laboratory animals.

Hargreave, F. E., Dolovich, J., Robertson, D. G., and Kerigan, A. T. II.   The late asthmatic response. *CMA Journal* 110:415–424, 1974.
Review of late asthmatic responses.

Hill, D. H.   Inter-relation of immediate and late asthmatic reactions in childhood. *Allergy* 36:549–554, 1981.
Report on a study of patterns of asthmatic responses in allergic children following bronchial provocation testing.

Kay, A. B., and Lee, T. H.   Neutrophil chemotactic factor of anaphylaxis. *J. Allergy Clin. Immunol.* 70(5):317–320, 1982.
Review of the mast cell mediator neutrophil chemotactic factor of anaphylaxis and relevance to clinic medicine.

Metzger, W. J., Donnelly, A., and Richerson, H. B.   Modification of late asthmatic responses during immunotherapy for alternaria-induced asthma (Abstr.). *J. Allergy Clin. Immunol.* 1:119, 1983.
Study report of immunotherapy for mold asthma.

Metzger, W. J., Dorminey, H. C., Robbins, D., and Richerson, H. B.   Late asthmatic responses during bronchial provocation. Correlation with specific IgE and symptoms (abstr.) *J. Allergy Clin. Immunol.* 67:11, 1981.
Study report of late asthmatic responses to mold.

Pepys, J.   Clinical and therapeutic significance of patterns of allergic reactions of the lungs to extrinsic agents. *Am. Rev. Respir. Dis.* 116:573–588, 1977.
Review article on various patterns of allergic pulmonary responses.

Pepys, J.   The effect of inhaled beclomethasone dipropionate (Becotide) and sodium cromoglycate on asthmatic reactions to provocation tests. *Clin. Allergy* 4:13–24, 1974.
Study report on usage of medication in altering asthmatic responses.

Pepys, J., and Hutchcroft, B. J.   Bronchial provocation tests in etiologic diagnosis and analysis of asthma. *Am. Rev. Respir. Dis.* 112:829–859, 1975.
Review article on use of bronchial provocation testing in asthma.

Price, J. F., Hey, E. N., and Soothill, J. F.   Antigen provocation to the skin, nose and lung in children with asthma: Immediate and dual hypersensitivity reactions. *Clin. Exp. Immunol.* 47:587–594, 1982.
Report on a study comparing patterns of responses in skin, nose, and lungs in asthmatic children.

Rebuck, A. S.   Symposium on allergic lung disease I. The clinical picture of asthma. *CMA Journal* 110:409–413, 1974.
Reviews the clinical features of asthma.

Robertson, D. G., et al.   Late asthmatic responses induced by ragweed pollen allergen. *J. Allergy Clin. Immunol.* 54:244–254, 1974.
Report of a study on ragweed pollen allergy in adults.

Shampain, M. P., et al.   Animal model of late pulmonary responses to *Alternaria* challenge. *Am. Rev. Respir. Dis.* 126:493–498, 1982.
Presentation of an animal model used to investigate the pathophysiology of the late asthmatic response.

Stevens, F. A.   A comparison of pulmonary and dermal sensitivity to inhaled substances. *J. Allergy* 5:285–288, 1934.
Reports on the use of bronchial provocation testing in asthmatic patients.

Van Lookeran Champaigne, J. G., Knol, K., and DeVries, K.   House dust provocation in children. *Scand. J. Respir. Disease* 50:76–85, 1969.
Reports a study on house dust allergy in children.

Warner, J. O.   Significance of late reactions after bronchial challenge with house dust mite. *Arch. Dis. Child.* 51:905–911, 1976.
Reports a study on house dust mite allergy in children.

Warner, J. O., Soothill, J. F., Price, J. F., and Hey, E. N.   Controlled trial of hyposensitization to Dermatophagoides pteronyssimus in children with asthma. *Lancet* 28:912–915, 1978.
Presents a study report of hyposensitization in mite allergic children.

27. PREGNANCY AND ASTHMA
Rajesh G. Bhagat

An estimated 0.4 to 1.3% of pregnancies in the United States are complicated by asthma. In 15 to 20% of such pregnancies, asthma is severe enough to require hospitalization, making this a common medical management problem.

A review of various studies suggests that there is no consistent effect of pregnancy on the status of asthma. It is difficult to predict whether asthma will improve, worsen, or remain unchanged in a given patient, though there is some suggestion of worsening of asthma in patients who have severe asthma prior to the pregnancy. Pregnant asthmatic patients seem likely to repeat the same pattern during subsequent pregnancies (i.e., if the status of asthma improved during the first pregnancy, it will improve during the subsequent pregnancies).

In general, the incidence of premature labor and perinatal mortality are somewhat higher in asthmatic pregnancies than in nonasthmatic pregnancies. These complications are more likely to occur in patients whose asthma is under poor control although the reasons for this are unclear. In a study of severe, corticosteroid requiring asthmatic patients, the incidence of these complications was not significantly different from those occurring in nonasthmatic pregnancies, probably because of better asthma control and close follow-up. Thus there seem to be compelling reasons to keep pregnant asthmatic patients under good control.

Theophylline is a relatively safe drug for the control of asthma in pregnant women. Although theophylline is presumed to cross the placenta, there have been no cases of fetal malformation or any other complication in infants caused by chronic maternal ingestion of theophylline during pregnancy.

The data regarding the frequent use of epinephrine in pregnant asthmatic patients are not clear. A recent study associated fetal malformations with epinephrine use. It is likely that these malformations were associated with the severe unstable asthma that required the use of epinephrine, not with the use of epinephrine itself.

Sufficient data have not been collected to clearly establish whether or not terbutaline, metaproterenol, salbutamol, and cromolyn can be used safely. It should be noted, however, that terbutaline is frequently used to inhibit uterine activity during labor, and there are several reports of the occurrence of pulmonary edema in mothers receiving intravenous terbutaline to prevent the progression of labor.

Neither oral nor inhaled corticosteroids administered during pregnancy have a harmful effect on the outcome of pregnancy. It is safer to use corticosteroids in mothers with severe asthmatic symptoms not responsive to bronchodilators, than to risk the fetal damage associated with severe maternal asthma with resultant hypoxia.

Immunotherapy during pregnancy does not appear to be harmful to the fetus. Most authorities will continue maintenance immunotherapy in a pregnant asthmatic patient. Sufficient data are not available at the present time regarding the safety of starting immunotherapy during pregnancy.

Antihistamines may be required to control various allergic symptoms (i.e., urticaria, angioedema, drug reaction, allergic and vasomotor rhinitis) in some pregnant women. Although the judicious use of diphenhydramine, tripelennamine, and chlorpheniramine is safe during pregnancy, brompheniramine should be avoided because of its possible teratogenic effect. Sufficient data regarding the safety of hydroxyzine, cyprohepatidine, and triprolidine are not available at the present time; therefore, these drugs should be used with great caution, if at all, during pregnancy.

The available data indicate that cautious use of phenylephrine is justified if absolutely necessary to control nasal symptoms. The use of other decongestants is not recommended, either because of possible risk of fetal malformation or lack of sufficient data at the present time.

Although current knowledge regarding **management of asthma** during pregnancy suggests major alterations in the therapeutic regimen are unnecessary, the following points should be kept in mind while managing such patients:

1. Throughout the pregnancy the primary concern should be the control of the patient's asthma and avoidance of maternal hypoxemia and hypocapnia. It is well established that oxygen delivery to the fetal tissues is relatively well

preserved even when oxygen concentration of the inspired air to the mother falls to 10 to 15%. A further decrease in maternal oxygen supply, however, may render the fetus hypoxic. Moreover, maternal alkalosis (pH $\geq$ 7.6 or $PCO_2 \leq 17$ mm Hg) reduces fetal oxygenation by (a) constricting uterine vessels and (b) increasing maternal hemoglobin affinity for oxygen, thereby reducing the oxygen delivery to the fetus. The mechanical effect of forced hyperventilation also decreases the uterine blood flow; therefore, to ensure adequate fetal oxygenation, maternal hypoxemia and alkalosis should be avoided by optimal control of asthma in pregnant women.

2. Judicious use of steroids may be required to achieve the proper control of asthma in some patients.
3. Medications used during the first trimester should be limited to those absolutely necessary for the patient's well-being.
4. Bronchodilator combinations containing iodides (e.g., Ornade, Quadrinol) should be avoided because of the risk of congenital goiter and hypothyroidism.
5. Immunotherapy should be cautiously continued—without increasing the dose—in order to avoid localized and generalized reactions to this mode of therapy.

The following points should be considered while **managing labor and delivery** of a pregnant asthmatic patient:

1. Terbutaline is relatively contraindicated near term because of its inhibitory effect on labor.
2. Other antiasthmatic medications can be continued to control asthmatic symptoms during this critical period.
3. Narcotic analgesics should be avoided if possible or used cautiously because they may inhibit cough reflex, dry the secretions, release histamine, and provoke bronchospasm.
4. Prostaglandins commonly used to induce labor after an incomplete abortion or after fetal death has occurred should not be used in asthmatic patients because of the likelihood of provoking severe bronchospasm.
5. If anesthesia is required, epidural block, saddle block, pudendal block, or local anesthesia is recommended.
6. If general anesthesia is needed (e.g., for cesarean section) halogenated agents that possess bronchodilating properties should be used. Cyclopropane should be avoided because of its bronchospastic action. Ether should be avoided because of irritating action on the bronchial mucosa. (See Chap. 26 for more details).
7. Corticosteroid-requiring pregnant asthmatic patients may have suppressed adrenal function, and therefore should be given supplemental corticosteroids during labor to counter the stress of labor and delivery. The current dosage recommendation is 100 mg hydrocortisone IM at the time of admission to the delivery room followed by 100 mg IM every 8 hours for 24 hours or until absence of puerperal complication is established.

Theophylline ingested by the mother is ultimately secreted in the breast milk, resulting in milk levels of about 75% of that simultaneously measured in the mother's serum. Usually the infant does not ingest more than 8 mg of theophylline per L of milk and this amount of theophylline does not cause symptoms. Occasional cases of hyperirritability of an infant following ingestion of breast milk containing theophylline are reported. If there is any question of drug effect on the nursing infant, the amount of theophylline in breast milk can be reduced by postponing ingestion of short-acting theophylline preparations until just after nursing.

Beta-adrenergic agents are secreted into the breast milk in amounts of less than 1% of the administered dose. Antihistamines and corticosteroids are also secreted into the breast milk in trace amounts; therefore, these drugs do not generally cause problems in nursing infants.

Nebulized atropine used to control asthma in some patients also seems to be excreted in the breast milk in negligible amounts; therefore, nebulized atropine can be used in the nursing asthmatic patient if necessary.

Gluck, J. C., and Gluck, P. A.   The effects of pregnancy on asthma: A prospective study. *Ann. Allergy* 37:164–168, 1976.
A study of 47 patients showing that status of asthma worsened in 43% of patients, remained unchanged in 43%, and improved in 14% of patients during pregnancy. Patients with severe asthma were likely to worsen during pregnancy.

Greenberger, P. A., and Patterson, R.   Safety of therapy for allergic symptoms during pregnancy. *Ann. Intern. Med.* 89:234–237, 1978.
A concise review of the literature regarding the safety of various classes of medications used to control allergic symptoms (i.e., bronchodilators, antihistamines, decongestants, steroids, cromolyn, and so on) during pregnancy.

Greenberger, P. A., and Patterson, R.   Beclomethasone dipropionate for severe asthma during pregnancy. *Ann. Int. Med.* 98:478–480, 1983.
When used in recommended doses, this drug is safe for use in pregnancy.

McKenzie, S. A., Selly, J. A., and Agnew, J. E.   Secretion of prednisolone into breast milk. *Arch. Dis. Child.* 50:894–896, 1975.
The secretion of radiolabelled prednisolone in the breast milk of seven volunteers was studied over a period of about 48 hours following oral administration of 5 mg of radiolabelled prednisolone. A range of only 0.07 to 0.23% (ave. 0.14%) of the dose per liter was recovered.

Metzger, W. J., Turner, E., and Patterson, R.   The safety of immunotherapy during pregnancy. *J. Allergy Clin. Immunol.* 61:268–272, 1978.
Retrospective study of 121 pregnancies from 90 atopic mothers receiving immunotherapy suggested that maternal or fetal complications in such patients were similar to those occurring in atopic pregnant women not receiving immunotherapy. Therefore cautious continuation of immunotherapy is recommended during pregnancy.

Moya, F., Morishima, H. O., Shnider, S. M., and James, L. S.   Influence of maternal hyperventilation on the newborn infant. *Am. J. Obstet. Gynecol.* 91:76–84, 1965.
A study of pregnant asthmatic patients undergoing hyperventilation suggested that maternal alkalosis (pH $\geq$ 7.6 and PCO_2 $\leq$ 17 mm Hg) causes depression of fetal respiration and low Apgar scores.

Nelson, H. S.   Pregnancy and Allergic Diseases. In C. W. Bierman and D. S. Pearlman (Eds.), *Allergic Diseases of Infancy, Childhood and Adolescence.* Philadelphia: Saunders, 1980. Pp. 675–685.
An excellent review of this subject.

Schatz, M., et al.   Corticosteroid therapy for pregnant asthmatic patient. *J.A.M.A.* 233:804–807, 1975.
The study showed that incidence of maternal and fetal complications were not significantly different among 55 steroid-dependent asthmatic pregnant women than in nonasthmatic pregnant women.

Sims, C. D., Chamberlin, C. V. P., and De Sweit, M.   Lung function tests in bronchial asthma during and after pregnancy. *Br. J. Obstet. Gynaecol.* 83:434–437, 1976.
This study also suggested that there was no consistent effect of pregnancy on the status of asthma, as evidenced from serial measurements of lung functions during and after pregnancy.

Turner, E. S., Greenberger, P. A., and Patterson, R.   Management of the pregnant asthmatic patient. *Ann. Intern. Med.* 93:905–918, 1980.
An excellent up-to-date review of all the aspects of management of pregnant asthmatic patients.

Wulf, K. H., Kunzel, W. and Lehman, V.   Clinical Aspect of Placental Gas Exchange. In L. D. Longo and H. Barkels (Eds.), *Respiratory Gas Exchange and Blood Flow in the Placenta.* National Institute of Health, Public Health Service, U.S. Department of Health, Education and Welfare, 63–74, 1972.
The oxygen delivery to fetal tissues is relatively well preserved when oxygen concentration

of inspired air to the mother falls to around 10 to 15% and maternal PO_2 is around 50 mm Hg.

Yurchak, A. M., and Jusko, W. J. Theophylline secretion into breast milk. *Pediatrics* 57:518–520, 1976.

The authors studied theophylline pharmacokinetics in five nursing mothers and correlated their findings to the concentration of theophylline in breast milk. They concluded that in general on a body weight basis the infants would receive an inconsequential amount of the drug through breast milk.

28. ANESTHESIA AND SURGERY IN THE ASTHMATIC PATIENT
Mary Shields

The decision to perform surgery on a patient who has asthma must include an evaluation of the risks that the asthma adds to the usual risks of surgery. In order to effectively evaluate the added risks, the control of pulmonary status at the time of surgery as well as the history of the disease and the medications needed to control it must be considered.

Preoperative evaluation and management are of crucial importance in the surgical approach to the asthmatic patient. The preoperative assessment is important to planning: known allergens and irritants must be identified so that they can be avoided. As in other patients, allergic reactions to drugs must be clearly documented. In addition, a thorough history of drugs needed to control asthmatic symptoms should be obtained. It is especially important to obtain a history of previous steroid use. A normal examination of the chest does not rule out the presence of major abnormalities in pulmonary physiology, therefore, pulmonary function studies must be obtained preoperatively to provide both an objective method for detection of subtle abnormalities in pulmonary status and a baseline with which to compare postoperative lung functions. The results of the preoperative pulmonary function studies may also help identify patients who may have problems in the postoperative period. In a study by Stein and colleagues (1962) 63 preoperative patients were randomly chosen to receive preoperative pulmonary evaluation. Among the 33 patients with normal pulmonary function parameters, only 1 had postoperative pulmonary complications. Among the 30 patients with abnormal results in pulmonary functions, 21 had postoperative pulmonary complications. An abnormal maximal expiratory flow rate was the best predictor of complications, perhaps because it predicts the ability to cough effectively. FEV_1 and the RV/TLC ratio, an indicator of hyperinflation, were of less value.

A patient with a history of mild asthma who has recently done well clinically and has normal pulmonary functions may not require bronchodilators during the preoperative period. A patient with moderate or severe asthma and pulmonary function abnormalities requires optimal bronchodilator therapy before surgery in an attempt to reduce operative risk. Bronchodilators, both intravenous (aminophylline) and inhaled (beta sympathomimetics given by nebulization), should be used during surgery to attain optimal bronchopulmonary status.

The **use of steroids** in asthmatic patients at the time of surgery is often a subject of debate; however, it is generally accepted that all patients who needed steroids for control of asthma in the recent period before surgery must have steroids prior to, during, and immediately after the surgical procedure because of the possibility of adrenal crisis resulting from a suppressed adrenal-pituitary axis that is not responsive to the stress of surgery. If corticosteroids have been needed to control asthma in the period immediately before surgery, the amount of steroid should be increased and given daily in divided doses during and after surgery, and then tapered back to the baseline levels depending on the patient's status. If corticosteroids have been needed in the past but were not necessary for clinical control in the period immediately before surgery, steroids can be discontinued quickly after the stress of surgery is over.

How long a patient must have been off steroids to no longer require steroid coverage is debatable. Two studies provide an interesting contrast in how long the hypothalamic-pituitary-adrenal axis might take to recover following cessation of corticosteroid therapy. In the first study, 14 patients were monitored with plasma ACTH and 17-hydroxycorticosteroid levels at various intervals following the elimination of steroid therapy. Six of these patients had been treated with "supraphysiologic" (exact dose not delineated) doses for 1 to 10 years. The remaining eight patients were monitored following excision of adrenocortical tumors causing Cushing's syndrome. Corticosteroid levels and plasma ACTH levels did not return to normal until 9 months after the elimination of excessive steroid therapy. In the second study 24 asthmatic children were followed after their steroid therapy, which was an average of 2 year's duration, had been tapered. Three methods of evaluation of the adrenal pituitary axis were utilized: urinary 17-hydroxycorticosteroid response to oral metyrapone; plasma cortisol response to insulin-induced hypoglycemia; and resting morning plasma cortisol concentrations. Normal response to all three methods of testing was found 4 to 8 weeks after discontinuation of steroids or lowering steroids to minimal dosages. Therefore, the most conservative recommendation is that patients should be "covered" for surgical procedures within 1 year following cessation of corticosteroid therapy.

Although different coverage protocols are recommended, the most commonly used regimen includes 200 mg of cortisone per 24 hours both the day of and the day after surgical procedure. Tapering following this increase has not been proved necessary from an endocrinologic standpoint, but many physicians prefer to do so.

This conservative approach is generally reasonable, provided that the asthma is mild with no clinical symptoms when the patient is off steroids and pulmonary functions are normal. It is important to emphasize that the patient should have the best pulmonary functions possible in order to have the fewest complications from the surgery. Pulmonary functions must be performed and treatment provided to reverse any abnormalities. This treatment should include steroids if necessary even if the patient has not been on steroids for long periods prior to the surgery. The importance of pulmonary functions cannot be overemphasized in evaluating the need for steroids to control asthma.

The anesthesia literature contains few controlled studies of **preoperative medications** in asthmatic patients. Antihistamines seem to provide both drying of secretions and effective sedation. Atropine decreases secretions, lowers pulmonary resistance, and increases mucociliary transport. Morphine causes release of histamine that theoretically may result in smooth muscle spasm, although many clinicians believe morphine has little if any bronchospastic actions.

If possible, reflex bronchoconstriction from stimulation of vagal receptors should be avoided during anesthetic induction. Cough reflex stimulation is also best avoided. Diazepam has been used intravenously to facilitate slow induction without histamine release.

Among inhalation agents, diethyl ether was used as a bronchodilator for years, but it created increased secretions and was explosive. Halothane has bronchodilating properties as an anesthetic agent, but has been reported in canine studies to be associated with increased cardiac arrhythmias when administered during or after high dosages of intravenous aminophylline. Ketamine was originally thought to be a good agent for use in asthmatic patients because of bronchodilating properties, but several recent reports have indicated that it may precipitate bronchospasm in some asthmatic patients. In general, the best agent is probably isoflurane because it is a good bronchodilator and has effective muscle relaxant properties with fewer associated arrhythmias than halothane.

Intraoperative bronchospasm is best treated by elimination of precipitating stimuli such as traction on the peritoneum. Increasing depth of anesthesia with use of bronchodilating agents and avoiding histamine releasers can help avert bronchospasm.

Atelectasis is the most common postoperative pulmonary complication. Postoperative difficulties vary with the type of anesthetic, with intubation, and with type and duration of surgery. While preoperative assessment is important in predicting pulmonary complications, the value of adequate chest physiotherapy and bronchodilator use in the postoperative period cannot be overemphasized.

Changes in pulmonary mechanics that can be seen postoperatively include decreases in total lung capacity, functional residual capacity, and compliance. The changes are probably all related to atelectasis and can all increase problems caused by asthma. Voluntary maximal inhalation—deep breathing with sustained inspiration—has been found to assist with the inflation of collapsed alveoli and prevention of postoperative pulmonary complications, and this technique should be stressed in the postoperative management of asthmatic patients.

The risks and benefits of a surgical procedure must be clearly weighed in every patient. The asthmatic patient with current symptoms is clearly at increased risk, but meticulous management of asthma can reduce the risk to an acceptable level to allow surgery.

Bartlett, R. H., Garzzaniga, A. B., and Geraghty, T. R.   Respiratory maneuvers to prevent postoperative pulmonary complications. A critical review. *J.A.M.A.* 224:1017–1021, 1973.
Review of postoperative pulmonary physiology and its correlation with maneuvers to prevent postoperative complications.
Benatar, S. R.   Anaesthesia for the asthmatic. *S. Afr. Med. J.* 59:409–412, 1981.
Good discussion of pertinent factors in pulmonary care of surgical asthmatic patients.
Fass, B.   Glucocorticoid therapy for nonendocrine disorders: Withdrawal and "coverage". *Pediatr. Clin. North Am.* 26:251–256, 1979.
A review of management problems concerning stress "coverage" of pediatric patients maintained on steroids; includes suggested therapeutic regimens.
Gold, M. I.   Current concepts in the management of asthmatic patients for surgical anesthesia. *Weekly Anesth. Update* 2:2–7, 1979.
This article includes physiologic factors in plan for management of asthmatic patients undergoing surgical anesthesia.
Graber, A. L., et al.   Natural history of pituitary-adrenal recovery following long-term suppression with corticosteroids. *J. Clin. Endocrinol. Metab.* 25:11–16, 1965.
Significant observations concerning recovery of adrenal responsiveness following prolonged suppression by "supraphysiologic" doses of corticosteroids.
Hodgkin, J. E., Dines, D. E., and Didier, E. P.   Preoperative evaluation of the patient with pulmonary disease. *Mayo Clin. Proc.* 48:114–118, 1973
Indicates importance of baseline pulmonary function parameters prior to surgery.
Jasani, M. K., et al.   Studies of rise of 11-OHCS in corticosteroid-treated patients with rheumatoid arthritis during surgery. Correlations with the functional integrity of the hypothalamo-pituitary-adrenal axis. *Q. J. Med.* 37:407–421, 1968.
Study documented subnormal response of circulating 11-OHCS levels to corticotropin following prolonged oral corticosteroid administration in rheumatoid arthritic patients requiring surgery.
McFadden, E. R., Kiser, R., and deGroot, W. J.   Acute bronchial asthma: Relationships between clinical and physiologic manifestations. *N. Engl. J. Med.* 288:221–225, 1973.
A description of the relationship between clinical and physiologic abnormalities associated with acute episodes of asthma.
Morris, H. G., and Jorgensen, J. R.   Recovery of endogenous pituitary-adrenal function in corticosteroid-treated children. *J. Pediatr.* 79:480–488, 1971.
Observations of adrenal response in group of asthmatic children requiring corticosteroid

therapy for an average of 2 years; study controlled with children not receiving steroids for 1 year.

Potgieter, P. D.   Postoperative pulmonary morbidity. *S. Afr. Med. J.* 59:412–416, 1981.
Suggestion that postoperative pulmonary morbidity could be decreased with the use of voluntary maximal inhalation exercises.

Rodriguez, R., and Gold, M. I.   Enflurane as a primary anesthetic agent for patients with chronic obstructive pulmonary disease. *Anesth. Analg.* 55:806–809, 1976.
Enflurane may be the anesthetic of choice in COPD.

Sprague, D.   Intraanesthetic bronchospasm. *Weekly Anesth. Update* 2:2, 1978.
Emphasizes individualized treatment of intraanesthetic bronchospasm when it occurs.

Stein, M., Koota, G. M., Simon, M., and Frank, H. A.   Pulmonary evaluation of surgical patients. *J.A.M.A.* 181:765–770, 1962.
Review of predictive aspects of preoperative pulmonary function tests in the surgical population.

Stirt, J. A., et al.   Halothane-induced cardiac arrhythmias following administration of aminophylline in experimental animals. *Anesth. Analg.* 60:517–520, 1981.
A review of the potential cardiac toxicity of aminophylline during anesthesia.

29. PSYCHOLOGICAL CONSIDERATIONS IN ASTHMA
Geri S. Wolfson

Knowledge of the interplay of psychological and organic factors in illness has a long and complicated history. Historically, there have been three approaches to understanding this interplay—the psychogenic, the somatopsychic, and, more recently, the psychomaintenance. Perhaps the most practical of these is the psychomaintenance hypothesis that psychological factors can maintain, exacerbate, or exaggerate physical illness. Begging the issue of whether or not the genesis of an illness can be primarily psychological, and acknowledging that somatic variables can cause psychological problems, this chapter will focus on how psychological factors perpetuate asthma in people whose medical management should not, from the objective parameters of the illness, be complicated.

To understand psychomaintenance variables one must examine the possible mechanisms involved. Compliance, a major problem facing medical health caregivers, significantly contributes to treatment failures. Failure to comply, conservatively estimated at 50% for long-term treatment regimens, is manifested by not following the physician's instructions, missing appointments, delay in seeking care, misusing p.r.n. medications, or misrepresenting symptoms. It has been repeatedly demonstrated that compliance correlates to satisfaction with, and comprehension of, the physician's communications. Consider 14-year-old Beth, who was resentful that she could not understand her doctor's explanation for prescribing asthma medications, yet was too intimidated by him to ask. To avoid his ire, she lied about her compliance and avoided interaction with him whenever possible.

Mechanisms other than poor doctor-patient communication that can lead to noncompliance include personality and developmental considerations. Personality traits influence the way one presents oneself to a physician, which in turn influences the physician's judgment. Everyone has seen the patient who habitually underestimates and denies his or her pain and distress. Research has demonstrated that such low panic-fear personality types are likely to be undermedicated and underuse p.r.n. medications (Jones et al., 1979). Consequently, they are hospitalized at approximately twice the usual rate.

Developmental considerations greatly affect a child's ability for self-care. Medical mismanagement—hence, psychomaintenance—is often the result of expecta-

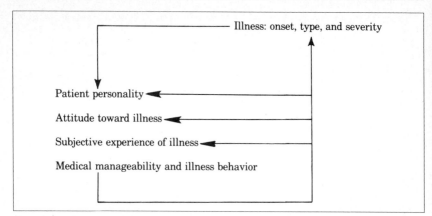

Fig. 11. Psychomaintenance in adults. A conceptual framework to facilitate consideration of factors that may perpetuate illness in adult patients. Adapted from J. Dirks and J. Schraa, Psychosocial assessment in chronic asthma. *J. Respir. Dis.* 3(8):24–36, 1982.

tions that exceed the child's ability. Allowing a child with dubious time-telling skills to assume responsibility for taking medications is obviously doomed to fail.

As Figure 11 illustrates, the interaction of the objective medical parameters of the disease with personality variables affects the patient's attitudes toward and experience of the asthma. The resulting illness behavior influences the medical manageability or intractability of asthma. How well managed the illness is affects both the objective medical illness and the patient's psychological functioning, completing the feedback loop.

Psychologists at National Jewish Hospital/National Asthma Center have developed the Battery of Asthma Illness Behavior (BAIB) to measure each of the psychological dimensions represented in the scheme (see Figure 11). Their research on more than 600 asthma patients has consistently demonstrated a relationship between BAIB scores and medical outcome variables, including rehospitalization rates, days hospitalized, and intensity of medical regimen prescribed. What makes these findings especially impressive is that these relationships have been upheld independent of longitudinal spirometric pulmonary function, age of asthma onset, and duration of asthma. In combination with objective measures of illness severity, the predictions are even stronger. Obviously, not every physician has access to the psychological information obtainable from the BAIB. An understanding of the concepts it taps, however, can have valuable clinical implications.

The tests measure three levels of psychological functioning: (a) personality, (b) attitudes, and (c) experience of illness.

Personality. High or low scores on "panic-fear," a variable derived from the Minnesota Multi-Phasic Personality Inventory (MMPI), have consistently been shown to relate to psychomaintenance of asthma in adult patients. High panic-fear patients present as being excessively dependent, emotionally labile, helpless, demanding, and prone to give up quickly when things go wrong. Their basic personality is characterized by chronic, anxious dependence. These patients exhibit numerous behaviors that bode poorly for medical manageability. They tend to exaggerate their symptoms, use both prescribed and p.r.n. medications excessively, and hyperventilate when having an asthma attack. They are also excessively dependent on their medical caregivers and unwilling to assume an appropriate amount of responsibility for their self-care.

Low panic-fear personalities have already been alluded to as patients who habitually minimize their symptoms, fail to seek medical attention, and maintain an independent "it-doesn't-bother-me" stance. Patients with this personality constellation may contribute to the psychomaintenance of their illlness by underusing medications and denying symptoms until hospitalization is unavoidable. Frequently these patients are undermedicated because of the way they present themselves to their physicians.

Attitudes. It is important to ascertain patients' perceptions of their illness as these preceptions significantly affect how they care for themselves. That is, what does the illness mean to the individual? What is the understanding of its etiology, course, and prognosis? How stigmatizing is the illness? How much does it interfere with the patient's functioning?

Attitudinal patterns that have been demonstrated to relate to the psychomaintenance of asthma include two extremes—optimism or pessimism—about prognosis. Patients who exhibit extreme pessimism about the possibility of medical control also frequently attribute most of life's difficulties to their illness. Thus, asthma allows them to deny responsibility for problems such as poor work performance and poor marital adjustment. Frequently these patients exacerbate their disease by their lack of motivation to comply with the prescribed treatment. Their pessimistic and often depressed demeanor may lead the physician to judge their illness as more severe than it is.

When patients are angry in addition to being pessimistic another set of management problems emerges. These patients blame their physicians for their lack of control and are often "doctor-shoppers." Justifying their noncompliance by lack of trust in their physician's competence, these patients are among the most difficult to manage.

An attitude of overoptimism about one's ability to control his or her asthma also may lead to illness exacerbation. Seeing asthma through rose-colored glasses typifies these patients and results in underusing medications and medical services. Physicians can be easily swayed by this cheery outlook and consequently often undermedicate these patients.

Experience of Illness. Each patient subjectively experiences respiratory distress somewhat differently. The amount of anxiety focused on the illness and the frequency with which patients mislabel nonairway obstruction symptoms as asthma can contribute to psychomaintenance.

Illness-focused, not generalized, anxiety, is adaptive. It signals the patient to take early intervention steps to ameliorate the symptoms. Too little anxiety during respiratory distress, however, can result in minimization or denial of symptoms. Consequently, patients with low illness-specific anxiety typically fail to take appropriate p.r.n. medications and delay too long before seeking medical attention.

Mislabeling nonairway obstruction symptoms such as fatigue, anxiety, or rapid breathing as asthma has obvious negative consequences. The patient may treat the "asthma" with p.r.n. medication unnecessarily. Additionally, the unaware physician may respond to what is reported by the patient as an acute exacerbation with increased medication or even hospitalization.

An additional consideration that can lead to noncompliance is the correlation between long-term corticosteroids and short-term memory deficits. Chronically forgetting to take medications will obviously have a detrimental effect on illness control.

The same issues are important in pediatric patients but they are complicated by other considerations unique to children. Outside influences, especially family, are a much more cogent force for children than adults. Developmental factors pose problems because of the discrepancy in expectations across ages. What may

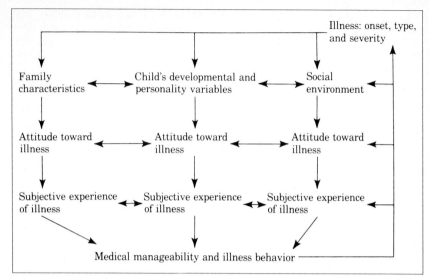

Fig. 12. Psychomaintenance in pediatrics. A conceptual framework to facilitate consideration of factors that may perpetuate illness in pediatric patients.

be seen as age appropriate in a 6-year-old is poor adjustment in a 10-year-old. Figure 12 depicts a model of psychomaintenance in children. Included are the numerous social, personality, familial, medical, and developmental factors that influence a child's adjustment to chronic illness. Like the adult model, it is a giant feedback loop reflecting the self-perpetuating nature of disease adjustment and maladjustment.

The facets that have been considered in adults—personality variables, attitude toward and experience of the illness—are also applicable to children. A child's psychological defenses and personality style can affect illness management. Consider the asthmatic child whose major defenses are denial and avoidance. Although this might be an acceptable way to handle a classmate's taunting, when it extends to illness symptoms, this child is in danger of exacerbating asthma by not attending to early warning signs of wheezing.

Children's attitudes toward and understanding of their illness are often a significant psychomaintenance variable. Explanations that children have for things they do not understand are typically illogical and fanciful. Thus, 6-year-old Jack spent his free time outside because of his total magical belief in a cure for asthma. Similarly, 12-year-old Marcia stopped taking corticosteroids because she thought "they made kids not like you."

When treating children, it is crucial to take family variables into consideration. How much weight is given to family dimensions as possible contributors to psychomaintenance depends primarily on the age of the child. With a young child, family factors are obviously most significant because it is the parents, not the child, who assume responsibility for administering medications, determining when medical help is needed, and so on. As a child grows older the interactive balance switches slowly until the burden of care rests completely with the child.

Family characteristics include its composition, parents' socioeconomic and marital status, as well as parents' and siblings' personality factors (i.e., caring, demanding, withholding, or affectionate). Each of these factors can affect the asthma by influencing the family's attitudes and experience of the patient and the illness. Clearly if the family believes a child is manipulative with his or her asthma, they respond differently to episodes of wheezing. Similarly, if parents can avoid marital strife by focusing on their child's sickness, they may have a vested interest in maintaining the illness. For example, twelve-year-old Chris's mother was convinced that her son had severe asthma. When he wheezed, she panicked and frequently overreacted, taking him to hospital emergency rooms unnecessarily. She treated Chris as a helpless victim, keeping him in a dependent state. Her exaggeration of his symptoms resulted in overmedication and overhospitalization. When this pattern was pointed out and the dysfunctional family system disrupted, the father became chronically ill, relieving his son of the illness role needed to maintain the family dynamics.

A crucial factor is the **social milieu** in which the child lives. Physical characteristics (e.g., urban, rural, army base) and pervasive attitudes (e.g., liberal or conservative, accepting or condemning) come under this rubric and can have a cogent effect on illness adjustment. Children from families that tend to "tough it out," would be likely to adapt the machismo creed of their milieu and deny illness symptoms. Children from families that accept, and even at times indulge illness, may be overmedicated and over-protected.

How can a primary care physician ascertain which, if any, psychomaintenance variables are in operation? It is of course desirable to have precise measurements but, even without access to psychological services, the concepts have practical utility. If a patient is difficult to manage medically and one suspects contributing psychological factors, it is wise to keep the conceptual models in Figures 11 and 12 in mind. Questions in the Table 21 will help guide a patient interview to unexplored or problematic areas.

Once the problem areas have been assessed, **treatment** follows logically. Sometimes the process of clearly identifying areas of concern and the concomitant increase in physician-patient communication is enough to ameliorate the difficulty.

Two common mechanisms leading to psychomaintenance are poor physician-patient communication and insufficient knowledge. Both of these can be easily addressed and treated by the primary care physician and the nursing staff.

It is crucial to talk at a level patients understand and to ensure comprehension by having patients explain their treatment regimens. Asking open-ended questions (e.g., How are you feeling? Anything else you would like to talk about?) will encourage patients to air their concerns.

Education should be geared to patients and their caretakers. All patients need to know the reasons for their medications, any possible side effects, and the specifics of their disease (precipitants, course, probable prognosis).

Additionally, a patient and his family can benefit from frequent feedback as to how his coping styles may be maintaining his illness. For example, with a high panic-fear patient one may:

1. Instruct the patient that he or she tends to overreport symptoms. A mini-peak flowmeter with instructions not to take action unless the functions drop below a specified point may be considered.
2. Compare the patient's self-report with objective measures, which will reduce the likelihood of overmedicating these patients because of their self-presentation.
3. Excessively drill the patient in self-care steps during respiratory distress as these patients tend to panic and may think irrationally.
4. Teach the patient relaxation techniques and diaphragmatic breathing to help counteract anxiety and the tendency to hyperventilate.

Table 21. Interview guide to elucidate unexplored or problematic areas

ADULT

Personality level

Does this patient:

Consistently present as being in more distress than objective medical measurements would suggest?

Tend to be overly dramatic and prone to exaggeration?

Seem anxious and dependent, calling more than necessary?

If the answer to these questions is yes, suspect high panic-fear personality.

Does this patient:

Consistently underestimate his or her asthma?

Tend to "tough it out" and frequently delay too long before seeking medical advice?

If the answer to these questions is yes, suspect low panic-fear personality.

Attitude level

What does the illness mean to the patient—how stigmatized is he or she by it?

How does the patient see asthma interfering with his or her functioning?

How optimistic or pessimistic is the patient about the manageability of his or her asthma?

What are the patient's attitudes toward the medical caregivers—angry, distrustful?

Are there secondary gains for the patient from being sick?

Is memory a problem for the patient?

Experience

What is it like for the patient during an asthma attack? Is he or she afraid of dying, excessively anxious, angry?

Does this patient exacerbate an attack by hyperventilating?

CHILD

All the questions for adults apply to the pediatric patient. In addition, the physician should answer these questions about both the child, and the child's parents. Additional considerations include:

Developmental

What is this child's developmental level?

Is this child intelligent enough to understand medical instructions and the reasons for them?

Is memory a problem for the child?

How responsible can he or she be for self-care (e.g., time-telling skills, motor coordination)?

Attitudes

What is this child's attitude about asthma? Children frequently have idiosyncratic ways of understanding asthma. It is crucial to assess this. Innocently inquring What is asthma?, and How do you get it? will often provoke a long explanation of defective parts, punishments for being bad, magical cures, and meanings of the disease. Another way to get at this with a young child (6–10 years old) is to ask him or her to draw a picture of a person with and then without asthma. Comparing the two drawings can be enlightening.

Social environment

How do friends, classmates, teachers—especially physical education teachers—respond to the patient when he or she is sick?

What does the school nurse do?

5. Frequently reassure these patients that their asthma is manageable and encourage appropriate independence to help combat their anxiety, dependence, and pessimism about asthma.

With a low panic-fear personality one might:

1. Help the patient see how denying symptoms and delaying action exacerbates the illness causing increasing dependence as a result of attempts to be independent. A mini-peak flowmeter for home use might be considered.
2. Comparing the patient's self-report with objective measures, which will reduce likelihood of undermedicating these patients because of their presentations.
3. Remember that a friendly, straightforward style works best with these patients, who are quick to interpret others' actions as authoritarian and controlling.
4. Keep in mind that teaching relaxation techniques is generally contraindicated for these patients.

If problems persist after a reasonable attempt to elucidate them with your patient, then a referral is in order. The treatment modalities used in order of severity of impairment include discussion groups, psychotherapy interventions, and residential treatment centers. Discussion groups typically are led by mental health professionals with some knowledge of asthma and chronic illness, and focus on illness-specific concerns, feelings of alienation and isolation, coping methods, reactions of family and friends, and so on. Psychotherapy does not necessarily have to be long term and can consist of individual, group, or family treatment. Referrals should be specifically to a mental health professional with some expertise in this area. Finally, residential treatment can be recommended for those patients whose symptoms persist despite treatment attempts in less structured settings. Treatment usually entails a long-term stay in a facility with an array of interdisciplinary services designed to meet the numerous physical, emotional, and social needs of the patient.

Dirks, J. F., and Schraa, J. C.   How patient attitudes may foil asthma management. *J. Respir. Dis.* 3(8):24–36, 1982.
   An excellent review written for physicians of psychomaintenance issues in adults.
Jones, N., Kinsman, R., Dirks, J., and Dahlem, N.   Psychological contributions to chronicity in asthma: Patient response styles influencing medical treatment and its outcome. *Med. Care* 17:1103–1118, 1979.
   Review of the research relating response styles of asthmatic patients with medical treatment and outcome.
Kinsman, R., Dirks, J., and Jones, N.   Psychomaintenance of Chronic Physical Illness: Clinical Assessment of Personal Styles Affecting Medical Management. In T. Millon, C. Green, and R. Meagher (Eds.), *Handbook of Clinical Health Psychology.* New York: Plenum, 1982. Pp. 435–466.
   A comprehensive overview of psychological considerations in bronchial asthma with adult patients.
Kinsman, R., Dirks, J., Jones, N., and Dahlem, N.   Anxiety reduction in asthma: Four catches to general application. *Psychosom. Med.* 42:397–405, 1980.
   A closer look at relaxation training techniques for asthma patients, with suggestions when they should and should not be used.
Knapp, P.   Psychotherapeutic Management of Bronchial Asthma. In E. D. Wittkower and H. Warnes (Eds.), *Psychosomatic Medicine: Its Clinical Applications.* New York: Harper & Row, 1977. Pp. 210–219.
   Review of the different psychotherapeutic approaches in the treatment of bronchial asthma.
Matus, I.   Assessing the nature and clinical significance of psychological contributions to childhood asthma. *Am. J. Orthopsychiatry* 51:327–341, 1981.
   A well-written overview exploring how psychological factors can affect the course of asthma in children.

Pinkerton, P.   Psychosomatic inter-relationships in the management of childhood asthma. *Psychother. Psychosom.* 19:157–265, 1971.
Case examples illustrate how psychological factors may interfere with medical management in childhood asthma.

Sackett, D., and Haynes, R.   *Compliance with Therapeutic Regimens.* Johns Hopkins University Press: Baltimore, 1976.
A review of research looking at factors that contribute to noncompliance.

Schraa, J., and Dirks, J.   Improving patient recall and comprehension of the treatment regimen. *J. Asthma* 19:159–162, 1982.
Practical suggestions to improve patient understanding and retention of medical information.

THERAPEUTIC AGENTS USED IN THE TREATMENT
OF ASTHMA AND ALLERGIC DISEASE

Don A. Bukstein

Theophylline is an effective bronchodilator that has been in use since the 1930s. Theophylline is thought to produce bronchodilatation both directly, by producing smooth muscle relaxation, and indirectly by inhibiting the release of mediators from the mast cell (e.g., leukotrienes, histamine, ECF-A). Theophylline is believed to produce this effect by inhibiting cellular phosphodiesterase, thus increasing the level of cellular cyclic adenosine monophosphate (AMP). Recent research, however, suggests that theophylline's mechanism of action may be by affecting calcium flux across cell membranes. Theophylline also increases respiratory muscle (diaphragm and probably intercostal and accessory muscles) contractility and may have therapeutic and preventive implications on the development of respiratory muscle fatigue.

Pharmacokinetic studies have demonstrated that there are marked differences in the rate at which patients metabolize theophylline. Serum half-life ($t\frac{1}{2}$) may vary between 2.6 hours to 20 hours. Environmental factors such as smoking and diet are important in influencing the clearance rate of theophylline. Age is also an important factor; children metabolize theophylline much more rapidly than adults. Finally, because theophylline is primarily (90%) metabolized by the liver microsomal enzyme system, diseases or drugs that affect the liver will markedly increase the half-life of theophylline. For a summary of factors that influence theophylline metabolism, see Table 22.

Theophylline is metabolized to three major metabolites: 3-methylxanthine, 1, 3-dimethyl uric acid, and 1-methyl uric acid. There is some indication that the enzyme that metabolizes theophylline to 3-methylxanthine is saturable. Because of this, when the serum concentration is already high and the enzyme systems are near saturation, a small change in dose can result in a disproportionately high increase in serum concentration. This effect is primarily seen in children prior to puberty, and could also explain the marked differences in the extent to which viral infections affect theophylline metabolism.

The commonly used antibiotic erythromycin has been shown by many investigators to markedly decrease the metabolism of theophylline. Therefore, it is recommended that for those patients whose serum theophylline levels are between 15 to 20 μg/ml, a 25% reduction should be made in their theophylline dose while taking erythromycin.

Theophylline is only minimally excreted (10%) unchanged in the urine; therefore, theophylline may be safely given to patients with impaired renal function.

There are several general facts to consider when using theophylline intravenously. First, aminophylline, a salt of theophylline, is the intravenous form of theophylline. One mg of theophylline is equivalent to 1.2 mg of aminophylline. Second, rapid intravenous administration of aminophylline is contraindicated because of the risk of inducing a fatal cardiac arrhythmia. Fatal cardiac arrhythmias have also been caused by the infusion of aminophylline through a central venous-pressure catheter. An aminophylline bolus should be infused into a peripheral vein over a *minimum* of 20 minutes. And third, aminophylline reduces pulmonary vascular resistance and can thereby increase perfusion to underventilated portions of the lung. This increase can result in a decrease in arterial oxygen tension, even though the airway obstruction is improving. Therefore, a patient receiving a bolus of aminophylline intravenously should receive supplemental oxygen.

The goal of intravenous administration of aminophylline is to achieve a therapeutic level of theophylline as rapidly as possible, and then to maintain a con-

Table 22. Factors affecting theophylline metabolism

Increase	Decrease
Young age	Heart failure
Cigarette smoking	Liver disease
Charcoal-broiled beef	Influenza vaccine
High-protein diet	Viral infection
Treatment with phenobarbital	Cimetidine
(daily for 4 wk)	Troleandomycin (TAO)
	Erythromycin
	High carbohydrate/low protein diet
	Renal failure (minimal effect)

stant theophylline level within the therapeutic range (10–20 μg/ml). The most effective method of accomplishing these goals is to give a bolus of aminophylline to quickly achieve the desired serum concentration. Intermittent bolus infusions (usually every 6 hours) are less desirable, but are acceptable, and perhaps preferable if adequate technology (e.g., reliable equipment that provides a continuous rate of infusion) and trained personnel to monitor the infusion are not available. When using intermittent infusion, peak theophylline levels should be monitored to avoid toxicity. Trough levels should also be monitored if there is a suggestion that the clinical status of the patient will deteriorate at the end of the dosing interval.

In 1973 Mitenko and Ogilvie published data recommending an aminophylline loading dose of 5.6 mg/kg to be given over 20 minutes, followed by a maintenance dose of 0.9 mg/kg/hr. Subsequent studies have shown that for a large percentage of patients this dosing regimen will result in toxic levels while in other patients it would be inadequate to maintain therapeutic levels. As is obvious when examining Tables 22 and 23, there is no one dosage for maintenance therapy that can be recommended for all patients because of the wide variability in theophylline pharmacokinetics.

In some patients the history of prior experience with theophylline therapy is helpful in guiding maintenance therapy. For example, if the patient has experienced nausea or headache with low dosages of oral theophylline preparations, the maintenance intravenous dosage should also be low. In general, for maintenance therapy without serum theophylline levels as a guide, the dosages of intravenous aminophylline in adults and children are outlined in Table 23. Often such dosages may be suboptimal, but for the most part they are safe. However, even at

Table 23. Dosage of intravenous aminophylline

Age and clinical status	Rate of continuous IV infusion
Children aged 1–9 yr	1.0 mg/kg/hr
Children aged 9–16 and young adult smokers	0.8 mg/kg/hr
Otherwise healthy nonsmoking adults	0.5 mg/kg/hr
Older patients and patients with cor pulmonale	0.3 mg/kg/hr
Patients with congestive heart failure, liver disease	0.1–0.2 mg/kg/hr

Loading dose is 6 mg/kg for all patients
Initial maintenance dose varies widely depending on the age of the patient and the clinical situation.

Table 24. Calculations of loading doses and
adjustments in maintenance doses for continuous IV infusion

LOADING CALCULATION

Desired concentration − current concentration = change in concentration

Loading dose (mg) = change in concentration × kg body weight × V_D*
For example:

Current concentration	= 5 μg/ml
Desired concentration	= 15 μg/ml
Weight	= 33 kg
Loading dose	= (10 μg/ml)(0.5 L/kg)(33 kg)
	= 165 mg theophylline
	= 194 mg aminophylline

MAINTENANCE ADJUSTMENT

Clearance = current dose (mg/kg/hr) − current concentration (μg/ml)
For example:

Current concentration	= 10 μg/ml
Current dose	= 1.5 mg/kg/hr
Clearance	= 1.5 mg/kg/hr − 10 μg/ml
	= 150 ml/kg/hr

If desire to maintain 15 μg/ml after loading

For example: dose	= clearance × current concentration
	= 150 ml/kg/hr × 15 μg/ml
	= 2.25 mg theophylline/hr
	= 2.65 mg aminophylline/hr

*V_D = Volume of distribution, which is assumed to be approximately 0.5 L/kg.

these dosages toxicity may occur. One should be familiar with those factors that both increase and decrease theophylline metabolism (see Table 22). In the obese patient, the ideal body weight should be used in calculating the dosage of aminophylline.

There are several considerations in selecting a dose of intravenous aminophylline. If a patient has not had any theophylline compounds within the last 12 hours, a loading dose is indicated (6 mg aminophylline/kg; see Table 23). If a patient has taken any form of theophylline within the last 12 hours, it is best to first obtain a serum theophylline level, and then to select a loading dose that places the patient within the therapeutic range. One method of calculating a loading dose under these circumstances is shown in Table 24. The first approximation of a maintenance rate for IV infusion can be selected from Table 23. Adjustment of the maintenance rate requires measurement of a serum theophylline concentration and calculation of the approximate clearance rate from the dose being administered and the serum concentration achieved with that dose (see Table 24).

There are many forms of theophylline available. The efficacy of these drugs depends on their conversion to theophylline. It is therefore best to compare and dose all preparations based on their anhydrous theophylline content.

Theophylline is available orally in short-acting liquids and coated tablets, and in sustained-release preparations. Many liquid preparations are combined with alcohol. The addition of alcohol does *not* enhance the absorption of theophylline and has certain inherent disadvantages, such as unpleasant taste or CNS depression.

The uncoated tablets and liquid preparations are rapidly and completely absorbed from the gastrointestinal tract. Their main disadvantage is that in children and other patients who metabolize the drug rapidly marked fluctuations in peak and trough serum concentrations occur; thus, shorter dosing intervals are required to maintain therapeutic levels. The sustained-release preparations have been shown in many studies to decrease the fluctuation between peak and trough levels, thereby allowing the dosing intervals to be lengthened. This longer dosing interval will enhance compliance. Many sustained-release preparations recommend dosing every 12 hours. However, in most children, and in adults who metabolize the drug rapidly, an 8-hour dosing interval will produce less fluctuation in serum levels. Consistent absorption of sustained-release preparations depends on each dose remaining in the GI tract long enough to permit breakdown of the vehicle and absorption. This process is occasionally a problem in young children who tend to have variable GI transit times and thus variable absorption.

Children who cannot swallow a capsule or tablet can often be given granules from sustained-release capsules mixed with strained food or pudding. The granules should not be chewed because their sustained-release characteristics will be destroyed. Patients should not be directed to take portions of a capsule because many of the granules are only "fill" and contain no actual drug.

Numerous oral preparations contain both theophylline and ephedrine in a fixed ratio. The literature is mixed concerning whether or not there is an additive effect of the combination. Even when it seems clinically useful to combine these two drugs, most practitioners find that the ratio of the drugs in these preparations is such that in order for the patient to receive an adequate dose of theophylline, a toxic dose of ephedrine must be administered. Because the effects of theophylline and the beta$_2$-adrenergic agonists are mediated through different pathways, the combination of these two drug forms should have an additive effect, and there have been several studies which demonstrated this. Because of this additive effect, many practitioners recommend that theophylline and the beta$_2$-adrenergic agonists (e.g., metaproterenol, terbutaline) be used conjointly, but titrated individually. Although animal studies demonstrate that extremely high serum levels of theophylline increase the cardiotoxic potential of beta-adrenergic agonists, similar toxicity has not been demonstrated in man. In addition, use of the two drug forms together can allow maximum therapeutic effects without having to use either drug in maximum, potentially toxic, amounts.

Indications for Oral Theophylline Use

Oral theophylline is administered in two distinct situations: (1) an acute asthma episode and (2) chronic asthma. In the acute attack the goal is to achieve a therapeutic level of theophylline as rapidly as possible, and then to maintain a constant theophylline level within the therapeutic range until the attack resolves. This can be accomplished by administration of one-half to two-thirds the usual dose in a rapidly absorbed liquid form with the *initial* dose of a sustained release preparation. This is analogous to treating a patient intravenously with a loading bolus of aminophylline followed by a continuous infusion of aminophylline.

In the treatment of the chronic asthmatic patient, the goal of the theophylline therapy is to maximize pulmonary functions and to relieve symptoms with the least amount of side effects. Side effects such as nervousness, insomnia, irritability, and headaches can be minimized by slowly titrating the patient's dose into the therapeutic range. To accomplish this, Hendeles and co-workers (1977) have suggested the following approach: The patient is started at a dose of 16 mg/kg/day or 400 mg/day—whichever is less. If tolerated, the dose is increased in 25%

Table 25. Daily theophylline dosages for different age groups

Age (yr)	Total daily dosage (mg/kg/24 hr)
1–9	24
9–12	20
12–18	16
Older than 18	12 (or 900 mg/24hr, whichever is less)

increments every 3 days until age-determined mean dosages are reached (Table 25). At this time, a peak serum theophylline level is obtained, and final adjustments are made according to the schema outlined in Table 26. By using this schema, a minimum of theophylline levels will have to be obtained to determine the correct dose for chronic therapy. If the patient's pulmonary functions are maximized at a low level of theophylline, and if the patient is stable, the dose should not be increased solely to get the level into the therapeutic range.

Rectal solutions provide reliable absorption and are an acceptable route of theophylline administration. Peak serum levels occur 1 to 2 hours after administration of the solution. However, use of this form of therapy is rarely indicated. It should never be used as a route for chronic administration because of the psychological implications. While rectal solutions may be useful for administration during exacerbations associated with gastroenteritis and vomiting, theophylline toxicity must be eliminated as a cause of persistant vomiting before this form of therapy is used. In contrast to rectal solutions, **rectal suppositories** provide poor and erratic absorbtion of theophylline and, therefore, should never be used. An increased incidence of toxicity is associated with rectal suppositories compared with other dosage forms.

As mentioned previously, the **therapeutic range** of theophylline is between 10 and 20 μg/ml. Serum levels should be obtained yearly in adults. In children, levels should be obtained every 6 months. Theophylline levels should also be obtained if the response to a usual dosage is inadequate of if the symptoms of toxicity occur. Levels should be obtained when a patient is not ill and has no factors that might affect theophylline metabolism. Peak serum concentrations usually occur 1 to 2 hours after a rapidly absorbed preparation and 3 to 4 hours after the administration of a sustained-release preparation, however, maximum levels can be seen at any point (i.e., up to 8 or 10 hours) after the administration of a sustained-release preparation. If serum levels are markedly low on a usual dosage regimen, problems with compliance should be considered.

Toxic symptoms may occur at any level, but they increase sharply in frequency as the theophylline concentration exceeds 20 μg/ml. The common side effects are nausea, vomiting, diarrhea, nervousness, insomnia, and increasing diuresis. Seizures have been reported in adult patients with levels below 30 μg/ml, without any prodromal symptoms. Fatal cardiac arrhythmias have been associated with elevated theophylline levels.

Should an overdosage occur, the drug should be stopped immediately. If the patient was taking theophylline orally, an emetic should be administered followed by large amounts of activated charcoal. Mahutte et al. (1983) have shown that the charcoal significantly enhances the clearance of theophylline. A saline cathartic should be administered to decrease the gastrointestinal transit time.

If the theophylline level is excessive, the patient should be hospitalized, monitored carefully, and given supportive care. If the theophylline level is greater than 60 μg/ml, charcoal hemoperfusion or hemodialysis should be strongly con-

Table 26. Final adjustment of oral dose guided by
measurement of serum theophylline concentration*

Peak theophylline level (µg/ml)	Approximate adjustment in total daily dose	Comment
5	100% increase	If patient is asymptomatic, consider trial off drug; repeat measurement of serum
5–7.5	50% increase	concentration after dose adjustment
8–10	20% increase	Even if patient is asymptomatic at this level, an increased serum concentration may prevent symptoms during a viral upper respiratory tract infection (URI), or heavy exposure to an inhalant allergen, or vigorous exertion
10–13	Cautious 10% increase if clinically indicated	If patient is asymptomatic, no increase is necessary; if symptoms occur during URI or exercise, increase as indicated. Care must be taken if patient has ongoing viral infection as basal metabolism may be affected
	None	If "breakthrough" in asthmatic symptoms occurs at the end of dosing interval, change to sustained-release product and repeat serum level measurement
14–20	Occasional intolerance requires a 10% decrease	If side effects occur, decrease total daily dose
21–25	10% decrease	Even if side effects are absent
26–30	25%–33% decrease	Even if side effects are absent, omit next dose and decrease total daily dose as indicated; repeat measurement of serum concentration
35	50% decrease	Omit next two doses, decrease as indicated, and repeat measurement of serum concentration

*To avoid potential toxic reaction (1) ensure that the sample represents a peak level obtained at steady state (e.g., no missed or extra doses with close approximation of described dosing intervals during previous 48 hours); (2) repeat laboratory determination if not initially performed in duplicate; (3) the increase of 50% or 100% should be made in 5% increments at 2-day intervals to further ensure safety and tolerance.

sidered. If the level is below 40 µg/ml, charcoal hemoperfusion is probably not indicated. It is not yet clearly defined whether charcoal hemoperfusion should be instituted with patients whose levels fall between 40 and 60 µg/ml and have CNS symptoms.

Banner, A. S., Sunderrajan, E. V., Agarwal, M. K., and Addington, W. W.   Arrhythmogenic effects of orally administered bronchodilators. *Arch. Intern. Med.* 139:434–437, 1979.
Serious arrhythmias are uncommon with theophylline therapy, but can occur in patients with preexisting ventricular extrasystoles.
Godfrey, S., and Konig, P. Suppression of exercise-induced asthma by salbutamol, theophylline, atropine, cromolyn, and placebo in a group of asthmatic children. *Pediatrics* 56:930–934, 1975.
An excellent review and comparison of ability of theophylline to other drugs in preventing exercise-induced asthma.

Hendeles, L., and Weinberger, M. Theophylline and Derivatives. In E. Middleton, C. E. Reed, and E. F. Ellis (Eds.), *Allergy: Principles and Practice* (2nd ed.). St. Louis: Mosby, 1983. Pp. 535–574.
An exhaustive review of 102 cases of serious theophylline toxicity from 1943 to 1980.

Hendeles, L., Weinberger, M., and Bighley, L. Absolute bioavailability of oral theophylline. *Am. J. Hosp. Pharm.* 34:525–527, 1977.
Study showing plain, uncoated theophylline tablets are completely (96%) absorbed after oral administration.

Jacobs, M. H., Senior, R. M., and Kessler, G. Clinical experience with theophylline. Relationships between dosage, serum concentration, and toxicity. *J.A.M.A.* 235:1983–1986, 1976.
A review of the most frequent adverse effects of theophylline therapy. Nausea, anorexia, vomiting, and headaches are related to serum level of theophylline.

LaForce, C. F., Miller, M. F., and Chai, H. Effect of erythromycin on theophylline clearance in asthmatic children. *J. Pediatr.* 99:153–156, 1981.
Continuous intravenous administration of theophylline was associated with a 26% decrease in theophylline clearance and correspondingly higher steady-state serum concentrations after a 1-week course of erythromycin ethylsuccinate in 15 children with chronic asthma.

Levy, G., and Koysooko, R. Pharmacokinetic analysis of the effect of theophylline on pulmonary function in asthmatic children. *J. Pediatr.* 86:789–793, 1975.
One of many studies demonstrating that children metabolize theophylline faster than do adults, with mean half-lifes related to age.

Lillehei, J. P. Aminophylline, oral vs rectal administration. *J.A.M.A.* 205:530–533, 1968.
Theophylline suppositories may be dangerous because they are erratically and unreliably absorbed. Rectal solutions are more rapidly and reliably absorbed.

Mahutte, C. F., et al. Increase of serum theophylline clearance with orally administered activated charcoal. *Am. Rev. Respir. Dis.* 128:820–822, 1983.
This article discussed a new therapeutic modality in the treatment of theophylline toxicity.

Mitendo, P. A., and Ogilvie, R. I. Rational intravenous doses of theophylline. *N. Engl. J. Med.* 289–600, 1973.
This is the most often quoted study on the pharmocokinetics of intravenous theophylline.

Ogilvie, R. I. Clinical pharmacokinetics of theophylline. *Clin. Pharmacokinet.* 3:267–293, 1978.
An exhaustive review of the pharmacokinetics of theophylline and the important factors to consider in planning theophylline therapy.

Powell, J. R., et al. Theophylline disposition in acutely ill hospitalized patients. The effect of smoking, heart failure, severe airway obstruction, and pneumonia. *Am. Rev. Respir. Dis.* 118:229–238, 1978.
A study examining a few of the multiple factors that have been shown to alter theophylline half-life and the practical implications of these factors on therapy.

Russo, M. E. Management of theophylline intoxication with charcoal-column hemoperfusion. *N. Engl. J. Med.* 300:24–27, 1979.
An effective form of treatment for theophylline toxicity is resin hemodialysis or charcoal perfusion.

vanDellen, R. G. Theophylline: Practical application of new knowledge. *Mayo Clin. Proc.* 54:733–745, 1979.
The best review on all aspects of theophylline clinical pharmacology.

Vozeh, S., et al. Changes in theophylline clearance during acute illness. *J.A.M.A.* 240:1882–1884, 1978.
Theophylline pharmacokinetics may change in the same patient with changes in disease state (e.g., congestive heart failure, liver disease).

Weinberger, M., and Ginchansky, E. Dose-dependent kinetics of theophylline disposition in asthmatic children. *J. Pediatr.* 91:820–824, 1977.
Increases in dosage of theophylline are associated with serum concentrations greater than expected, suggesting that the clearance rate of theophylline was dose dependent.

Weingerger, M., Hendeles, L., and Bighley, L. The relation of product formulation to absorption of oral theophylline. *N. Engl. J. Med.* 199:852–857, 1978.
The most commonly quoted comparison of a few of the many sustained-release theophylline preparations on the market today.

31. ADRENERGIC AGENTS
Don A. Bukstein

Adrenergic sympathomimetic bronchodilators are useful in the treatment of asthma. These agents stimulate $beta_2$ receptors, and thus relax bronchial smooth muscle, improve mucociliary transport, and inhibit release of mediators of immediate hypersensitivity from mast cells. The pharmacologic treatment of asthma and chronic respiratory disease has been greatly improved by the relatively recent introduction of the beta-adrenergic agents that have greater specificity for $beta_2$ receptors, longer duration of action, and efficacy by the oral route.

The phenylethylamine structure is the nucleus for all the naturally occurring catecholamines as well as the synthetic compounds available for the treatment of asthma. Variations in pharmacologic activity have been produced by alterations of this structure by changing substituents on the benzene ring, on the alpha carbon, or at the terminal nitrogen (Fig. 13).

The physiologic effects of these compounds are mediated by type of adrenergic receptors within the tissues. Two types of adrenergic receptors have been defined: alpha and beta. The beta receptors have been divided into two subclasses: $beta_1$ (stimulating) and $beta_2$ (inhibitory). $Beta_2$ receptors are found in bronchial smooth muscle as well as in vascular smooth muscle and skeletal muscles. $Beta_1$ receptors predominate in cardiac muscle and are responsible for both chronotropic and inotropic effects. The ideal bronchodilator would be purely $beta_2$, eliminating all direct cardiac stimulating properties. The relative $beta_1$ and $beta_2$ stimulating effects of various adrenergic agents are functions of their molecular configuration. Modification of the molecular side chain by increasing the bulk adjacent to the nitrogen increases $beta_2$ specificity.

$Beta_2$ adrenergic effects appear to be mediated by stimulation of adenylate cyclase, with a consequent rise in intracellular cyclic adenosine monophosphate (cAMP). This increase in cAMP antagonizes the action of vasoactive substances derived from mast cells, thus inhibiting the bronchial smooth muscle spasm in asthma.

Monamine oxidase (MAO) and catechol-O-methyl-transferase are two enzymes responsible for metabolic transformation of the catecholamines. The highest concentrations of these enzymes are in the liver and the kidney. Epinephrine, isoproterenol, and isoetharine are not effective oral agents because of their rapid destruction in the gastrointestinal tract and their rapid conjugation and oxidation in the liver. Increasing the molecular bulk adjacent to the nitrogen to enhance $beta_2$ specificity also reduces susceptibility to degradation by MAO. Change in the position of the hydroxyl groups on the benzene ring or substitution for them to change the molecule into a noncatecholamine prevents degradation by catechol-O-methyl-transferase (see Fig. 13). Noncatecholamines have a longer duration of action and a greater oral bioavailability because of their resistance to inactivating enzymes of the liver and other tissues. Because of the alteration in degradation, these drugs are effective when taken orally. A significant amount of ad-

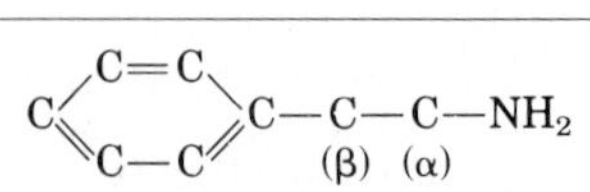

Fig. 13. Phenylethylamine structure that is the nucleus for all catecholamines.

ministered drug is excreted in the urine. Noncatecholamines can be further classified on the basis of chemical substitutions into resorcinols (metaproterenol, terbutaline, and fenoterol) and salijenins (albuterol) (Table 27).

Clinical Use of Beta-Adrenergic Agents

In the treatment of asthma, beta-adrenergic agents are used by oral, parenteral, and inhaled routes. Many clinical studies have investigated the efficacy, duration of action, and comparative value of these agents by various routes. Interpretation of these clinical investigations has been hampered by (1) differences in study design; (2) problems in selecting equipotent (equimolar) doses of the drugs; (3) variations in dosage and routes of administration; (4) lack of objective measures of patient improvement; (5) lack of consideration of the potentiating or inhibiting effects of other medications; and (6) lack of consideration of the development of resistance.

Beta-adrenergic agonists are extensively used in the treatment of acute and chronic asthma because of their ability to produce bronchodilatation through stimulation of $beta_2$-adrenergic receptors in the lungs. Beta-adrenergic agonists can be used in small amounts and are generally well tolerated, especially when given by inhalation. New agents with improved $beta_2$ specificity have been recently synthesized, and many are in use or are undergoing clinical trials, principally in Europe. At this writing, the drugs with the greatest $beta_2$ activity available in the United States are isoproterenol, metaproterenol, terbutaline, and albuterol; however, isoproterenol is not $beta_2$ selective, and metaproterenol is less $beta_2$ selective than terbutaline and albuterol.

Routine measurement of serum or plasma levels for beta agents is not currently available. Therefore, unlike serum theophylline levels, comparisons between serum drug levels and pulmonary function are not possible. Dosages and duration of action for these agents are not well established, especially when the agents are given by inhalation. Therefore, administered doses have been established on the basis of clinical response rather than by pharmacokinetic studies.

Oral Bronchodilators

The recent development and clinical use of newer $beta_2$-adrenergic receptor agents have added a new dimension to the treatment of asthma and other chronic respiratory diseases. These newer agents have greater specificity, longer duration, and efficacy by the oral route. New oral bronchodilators such as metaproterenol, terbutaline, and albuterol can provide bronchodilator therapy in the form of tablets, capsules, and liquids. With systemic absorption, the bronchodilator is available to all parts of the respiratory tree. The therapeutic efficacy of currently available oral beta-adrenergic agents is limited by systemic side effects (such as tremors); unfortunately, these side effects often begin to appear even at doses that are required for moderate degrees of bronchodilation. Although serum levels (which are not routinely available) peak within 30 minutes and may last 4 to 5 hours, many of the selective oral $beta_2$ agents have a bronchodilatory effect that may last for 6 to 8 hours. Some patients may require an even shorter dosing interval to provide a continuous effect.

Parenteral Bronchodilators

Epinephrine has been the mainstay of therapy for acute exacerbations of asthma. Though epinephrine has a powerful bronchodilatory action, its nonselective action of both alpha and beta receptors may very often produce undesirable cardiovascular side effects. Use of newer $beta_2$ agonists such as terbutaline may eliminate some of these cardiovascular side effects, although most studies comparing terbutaline to epinephrine have shown that both drugs cause the same degree of tachycardia. In any event, side effects from these drugs are usually very

Table 27. Recommended dosages of adrenergic bronchodilators

Drug name	Adrenergic specificity	Route of administration	Typical adult dosage	Pediatric dosage
Epinephrine	α, β, β_2	Oral Injection	25 mg q.i.d. 0.3 mg, 1 : 1000 dilution sc q. 20 min × 3	0.75 mg/kg, q. 4–6 hr 0.01 ml/kg, 1 : 1000 dilution sc, maximum 0.3 ml, q. 20 min × 3
Epinephrine suspension	α, β_1, β_2	Injection	0.15 to 0.3 ml, 1 : 200 dilution sc, q. 6 hr	0.005 ml/kg, 1 : 200 dilution sc, maximum 0.15 ml, q. 6 hr
Isoetharine	β_2	Nebulization[a] Metered-dose inhaler	0.25 to 1.0 ml, q. 2 hr 1 or 2 actuations, q. 2 hr	25–50 lb: 0.3 ml; 50–100 lb: 0.5 ml, q.2–4 hr Not recommended[b]
Metaproterenol	β_1, β_2	Nebulization[a] Metered-dose inhaler Tablet or syrup	0.3 ml, q. 2–4 hr 1 or 2 actuations, q. 2–4 hr 20 mg q.i.d.	25–50 lb: 0.1 ml; 50–100 lb: 0.2 ml, q. 2–4 hr Not recommended[b] 6–9 yr or under 60 lb: 10 mg q.i.d.; 9–12 yr or over 60 lb: 20 mg q.i.d.

Terbutaline	β_2	Tablet	5 mg t.i.d.	Not recommended[c]
		Injection	0.3 ml sc, q. 20 min × 3	0.01 mg/kg sc, maximum 0.3 ml, q. 20 min × 3
		Inhaled (injection solution)	2 ml, q. 2–4 hr	25–50 lb: 1 ml; 50–100 lb: 2 ml; q. 2–4 hr
		Metered-dose inhaler	2 actuations, q. 4–6 hr	Not recommended
Albuterol	β_2	Tablet or syrup	2–4 mg t.i.d. initially; maximum 8 mg t.i.d.	Recommended only for children 12 yr of age or older[d]
		Metered-dose inhaler	2 actuations, q. 4–6 hr	Not recommended[b]
Fenoterol[e]	β_2	Metered-dose inhaler	2 actuations, q. 6–8 hr	Not recommended

[a]Inhalation of solutions with low osmolarity (such as distilled water) can be irritating and produce cough. Solutions used for nebulization should be approximately isosmolar (330 mOsm/L; slightly below isosmolar is better than above). For example, metaproterenol (Alupent) 0.5 ml, and water, 0.5 ml, has an osmolarity of 241 mOsm/L; therefore, Alupent needs to be diluted with normal saline. Alupent, 0.5 ml, and normal saline, 0.5 ml, has an osmolarity of 241 mOsm/L.

[b]Although isoetharine, metaproterenol, and albuterol metered-dose inhalers are not officially recommended for use in children, they are commonly prescribed for children as young as 5 years of age, using doses similar for adults. They are useful in both preventing and treating bronchospasm. Side effects are similar to those described in adults. Clinicians prescribing these drugs should document that other forms of treatment are not optimal and then inform the patient and the parent that an approved drug is being used in a nonapproved manner.

[c]Oral terbutaline has been used in children. Similar to the use of metered-dose inhalers, other drugs must first be tried and documentation provided that use of these drugs was not optimal. The dose of terbutaline in children (5 years of age and older) is 50 to 100 μg/kg/dose, which produced significant bronchodilatation for at least 6 hours (Ardal, B, et al. *J. Pediatr.* 93:305–307, 1978). This dose can probably be used up to three times per day.

[d]Rachelefsky and co-workers (*Pediatrics* 69:397–403, 1982) have demonstrated that tablets or syrup were effective in treatment of asthmatic children 6 to 12 years of age and recommended 4 mg albuterol syrup (2 mg/5 ml) be given four times a day.

[e]Scheduled for release by the FDA in late 1983.

transient and can be controlled by adjusting the dose. **Subcutaneous terbutaline** or **epinephrine** is especially useful when a patient is too dyspneic to take a deep breath or too nauseated to take oral medication; these drugs are thus highly effective therapy for acute exacerbations of asthma. Theoretically, terbutaline should have a longer duration of action than epinephrine but comparative studies have not demonstrated a large difference in magnitude or duration of action of the two drugs. Epinephrine is the clear choice in the treatment of systemic anaphylaxis or acute urticaria because of the peripheral vasoconstrictor effects.

Intravenous therapy with beta-adrenergic agents is very hazardous and is rarely helpful in eliminating the need for mechanical ventilation. The use of intravenous isoproterenol in severe asthma has resulted in myocardial ischemia, infarction, and death (see Chap. 3). Although terbutaline and albuterol may be safer than isoproterenol for intravenous use, they are currently not approved in the United States for use for acute asthma. In addition, the experience with use of these drugs intravenously is much more limited than the experience with isoproterenol. Increased use may uncover problems with these drugs similar to the problems seen with intravenous isoproterenol.

Aerosol Bronchodilators
Whether or not selective beta$_2$-adrenergic aerosolized agents (both metered-dose and solutions) should be used routinely in mild to moderate asthma is debatable. The following arguments support the routine use of these agents:

1. Onset of action is rapid; thus, they usually provide immediate relief for the patient with bronchospasm and immediate protection for exercise in a patient with known exercise-induced bronchospasm.
2. The small dose inhaled and delivered to the target area (larger airways) often bypasses the significant systemic effects observed when the drug is administered orally or parenterally.
3. The efficacy of inhaled beta-adrenergic agents is superior to that of oral agents in blocking exercise-induced asthma.
4. The dosage needed is a fraction of the oral dose.
5. The routine use of aerosol bronchodilators before inhalation of cromolyn and beclomethasone optimizes the opening of small airways, enhancing delivery of these medications.

In contrast, the following arguments discourage the routine use of adrenergic aerosols:

1. Psychological dependence on this form of therapy may develop from dramatic and rapid bronchodilation.
2. The proper use of aerosol medication requires repeated instruction from well-trained personnel.
3. A potential risk exists for abuse and overuse.
4. The development of tachyphylaxis and subsequent tolerance may be increased, and may be associated with the reduction in number of available beta-adrenergic receptors and a reduced overall response with subsequent use of the drugs.
5. The potential irritative and bronchospastic effects of freon and cardiac toxicity of halogenated hydrocarbon propellants have been demonstrated in some animal studies.

The short duration of action and strong beta$_1$ effects of epinephrine metered-dose inhalers and aerosolized isoproterenol limit their value in chronic therapy. Terbutaline, albuterol, and fenoterol are selective beta$_2$ agonists with minimal beta$_1$ cardiovascular effects and prolonged duration of action (see Table 27).

The correct use of inhaled bronchodilators is of prime importance, and a great deal of the variability in effects of these inhaled agents probably can be explained by improper technique in their administration. This mishandling is especially true for the use of metered-dose inhalers. To ensure maximum value from use of the inhalers, patients should be educated thoroughly in proper technique when the devices are first prescribed. The technique should be checked on each patient visit, almost as if it were part of the physical examination.

An alternative to the use of hand-held, metered-dose inhaler devices is the use of aqueous solutions with hand-held bulb-nebulizers, or simple air pump units. These units are more cumbersome and annoying than the easier-to-use freon metered-dose cannister units and may reduce the potential for abuse. Compressor-driven nebulizers (DeVilbiss and Maximist) are effective in delivering inhaled medications to younger children and dyspneic patients.

Intermittent positive-pressure breathing devices are no more effective than metered-dose inhalers or air-driven nebulizers. These breathing devices increase the cost of medical care and increase the possibility of pneumothorax in a person with hyperexpanded lungs.

The therapeutic value of all these bronchodilators should be monitored for both symptomatic and functional improvement. Symptomatic improvement is usually very apparent in terms of reduced wheezing and increased activity level. Functional improvement can be best gauged by periodic spirometric pulmonary function testing.

The most common and troublesome **toxicity** of beta$_2$-adrenergic agents is neuromuscular stimulation. Most patients will initially have tremor with oral therapy. This tremor is secondary to direct action on peripheral skeletal muscle, and is not a central nervous system effect. Although tremor decreases as tolerance develops, it remains in approximately 30% of cases. The tremor, nervousness, and agitation that often accompany the oral use of the more selective beta$_2$ agents can be decreased by changing to the inhaled route.

The most significant beta$_1$ effect is cardiac stimulation. It is observed during use of all the agents, even the more selective beta$_2$ drugs. In general it is less of a problem when the drugs are given by inhalation and is most marked with subcutaneous or intravenous use of epinephrine and isoproterenol. In addition to the direct effect of the beta$_1$ agonists on the cardiac muscle, there is also a slight reflex tachycardia due to a fall in peripheral vascular resistance. Although the tachycardias may last for a considerable length of time, they rarely predispose to ventricular ectopic beats. Alpha stimulation may increase myocardial irritability and ischemia, while beta receptor stimulation may decrease blood pressure, causing dizziness and fainting. Other nonspecific side effects are headache, nausea, and vomiting.

Inhaled, subcutaneous, or intravenous beta-adrenergic agents may cause a drop in PaO$_2$ due to an alteration in the ventilation-perfusion ratio and increased perfusion to poorly oxygenated areas. The higher the pretreatment PaO$_2$, the greater the fall in PaO$_2$. Although this fall in oxygen tension tends to be small and is of short duration, O$_2$ should be given routinely when either injected or inhaled agents are given to patients in any significant respiratory distress.

Although in vitro tolerance to beta$_2$ effects can be demonstrated easily, the majority of studies have failed to show clinically significant acquired tolerance to beta$_2$ bronchodilation. However, a loss of approximately 30 to 50% in the duration of bronchodilatory activity with albuterol has been described by some investigators. Any tolerance that may develop is probably selective and nonprogressive, and probably rarely compromises treatment.

Ahlquist, R. P.   A study of the adenotropic receptors. *Am. J. Physiol.* 153:586–600, 1948.
The original description of adrenergic receptors and classification into alpha and beta groupings.

Banner, A. S., Sunderrajan, E. V., Agarwal, M. K., and Addington, W. N.   Arrhythmogenic effects of orally administered bronchodilators. *Arch. Intern. Med.* 139:434–437, 1979.
In patients with preexisting arrhythmias, terbutaline can increase prolonged ventricular ectopy.

Collins, J. M., McDevitt, D. G., and Shanks, R. G.   The cardio-toxicity of isoprenaline during hypoxia. *Br. J. Pharmacol.* 36:35–45, 1969.
One of the first descriptions of cardiotoxicity of adrenergic agents in patients with acute asthma.

Garra, B., et al.   A double-blind evaluation of the use of nebulized metaproterenol and isoproterenol in hospitalized asthmatic children and adolescents. *J. Allergy Clin. Immunol.* 60:63–68, 1977.
Metaproterenol seems to be more effective than isoproterenol in reversing bronchospasm in acutely ill asthmatic children.

Harper, T. B., and Strunk, R. C.   Techniques of administration of metered-dose aerosolized drugs in asthmatic children. *Am. J. Dis. Child.* 135:218–221, 1981.
Review of studies available and recommendations for most effective use of this form of therapy.

Knudson, R. T., and Constantine, H. P.   An effect of isoproterenol on ventilation-perfusion in asthmatic versus normal subjects. *J. Appl. Physiol.* 22:402–406, 1967.
The administration of isoproterenol to asthmatic patients increases ventilation of already well-ventilated portions of the lung to the detriment of poorly ventilated portions, further increasing unevenness of ventilation-perfusion distribution throughout the lung.

Matson, J. R., Gerald, M. L., and Strunk, R. C.   Myocardial ischemia complicating the use of isoproterenol in asthmatic children. *J. Pediatr.* 92:776–778, 1978.
Report of a 14-year-old boy who had chest pain accompanied by an ischemic pattern on EKG during use of IV isoproterenol. The ischemic pattern was not apparent on chest leads used to monitor rhythm but was seen with standard or 12-lead tracing.

McFadden, E. R.   Beta$_2$ receptor agonist: Metabolism and pharmacology. *J. Allergy Clin. Immunol.* 68:91–97, 1981.
A well-written overview of beta agonists, comparing their metabolism and pharmacologic usefulness.

Nelson, H. S.   Getting the most out of beta-adrenergics today. *J. Respir. Dis.* 3:11–19, 1982.
The role of adrenergic bronchodilator therapy in both the acute and chronic treatment of asthma is clearly and concisely explained.

Pang, L. M., Rodriguez-Martinez, F., Davis, W. J., and Mellins, R. B.   Terbutaline in the treatment of status asthmaticus. *Chest* 72:469–473, 1977.
Subcutaneous terbutaline is effective in the treatment of status asthmaticus with only modest effects on cardiovascular system.

Shenfied, G. M., and Paterson, J. W.   Clinical assessment of bronchodilator drugs delivered by aerosol. *Thorax* 28:124–128, 1973.
An excellent study comparing the efficacy of isoproterenol, terbutaline, and metaproterenol.

Svedmyr, L. V., Larsson, S. A., and Thiringer, G. K.   Development of "resistance" in beta adrenergic receptors of asthmatic patients. *Chest* 69:479–483, 1976.
Results of this study demonstrated that there was no deterioration in lung function with time when asthmatic patients were given terbutaline for 1 year. There was also no evidence of acquired tachyphylaxis to the pulmonary effects of isoproterenol.

Tai, E., and Read, J.   Response of blood gas tensions to aminophylline and isoprenaline in patients with asthma. *Thorax* 22:543–549, 1967.
Alterations in ventilation-perfusion ratios can occur with theophylline as well as isoproterenol.

Tandon, M. K.   Cardiopulmonary effects of fenoterol and salbutamol aerosols. *Chest* 77:429–431, 1980.
Salbutamol and fenoterol are compared as bronchodilators.

Weinberger, M., Hendeles, L., and Ahrens, R.   Clinical pharmacology of drugs used for asthma. *Ped. Clin. North Am.* 28:47–75, 1981.
Reviews pharmacology and clinical applications of all classes of bronchodilators.

Ziment, I.   *Respiratory Pharmacology and Therapeutics.* Philadelphia: Saunders, 1978. Pp. 190–218.
Contains many useful tables comparing the actions and side effects of the various agents, as well as the formulation of commercial preparations.

32. CROMOLYN SODIUM

Francine G. Andrews

Since its discovery and synthesis in 1965, cromolyn sodium (sodium cromogly-cate) has been recognized as an important mode of treatment for asthma. Nevertheless, some reluctance toward the use of cromolyn continues to exist in the United States. The purpose of this chapter is to review the basic pharmacology of cromolyn sodium and to clarify current indications for its clinical use. Potential future applications of cromolyn therapy and of its active analogues will also be discussed.

Cromolyn sodium was initially derived from the chromone khellin, a muscle relaxant found in the Middle Eastern herb ammi visnaga. Khellin was known to relieve angina pain and renal colic through specific smooth muscle relaxation. Coincidentally, khellin was also noted to have bronchodilator activity. Because of its severe gastrointestinal toxicity, researchers attempted to synthesize chemical derivatives with the same smooth muscle relaxing properties, but without such limiting adverse reactions. Cromolyn sodium was eventually developed by linking together two carboxychromone molecules. Because this substance was poorly absorbed orally and was insoluble in alcohol, the Turboinhaler (Spinhaler) was designed for drug administration. The drug is also now available as a solution that can be administered by a standard nebulizer.

Each cromolyn sodium capsule or vial of liquid contains 20 mg of cromolyn. The capsule also contains 20 mg of lactose powder as a carrier. Using either the Spinhaler or nebulized cromolyn, approximately 8% of the cromolyn reaches the respiratory tract. Some remains in the Spinhaler or nebulizer and the rest is either deposited in the upper airways or swallowed. Systemic absorption is minimal, with a mean plasma concentration of 9.2 ng/ml measured 15 minutes after inhalation of one capsule. Given orally only 1% of the drug is absorbed from the gastrointestinal tract. Cromolyn is excreted unchanged in the urine, bile, and feces. The plasma half-life after either inhalation or intravenous administration is 80 to 90 minutes. During this clearance time, cromolyn is bound to a plasma protein.

The major pharmacologic effect of cromolyn sodium appears to be stabilization of mast cell membranes. However, recent data have suggested that cromolyn may also modulate reflex-induced bronchoconstriction and perhaps even reduce nonspecific bronchial hyperreactivity. Early in vitro experiments demonstrated that cromolyn inhibited mast cell degranulation. Clinical studies also support the concept that cromolyn somehow inhibits mast cell degranulation, especially when the degranulation is triggered by IgE mechanisms, for prophylactic use of cromolyn before antigenic challenge prevents the usual immediate IgE-mediated bronchial reactions. Delayed or late-phase reactions are also inhibited by administration of cromolyn prior to antigenic challenge. These pharmacologic effects are apparently produced by prevention of the normal influx of calcium ions, which are required for mast cell degranulation. This may be accomplished by increasing the intracellular level of cyclic adenosine monophosphate (cAMP), which would then reduce calcium ion transport across the mast cell membrane. It has also been postulated that the hydrophilic nature of cromolyn may interfere directly with normal calcium influx.

Evidence has also emerged that cromolyn can prevent several types of reflex-induced asthma that do not appear to be dependent on mast cell mediator release. Two examples are the wheezing observed after challenges with hyperpnea or cold air or sulfur dioxide. This effect is presumably achieved by inhibiting a pathophysiologic pathway unrelated to mast cell–derived chemical mediators. Therapy over an extended period of time also appears to decrease nonspecific bronchial hyperactivity found in most asthmatic patients.

Despite the proved benefits associated with cromolyn therapy, many physicians are not adequately informed about its proper role in the treatment of asthma. According to numerous clinical studies, approximately 70% of all asthmatic patients will improve with use of cromolyn sodium. Contrary to early reports, factors such as age, degree of atopy, and severity of disease are not reliable in predicting individual patient response. In other words, both intrinsic and extrinsic asthmatic patients may benefit from cromolyn therapy. In order to ascertain its effectiveness a therapeutic trial of 1 to 2 months is necessary.

Although its efficacy can not be individually anticipated, there are certain clinical situations in which cromolyn therapy should be considered. Cromolyn appears to be as effective as theophylline for the initial therapy of mild to moderate asthma. This is particularly true in young children who either cannot tolerate theophylline because of the side effects or who cannot use sustained-released theophylline preparations because of irratic absorption of the drug caused by the variable gastrointestinal transit times that often occur. Because cromolyn is an effective agent for inhibition of pollen-induced bronchoconstriction, it is an excellent medication during peak pollen seasons, either used alone or as an adjunct to immunotherapy. Patients sensitive to animal dander or to various occupational exposures are often best managed by using cromolyn prophylactically. Inhibition of exercise-induced bronchospasm can be effectively achieved with prophylactic use of cromolyn. All patients with chronic perennial asthma should have a trial on cromolyn prior to use of long-term oral or inhaled steroids. Cromolyn therapy can significantly reduce steroid requirements in patients with aspirin intolerance and nasal polyps.

In order to achieve maximum therapeutic improvement, several points on cromolyn use need to be stressed. Most important is proper initial instruction and demonstration on its use. The prophylactic nature of its effect and need for regular use must also be emphasized. Initially, the dosage should be 20 mg (1 capsule or vial of liquid) four times a day. The dosage may then be tapered to two or three times a day depending on clinical course. In general, the dosage should never be lower than 20 mg twice a day. Effectiveness should be assessed only after a clinical trial of 3 to 4 weeks. Patients should also be encouraged to use cromolyn prior to exercise and exposure to known allergens.

The effect of cromolyn therapy on other concomitant treatment has been investigated. Addition of cromolyn sodium to the medication regimen in steroid-dependent asthmatic patients occasionally allows for reduction of steroid use. This "steroid-sparing" effect is apparently a consequence of the drug's direct antiasthmatic effect. Other studies have also shown significant reduction in need for both oral and inhaled bronchodilators when cromolyn is added to the medical regimen.

Choice of the mode of therapy for cromolyn, the Spinhaler or nebulization of the liquid, depends on the age of the patient and the remainder of the therapeutic regimen. For example, young children cannot use the Spinhaler effectively and must use the nebulized solution. Recent studies have demonstrated the effectiveness of this treatment modality in children younger than 6 years of age. In general patients older than 6 years can use a Spinhaler effectively. If these patients are using an inhaled bronchodilator routinely, the Spinhaler should be used after the bronchodilator to improve the entry into the airway and reduce irritation that may occur from the powder in patients with hyperreactive airways. For patients using regular nebulized treatment, the cromolyn liquid may be added to the other liquids being used.

Cromolyn has been shown to be beneficial in several other conditions. Both perennial and seasonal allergic rhinitis can be improved by using cromolyn solution intranasally (marketed as Nasalcrom) or by using direct inhalation of the powder intranasally. Use of a cromolyn solution for allergic conjunctivitis has also been helpful in some patients, although the cromolyn solutions available commercially are not approved for this use. Symptoms from certain nonatopic conditions may also be alleviated. Preliminary studies have indicated pain associated with aphthous ulcers can be reduced by using topical cromolyn. Diarrhea caused by systemic mastocytosis has reportedly been controlled with massive oral administation of cromolyn sodium. Similarly, ulcerative colitis and chronic proctitis have been treated with oral and rectal cromolyn sodium; in several cases both clinical symptom scores and rectal biopsies improved significantly. Inhibition of gastrointestinal symptoms found with milk protein allergy has been achieved with large doses of oral cromolyn sodium.

One of the major advantages of cromolyn therapy compared with other antiasthmatic therapies is the paucity of adverse reactions. The most frequent side effects are coughing and transient reflex bronchospasm after inhalation of the powder. These effects are often exaggerated during an exacerbation or in patients with very reactive airways. The irritation caused by the cromolyn powder can be minimized by proper inhalation technique or by having the patient use an inhaled bronchodilator before inhaling the powder. Unlike the powder, inhalation of cromolyn by nebulization is not irritating. In the past the use of cromolyn was commonly discontinued during exacerbations of asthma because of the irritation of the drug; however, using inhaled bronchodilators before the powder will allow continuation of cromolyn during most episodes of wheezing. If irritation is still a problem, the drug can be taken by nebulization without difficulty. Another problem that patients occasionally complain of is pharyngeal irritation, which can usually be avoided by drinking water immediately after inhalation. There have been a few isolated reports of apparent allergic reactions to cromolyn including urticaria, angioedema, and maculopapular rashes. Documented pulmonary infiltrates with eosinophilia have been reported on three occasions in patients on cromolyn therapy, but a causative effect of the cromolyn has not been demonstrated. Overall, the risk-to-benefit ratio of cromolyn sodium therapy is excellent.

Current research is aimed at finding a cromolynlike drug that could be administered and absorbed orally. Obviously, patient compliance may be improved with an orally active analogue. Several compounds have been synthesized, however, they have had limited clinical testing. For example, doxantrazole is a synthetic monocromone, which is readily absorbed from the gastrointestinal tract, that can inhibit mediator release in vitro. Clinically it does inhibit bronchoconstriction induced by allergen exposure; however, it is not as effective as cromolyn. A methylxanthine analogue has also been developed that may combine both cromolyn and theophyllinelike properties.

In conclusion, cromolyn sodium provides an important mode of treating asthma. Its pharmacologic effects are more encompassing than originally thought. Not only does cromolyn inhibit mast cell–mediator release, it also reduces bronchial hyperactivity and interferes with reflex-mediated asthma. The scope of its function may be further broadened as additional pharmacologic activities are identified and as new derivatives are synthesized.

Bernstein, I. L.   Cromolyn sodium in the treatment of asthma: Changing concepts. *J. Allergy Clin. Immunol.* 68:247–253, 1981.
   State-of-the-art, worthwhile review stimulating American physicians to rethink the usefulness of cromolyn.
Bernstein, I. L., Johnson, C. L., and Tse, C. S. T.   Therapy with cromolyn sodium. *Ann. Intern. Med.* 89:228–233, 1978.
   One of the earlier reviews of the usefulness of cromolyn in asthma and other diseases.
Drug Committee of the American Academy of Allergy.   A controlled study of cromolyn sodium. *J. Allergy Clin. Immunol.* 50:235–245, 1972.

Presents the first major study of cromolyn in the United States. Carry-over effect noted for as long as 4 weeks after the drug was stopped.

Geller-Bernstein, C., and Sneh, N. The management of bronchial asthma in children under the age of 3½ using Intal (sodium cromoglycate) administered by Spinhaler. *Clin. Allergy* 10 (Suppl.):503–508, 1980.

Although extensive education is required, the children are able to comply.

Gwin, E., Kerby, G. R., and Ruth, W. E. Cromolyn sodium in the treatment of asthma associated with aspirin hypersensitivity and nasal polyps. *Chest* 72:148–153, 1977.

A double-blind study demonstrating slight but significant improvement in pulmonary functions in this group of patients after 4 weeks of active treatment.

Hambleton, G., et al. Comparison of cromoglycate (cromolyn) and theophylline in controlling symptoms of chronic asthma. A collaborative study. *Lancet* 1:381–385, 1977.

Cromolyn and theophylline were equally effective in most patients. Only one patient who was able to be controlled on theophylline was not able to be controlled on cromolyn.

Hiller, E. J., Milner, A. D., and Lenney, W. Nebulized sodium cromoglycate in young asthmatic children. Double-blind trial. *Arch. Dis. Child.* 52:875–876, 1977.

A double-blind controlled trial showing significant difference in symptoms scores in children aged 2 to 5 years who were taking nebulized cromolyn versus placebo.

Johnson, H. G. Cromoglycate and other inhibitors of mediator release. In E. Middleton, C. E. Reed, and E. F. Ellis (Eds.), *Allergy: Principles and Practice* (2nd ed.). St. Louis: Mosby, 1983. Pp. 613–632.

Thorough review of uses and modes of action in all allergic diseases with an exhaustive reference list.

Mellon, M. H., Harden, K., and Zeiger, R. S. The effectiveness and safety of nebulizer cromolyn solution in the young childhood asthmatic. *Immunol. Allergy Practice* 4:168–172, 1982.

The nebulized form of drug is very useful.

Newth, C. J. L., Newth, C. V., and Turner, J. A. P. Comparison of nebulized sodium cromoglycate and oral theophylline in controlling symptoms of chronic asthma in preschool children: A double-blind study. *Aust. N.Z. J. Med.* 12:232–238, 1982.

Cromolyn was at least as effective as theophylline in controlling asthma symptoms in 1- to 6-year-old group.

Settipane, G. A., et al. Adverse reactions to cromolyn. *J.A.M.A.* 241:811–813, 1979.

The frequency of adverse reactions was 2%; all reactions were non-life-threatening and completely reversible.

Sheppard, D., Nadel, J. A., and Boushey, H. A. Inhibition of sulfur dioxide-induced bronchoconstriction by disodium cromoglycate in asthmatic subjects. *Am. Rev. Respir. Dis.* 124:257–259, 1981.

The findings suggest that SO_2 induces bronchoconstriction by stimulating release of mediators from mast cells or that cromolyn inhibits bronchoconstriction by a mechanism independent of its effect on mast cells.

---

33. ANTICHOLINERGIC AGENTS
Rajesh G. Bhagat

The bronchodilatory effects of anticholinergic agents have been recognized since the seventeenth century. Clinicians have been reluctant to use the drug for treatment of asthma because of the adverse side effects known to occur when the drugs are used by the parenteral route. The demonstration that these drugs had fewer side effects when used by the inhaled route has stimulated renewed interest in their use in asthma.

Asthma is provoked by both allergic and nonallergic triggers. Many of the nonallergic triggers (e.g., cold air, smoke, and so on) act by stimulating the vagal nerve endings located in the epithelium of the airways (see Fig. 14 for a diagram of the pathways involved). Stimulation of these nerve endings triggers the affer-

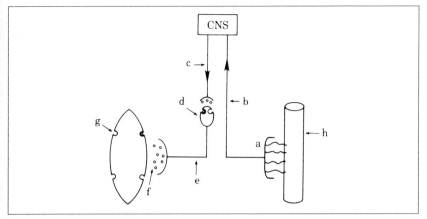

Fig. 14. The cholinergic pathways involved in asthma and the mechanism of action of the anticholinergic agents. a = vagal nerve endings; b = afferent vagus nerve; c = efferent vagus nerve; d = parasympathetic ganglion; e = postganglionic parasympathetic fibers; f = acetylcholine; g = receptor for acetylcholine on smooth muscles; h = bronchial tree.

ent vagus nerve, which carries on the impulse to the central nervous system. The efferent vagus nerve carries the impulse from the CNS to a parasympathetic ganglion located near the tracheobronchial tree. The subsequent activation of postganglionic parasympathetic fibers releases acetylcholine. When acetylcholine interacts with the receptor on the smooth muscle, contraction of the muscles occurs, which results in bronchospasm. The anticholinergic agents occupy the receptors for the acetylcholine preventing the bronchospasm induced by this pathway. Although the mechanism of histamine-induced bronchoconstriction is more complex, the vagus nerve may also be involved in its mediation, for histamine may stimulate vagal sensory nerve endings located in the airways. Therefore, anticholinergic agents may also be helpful in preventing histamine-induced bronchoconstriction in some patients.

The **anticholinergic agents** available for clinical use are atropine sulfate, atropine methylnitrate, and ipratropium bromide (SCH-1000). Atropine methylnitrate and ipratropium bromide are quaternary ammonium derivatives of atropine. These two agents have the advantage of not crossing the blood-brain barrier; thus, they do not cause as many side effects as atropine. Ipratropium bromide has the additional advantage of being available in the form of metered-dose inhaler. This metered-dose form is used extensively in Europe, but is currently not available in the United States. Atropine methylnitrate is also less readily available than atropine sulfate; therefore, atropine sulfate is a logical choice in most instances. None of these agents are yet approved by the FDA for the use in management of reactive airway diseases, however, there is no valid contraindication to their use by knowledgeable physicians as secondary agents in the management of these disorders.

Systemic administration of anticholinergic agents to alleviate bronchospasm results in many adverse effects. Administration by **nebulization** avoids the high systemic concentration of the drug while still keeping a high concentration in the tracheobronchial tree. This method reduces the systemic adverse effects without reducing the efficacy in the airways. Therefore, only administration of the aerosolized form is recommended in the management of chronic asthmatic patients.

The administration of aerosolized atropine sulfate in the dose recommended results in detectable serum concentrations. In most subjects these levels are negligible and the adverse effects are minimal—almost always only locally in the eyes and mouth. Occasionally, a patient may achieve a high serum concentration with resultant significant adverse effects occurring both locally and systemically. Because the occurrence of such a phenomenon in a given patient is impossible to predict, it is safer to begin the therapy with a smaller dose, increasing it gradually to the maximum tolerated dose. It should also be remembered that the degree of bronchodilation is dose dependent up to a certain limit (i.e., the greater the dose the greater the degree of bronchodilation). The dose should therefore be individualized.

A recent study recommends a **dose range** for atropine sulfate of 0.005 mg/kg/dose to 0.05 mg/kg/dose in children. Adults seem to tolerate a maximum of 0.025 mg/kg/dose without noticeable adverse effects. The inhalation of these agents is usually given four times a day.

The dose range of ipratropium bromide is 10 to 80 μg/dose. The average recommended dose for adults and children is 20 to 40 μg (i.e., 1–2 puffs of metered-dose aerosol) three to four times a day.

Atropine sulfate solution for nebulization can be prepared by dissolving atropine sulfate powder in physiologic saline to yield a concentration of 2 mg/ml of atropine sulfate. A higher concentration of 5 mg/ml can be administered to adolescent or adult patients, allowing the larger amount of medication to be delivered in less volume. Solutions of atropine sulfate should be refrigerated in brown bottles to prevent denaturation of atropine by light. The solution should not be used for longer than 30 days after preparation because of the possibility of bacterial contamination.

The **adverse effects** of these agents when administered *systemically* are well recognized and include bradycardia, dryness of mouth, and dilation of pupils with lower doses. The adverse effects seen with larger doses include tachycardia, palpitations, speech disturbance, difficulty swallowing, restlessness and fatigue, headaches, hot dry skin, difficulty in urination, decreased intestinal motility, blurred vision, ataxia, restlessness, excitement, hallucination, delirium, and coma.

Although the recommended dose of nebulized atropine is approximately five to ten times higher than the amounts of the drug used systemically, the side effects from nebulized atropine have been limited to mild dryness of the mouth, dilation of the pupils, and tachycardia. Physicians using aerosolized atropine, however, should be aware of the complete list of adverse effects, for an occasional patient may have a significant systemic absorption and may have some of the more serious adverse effects.

Although it is often stated that atropine increases the viscosity of bronchial secretions and impairs ciliary clearance, there is little evidence that such effects occur. More recent studies indicate that drying effects are found only in a certain subgroup of patients with excessive airway secretions and that these drying effects may have therapeutic benefit in these patients.

Several studies of **efficacy** have shown that these agents are effective bronchodilators. They have a more gradual onset of action (within 15 minutes after administration) than the aerosolized beta-adrenergic agents, but the action is sustained for up to 4 to 6 hours. Therefore, these agents appear more suitable for regular prophylactic use than for rapid symptomatic relief of acute bronchospasm.

The studies of efficacy of aerosolized anticholinergic agents administered to asthmatic patients on a chronic basis for longer than 6 months are not available, although isolated reports of chronic administration of these agents have shown that they are safe and continue to be effective in the management of asthma.

Because anticholinergic agents probably interfere with pathways involved in irritant-induced asthma better than those involved in allergen-induced asthma, one might speculate that patients with nonallergic asthma may be more responsive to these agents than patients with allergic asthma. Nevertheless, clinical studies with ipratropium bromide could not identify a subgroup of asthmatic patients that was more responsive to this agent. Therefore, these agents can be used in any asthmatic patient whose symptoms are not adequately controlled by routine use of theophylline and beta-adrenergic agents.

Because beta-adrenergic agonists and cholinergic antagonists act through different mechanisms, and possibly at different sites in the tracheobronchial tree, use of the two types of drugs together should be more potent than either alone. Clinical studies have shown that the combination does result in a small but significantly increased bronchodilation than either drug given alone. This small increase in bronchodilation may not be relevant in patients with mild asthma, but could be extremely useful in patients with severe asthma.

Although the FDA has not approved the use of anticholinergic agents in routine management of asthma, many European workers have found them to be safe and effective; therefore, knowledgeable physicians often use these agents for (1) steroid-dependent asthmatic patients whose symptoms are not adequately controlled by routine use of theophylline and beta-adrenergic agents. Use of anticholinergic agents in such patients may help achieve better control of asthma or decrease steroid requirements. (2) Patients in whom adverse effects of sympathomimetic agents such as tremors or palpitations are troublesome when the drugs are given in conventional dosage.

The following should be considered or documented prior to using these agents in any patient:

1. The therapy with these agents should be individualized to the patient as a special situation for a specific trial period.
2. The bronchodilators approved by the FDA should have failed to relieve the symptoms completely, or the risk/benefit ratios of these medications should be much higher than the risk/benefit ratio of atropine.
3. The efficacy as well as adverse effects of atropine must be reviewed with the patient.
4. It should be explained to the patient that the FDA has not approved these agents in the management of asthma, but his or her asthma is severe enough to warrant the use of such agents to control the symptoms.

Various studies have shown that these agents are effective in various **other respiratory diseases** like chronic bronchitis and cystic fibrosis, by alleviating the bronchospasm that is often associated with these diseases. Conflicting data exist regarding the efficacy of anticholinergic agents in the management of exercise-induced bronchospasm. These agents, when used in the accepted doses, are not uniformly effective in prevention of exercise-induced asthma.

Cavanaugh, M. J., and Cooper, D. M. Inhaled atropine sulfate: Dose response characteristics. *Am. Rev. Respir. Dis.* 114:517–524, 1976.
  The authors showed that response to inhaled atropine is dose dependent in children up to a certain limit. The optimal dose for children is 0.05 mg/kg/dose. Increasing the dose further did not increase the degree of bronchodilation.
Chamberlin, D. A., Musr, D. C. F., and Kennedy, K. P. Atropine methonitrate and isoprenaline in bronchial asthma. *Lancet* 283:1019–1021, 1962.
  The combination of these two agents had greater bronchodilator effects than either of the drugs alone.
Cropp, G. J. A. The role of parasympathetic nervous system in the maintenance of chronic airway obstruction in asthmatic children. *Am. Rev. Respir. Dis.* 112:599–605, 1975.
  Administration of aerosolized atropine sulfate (0.07 mg–0.08 mg/kg) and isoproterenol (1.5 mg) on separate occasions improved forced expiratory flow and SGaw to a similar

degree in 18 asthmatic children. The improvement in residual volume, total lung capacity, and functional residual capacity was more marked with atropine sulfate than with isoproterenol.

Boushey, H. A., and Gold, W. M.   Anti-cholinergic Agents. In E. Middleton, C. Reed, and E. Ellis, *Allergy: Principles and Practice* (2nd ed.). St. Louis: Mosby, 1983. Pp. 633–652.
An excellent discussion on the role of vagally mediated mechanisms in asthma and the role of anticholinergic agents in this disease.

Klock, L. E., et al.   A comparative study of atropine sulfate and isoproterenol hydrochloride in chronic bronchitis. *Am. Rev. Respir. Dis.* 112:371–376, 1975.
This study suggested that there was no significant difference in sputum production, sputum thickness, or dryness of mouth between treatment with isoproterenol and nebulized atropine (1 mg). Forty-five percent of patients had mild hesitancy in urination that did not require a change in dose of atropine.

Kradjan, W. A., et al.   Serum atropine concentration after inhalation of atropine sulfate. *Am. Rev. Respir. Dis.* 23:471–472, 1982.
The authors showed that after administration of 0.05 mg/kg of aerosolized atropine sulfate, measurable serum concentration occurred within 15 minutes and persisted for 4 hours. There appeared to be continued slow absorption of the drug throughout this time period. In most instances, the serum concentration of atropine was minimal with no systemic effects, but one patient obtained high serum concentrations of this drug with systemic side effects.

Larsen, G. L., Barron, R. J., Cotton, E. K., and Brooks, J. G.   A comparative study of inhaled atropine sulfate and isoproterenol hydrochloride in cystic fibrosis. *Am. Rev. Respir. Dis.* 119:399–407, 1979.
Nebulized atropine sulfate (0.1 mg/kg/dose) was found to be an effective bronchodilator in patients with cystic fibrosis.

Lopez-Vidriero, M. T., et al.   Effect of atropine on sputum production. *Thorax* 30:543–547, 1975.
A study suggesting that atropine has no effect on viscosity or volume of sputum in most patients. In some patients reduction of volume of sputum occurs mainly because of reduction in salivary secretion.

Marini, J. J., and Lakshiminarayan, S.   The effect of atropine inhalation in "irreversible" chronic bronchitis. *Chest* 77:591–596, 1980.
Nebulized atropine sulfate (0.05 mg/kg) was found to be an effective bronchodilator in patients with chronic bronchitis unresponsive to aerosolized isoproterenol.

Pak, C. C. F., Kradjan, W. A., Lakshiminarayan, S., and Marini, J. J.   Inhaled atropine sulfate—characteristics in adult patients with chronic air flow obstruction. *Am. Rev. Respir. Dis.* 125:331–334, 1982.
The response to nebulized atropine was dose dependent in adults. The optimal dose for adults was found to be 0.025 mg/kg/dose. Increasing the dose to 0.05 mg/kg/dose was associated with marginal benefit over 0.025 mg/kg/dose and was associated with significant adverse effects.

Pakes, G. E., et al.   Ipratropinum bromide: A review of its pharmacological properties and therapeutic efficacy in asthma and chronic bronchitis. *Drugs* 20:237–267, 1980.
Presents a detailed review on ipratropium bromide.

Ruffin, R. E., Fitzgerald, J. D., and Rebuck, A. S.   A comparison of bronchodilator activity of SCH-1000 and salbutamol. *J. Allergy Clin. Immunol.* 59:136–141, 1977.
In a single dose, double-blind crossover study with 200 mg of salbutamol and 40 mg of SCH-1000 (ipratropium bromide), salbutamol was found to be more effective than SCH-1000 during the initial 3 hours following the drug administration. There was no significant difference in effectiveness of both the drugs thereafter. SCH-1000 was effective both in atopic and nonatopic asthmatic patients.

Ruffin, R. E., et al.   Combination bronchodilator therapy in asthma. *J. Allergy Clin. Immunol.* 69:60–65, 1982.
In a double-blind crossover placebo controlled study, the combination of 60 mg of ipratropium bromide and 200 mg of fenoterol had a greater bronchodilator effect than either drug alone.

Tinkelman, D. G., Cavanaugh, M. J., and Cooper, D. M.   Inhibition of exercise-induced bronchospasm by atropine. *Am. Rev. Respir. Dis.* 114:87–94, 1976.
Prior treatment with nebulized atropine sulfate (0.1 mg/kg) blocked exercise-induced bronchospasm in 17 of the 18 children with exercise-induced asthma.

Weiner, N.   Atropine, Scopolamine and Related Antimuscarinic Drugs. In A. G. Gilman,

L. S. Goodman, and A. Gilman (Eds.), *The Pharmacological Basis of Therapeutics,* 6th edition. New York: Macmillan, 1980. Pp. 120–137.
A detailed review of various pharmacologic actions of systemically administered anticholinergic agents and their adverse effects on various systems.

Yeung, R., Nolan, G. M., and Levison, H.   Comparison of the effects of inhaled SCH-1000 and fenoterol on exercise induced bronchospasm in children. *Pediatrics* 66:109–114, 1980.
SCH-1000 was found to be less effective than fenoterol in controlling exercise-induced bronchospasm. It was found to be effective mainly in patients with less abnormal pulmonary functions and mild to moderately severe exercise-induced bronchospasm.

34. CORTICOSTEROIDS
Gerald L. Goldstein

Corticosteroids are effective in controlling symptoms of inflammatory and allergic diseases. Although the precise mechanisms of action in asthma and allergic disease are still unknown, there is considerable knowledge about the role of steroids in the inhibition of the immune response. Small doses of steroids suppress cell-mediated immunity; however, even large doses of steroids do not seem to affect the antibody response to an antigen. Steroids also affect the immune response by decreasing cellular migration, thereby reducing the accumulation of inflammatory cells at sites of inflammation, and by increasing the resistance of the capillary wall. Steroids inhibit prostaglandin formation by inhibiting the release of arachidonic acid from cell membranes. Steroids may also decrease production of mediators, potentiate the effect of catecholamines on cyclic adenosine monophosphate (cAMP) production, and decrease catabolism of cAMP. The end result of these actions is less edema, less accumulation of inflammatory cells, and less mucus formation.

Asthma
Corticosteroids have a potent, if gradual, antiasthmatic effect. In part this is due to decreased inflammation and mucus formation in the bronchi for the reasons already discussed. In addition, corticosteroids probably increase the cellular response to beta$_2$-adrenergic medications, and they may also decrease cholinergic reactivity. Corticosteroids may also stabilize mast cells and thus inhibit the release of mediators that can cause bronchoconstriction. A direct relaxation effect on smooth muscles has also been suggested.

Corticosteroids are indicated as adjunctive therapy in acute severe exacerbations of asthma that are not adequately controlled with optimal bronchodilator medications. This category includes all patients requiring hospitalization for the treatment of status asthmaticus. Early and aggressive use of systemic corticosteroids in the hospitalized patient reduces morbidity and may reduce mortality from the asthma attack. In view of the negligible risks associated with a short "burst" of high-dose corticosteroids and the 6 to 12 hours needed for response to occur, there is no reason to wait to see how the patient will do without them. An adequate dosage schedule for the hospitalized patient is methylprednisolone sodium succinate (Solu-Medrol), 1 mg/kg I.V. every 6 hours, or equivalent doses of another injectable corticosteroid. Higher doses do not seem to provide any additional benefit.

Short courses of high-dose steroids are also used on an outpatient basis to treat acute attacks not responding adequately to bronchodilators. In patients who have required frequent hospitalizations or emergency room visits, the early use of corticosteroids, before the attack is out of control, can often prevent a severe asthma attack. Ideally the patient should be seen prior to beginning corticosteroids so that the severity of the asthma can be assessed; then, if needed, immediate relief can be obtained with inhaled or injected bronchodilators. At this time, the presence of any concurrent infectious process (e.g., otitis media) can also be identified and treated along with the asthma. If a patient or parent is well educated and reliable, and the physician is satisfied that the asthma has not yet reached the point of requiring immediate relief but that it is getting progressively worse in spite of adequate nonsteroid medications, then corticosteroids may be started after a telephone consultation. There should be specific instructions for the patient to call back if there is increased respiratory distress, and the patient should be checked within the next 24 hours. Again, an adequate dose should be prescribed. There are few dose-related side effects for short-term use, although psychosis, hypertension, and sodium retention may occasionally be seen. Prednisone, 2 mg/kg/day, or its equivalent (up to a maximum of 60 mg/day), given in two or three divided doses for 3 to 5 days is generally adequate. It is important not to discontinue the steroids too quickly or the asthma may relapse. Ideally they should be discontinued when pulmonary functions have normalized. A brief 3- to 5-day course of corticosteroids even in high doses can be discontinued abruptly. A rapid taper may be used if 1 to 2 weeks of therapy have been required.

Although generally mild and transient, there are a few possible adverse effects from even brief courses of corticosteroids. Fluid retention with weight gain, edema, and decompensation of borderline congestive heart failure are possible. Thus, patients should be cautioned to reduce salt consumption. Elevated blood pressure may also result from fluid retention. Hypokalemia may be aggravated in patients taking diuretics. Occasionally depression, euphoria, or psychosis may accompany even short courses of high-dose steroids. Transient hyperglycemia and glycosuria, acute abdominal pain, and GI bleeding are other potential side effects. Loss of intradermal reactivity to purified protein derivative (PPD) in patients treated with as little as 1 mg/kg/day of prednisone for more than 4 days may occur, although this reaction usually requires about 2 weeks. The reactivity returns to presteroid levels within 1 week after steroids have been discontinued when the duration of steroid therapy was a week or less. There is no evidence that an occasional short course of steroids causes steroid dependency.

Prophylactic Steroids

Patients known, or suspected, to be unable to respond to stress with adequate endogenous cortisol output need to be made aware of the potential for adrenal crisis if subjected to stressful situations. Patients in this category are those on maintenance steroids, those who had been on long-term steroids but then had the steroids discontinued in the previous 9 months, or those who had completed a short course of high-dose steroids in the previous 2 weeks. In addition to understanding the potential risks, these patients should carry some identification of their risk (e.g., a bracelet or card). Adequate steroid coverage should be given to these patients in the event of an acute stressful situation, such as severe trauma, surgery, or a severe medical illness such as a gastroenteritis with loss of large amounts of fluids and electrolytes. Hydrocortisone hemisuccinate should be given intravenously every 6 hours. The dose should be in the range of 200 to 400 mg of hydrocortisone for adults, 25 mg for infants, and 75 mg for older children, and may be decreased rapidly as the stressful situation is resolved.

Severe anaphylactoid reactions to **iodinated radiocontrast dyes** are unpredictable and are not dose related. Patients who have had a systemic reaction are at increased risk to have a repeat reaction. If a repeat procedure is required, then prednisone, 50 mg (1 mg/kg in children) every 6 hours for three doses prior to the procedure is recommended. The last dose should be 1 hour prior to the procedure in conjunction with 50 mg IM diphenhydramine and 300 mg p.o. cimetidine. This regimen has been successful in preventing severe reactions in more than 90% of patients with a history of a previous severe anaphylactoid reaction. Those patients who did have a repeat reaction generally had only mild symptoms.

Occasionally the use of short-term high-dose systemic steroids may be justified to control a severe exacerbation of urticaria, angioedema, or contact or atopic dermatitis. A severe case of poison ivy is an example where morbidity can be greatly attenuated by the judicious use of a rapidly tapering, 5- to 7-day course of prednisone at 1 to 2 mg/kg/day. Rhinitis medicamentosa is another case where short-term steroids are beneficial in aiding patient withdrawal from nasal decongestant dependency. Although occasionally a short burst of oral corticosteroid may be helpful as initial therapy for severe allergic rhinitis, the use of depot steroid injections to control allergic rhinitis is not justified as the potential risks of the steroid therapy can be avoided by using other more conventional forms of therapy. A short course of high-dose corticosteroids, especially in conjunction with an appropriate antibiotic (amoxicillin, 40 mg/kg/day), may be effective in the treatment of persistent otitis media with effusion.

The Boston Collaborative Drug Surveillance Program.   Acute adverse reactions to prednisone in relation to dosage. *Clin. Pharmacol. Ther.* 13:694–698, 1972.
This study showed that 16.9% of 718 hospitalized patients suffered adverse reactions attributed to their high-dose steroid therapy. Psychiatric disturbances were dose related, but gastrointestinal symptoms (especially GI bleeding and pain), hyperglycemia, and superinfection were not.

Bovornkitti, S., Kangsadal, P., Sathirapat, P., and Oonsombatti, P.   Reversion and reconversion rate of tuberculin skin reactions in correlation with the use of prednisone. *Dis. Chest* 38:51–55, 1960.
Seventy intermediate-strength (5 tuberculin units) PPD-positive patients were treated with 40 mg prednisone/day as well as streptomycin and isoniazid. The PPD became negative in 14 ± 10 days after prednisone therapy was initiated and reconverted back to positive in 3 ± 6 days after the prednisone was discontinued.

Collins, J. V., Clark, T. J. H., Brown, D., and Townsend, J.   The use of corticosteroids in the treatment of acute asthma. *Q. J. Med.* 44:259–273, 1975.
Where steroids were the only therapy used most patients reported subjective improvement after 4 hours. Pulmonary function tests begin to improve at 6 hours, with marked improvement by 12 hours.

Ellul-Micallef, R., and Fenech, F. F.   Effect of intravenous prednisolone in asthmatics with diminished adrenergic responsiveness. *Lancet* 2:1269–1270, 1975.
The authors showed enhanced responsiveness to isoproterenol after a single dose of prednisolone in 8 of 10 patients.

Greenberger, P. A., et al.   Pretreatment of high-risk patients requiring radiographic contrast media studies. *J. Allergy Clin. Immunol.* 67:185–187, 1981.
Prednisone and diphenhydramine in the described protocol were given to 318 patients with a history of systemic reactions to radiographic contrast media. There was no adverse reaction in 92.5% of patients; 7.1% had mild reactions and 0.3% (one patient) had a moderately severe reaction.

Harfi, H., Hanissian, A. S., and Crawford, L. V.   Treatment of status asthmaticus in children with high doses and conventional doses of methylprednisolone. *Pediatrics* 61:829–831, 1978.
There was no significant difference in symptom scores or peak-flow improvement between the conventional dosage group (30 mg/m²) and the high-dose group (300 mg/m²) of methylprednisolone every 6 hours.

Kattan, M., Gurwitz, D., and Levison, H.   Corticosteroids in status asthmaticus. *J. Pediatr.* 96:596–599, 1980.
In this open study there was no apparent advantage in clinical score or peak-flow improvement in patients treated with corticosteroids versus those not treated with corticosteroids. This study included children who may have had relatively mild asthma.

Kirkpatrick, C. H.   Steroid therapy of allergic diseases. *Med. Clin. North Am.* 57:1309–1320, 1973.

A general review of the immunologic and pharmacologic effect of corticosteroids and their therapeutic implications with 60 references.

Loren, M. L., et al.   Corticosteroids in the treatment of acute exacerbations of asthma. *Ann. Allergy* 45:67–71, 1980.
In this double-blind, placebo-controlled study a short course of high-dose prednisone (2 mg/kg/day) produced significant improvement in symptoms and peak-flow rates as compared with placebo within 12 hours.

McFadden, E. R., et al.   A controlled study of the effects of single doses of hydrocortisone on the resolution of acute attacks of asthma. *Am. J. Med.* 60:52–59, 1976.
The authors were unable to detect any significant benefit from a single intravenous dose of hydrocortisone in the first 6 hours of therapy.

Oppenheimer, P.   Short term steroid therapy. Treatment of serous otitis media in children. *Arch. Otolaryng.* 88:138–140, 1968.
A 9-day tapering regimen of dexamethasone was three times more effective than a decongestant alone in normalizing ear drum appearance and audiograms in a group of 162 children.

Persico, M., Podoshun, L., and Fradis, M.   Otitis media with effusion: A steroid and antibiotic therapeutic trial before surgery. *Ann. Otol. Rhinol. Laryngol.* 87:191–196, 1978.
Fifty-three percent of the patients treated with both corticosteroid and ampicillin versus only 17% of those treated with ampicillin alone were cured by both clinical and audiometric criteria.

Pierson, W. E., Bierman, C. W., and Kelley, V. C.   A double-blind trial of corticosteroid therapy in status asthmaticus. *Pediatrics* 54:282–288, 1974.
Corticosteroid-treated patients had significantly less hypoxemia than the control group although there was no difference in pulmonary function or clinical scores.

Spiegel, R. J., et al.   Adrenal suppression after short-term corticosteroid therapy. *Lancet* 1:630–633, 1979.
Most, but not all, patients treated with high-dose corticosteroids for 1 to 4 weeks had recovery of adrenal function (as measured by a rapid corticotropin test) within 7 days of discontinuing therapy.

35. CHRONIC CORTICOSTEROIDS
Gerald L. Goldstein

Asthma
Chronic corticosteroid medications are indicated for those asthmatic patients who are not adequately controlled with nonsteroidal medications. These patients may have a significant inability to participate in normal activities, and they may have frequent severe asthma attacks. Their pulmonary function testing usually reveals persistently abnormal flow rates with incomplete reversibility following bronchodilator therapy. Chronic steroid medications will often allow these patients to lead a more normal life and to have less frequent severe attacks while normalizing their pulmonary functions. The type and dose of steroid must be chosen to achieve these goals while minimizing the risk of long-term steroid side effects. It is important to recognize the possibility that steroids may not significantly improve the control of asthma in some patients, especially those with extremely hyperreactive airways. Because these drugs have so many serious side effects, especially when used in high doses over long periods of time, it is imperative that the response to these drugs be documented by symptom records and frequent pulmonary function tests—ideally a combination of peak expiratory flow rates twice a day at home (using a mini-peak flowmeter such as that manufactured by Wright) and more complete spirometry in the office.

Fortunately there are now two approaches to the use of chronic steroids that do minimize long-term side effects. The first approach is alternate-day steroids, where a single morning dose is given every 48 hours. A short-acting steroid preparation such as prednisone, prednisolone, or methylprednisolone is required. Although the initial dose for adequate control may be three times higher than that previously required on a daily regimen, the side effects are less and a gradual recovery from the side effects of daily steroid therapy will occur. Side effects are not totally absent, however, and they are dose-related, so a gradual reduction in dosage should be attempted.

The other choice for long-term steroid management is beclomethasone. Beclomethasone is a potent topically active steroid with minimal systemic effects because of nearly complete inactivation in the liver on the first pass. However, systemic effects can be observed; they are dose-related and comparable to those of alternate-day steroids. Inhaled beclomethasone is poorly tolerated during acute wheezing because of irritation of the airways. It should not be used to treat acute asthma attacks. In fact, as soon as acute wheezing begins, beclomethasone must be temporarily stopped and systemic steroids, in high doses, substituted. Failure to substitute systemic steroids for beclomethasone during acute wheezing puts the patient at risk for serious complications because the need for steroids increases with the increased wheezing and stress of illness at the same time that the effective delivery of the beclomethasone is decreased by the respiratory distress. Beclomethasone therapy should be started only after asthma has been stabilized by systemic steroids, at the time when the systemic steroids are beginning to be withdrawn. It is wise to inform the patient that other conditions, such as atopic dermatitis, rhinitis, and allergic conjunctivitis, may reappear as systemic steroids are discontinued. The initial dose of beclomethasone should be in the range of 600 to 1200 µg/day, preferably given in four divided doses, although three divided doses may be acceptable. Higher doses may be required in some patients. Again, a gradual dosage reduction should be attempted to find the minimum dosage needed to control symptoms. If the patient is not adequately controlled by one of these regimens, the other should be tried. A few patients will remain whose asthma is not adequately controlled with either regimen. Be sure that their pulmonary functions have been normalized with 1 to 2 weeks of daily high-dose oral steroids before switching to either alternate-day oral therapy or inhaled therapy. If these patients still cannot be changed to either therapy, then a combination of these two methods should be tried. The systemic side effects of the alternate-day oral and inhaled therapies will be additive but are still preferable to the side effects that occur with long-term daily steroids, which are particularly severe in children.

Allergic Disease
Topical intranasal steroid sprays are now available for the treatment of perennial and seasonal **rhinitis.** A dexamethasone spray has been available for some time but its use is limited to short-term therapy because it is well absorbed and produces sytemic side effects. The new beclomethasone (Beconase, Glaxo; Vancenase, Schering) and flunisolide (Nasalide, Syntex) sprays have been shown to be potent topically with minimal systemic effects and appear safe for long-term use at the recommended dosages.

Steroid eye drops can be very helpful for severe allergic **conjunctivitis;** however, ophthalmologic consultation is required to ensure the absence of herpes keratitis and to monitor intraocular pressure before and during therapy.

Chronic systemic steroids are required infrequently to manage severe refractory chronic **urticaria.** An alternate-day regimen at the lowest possible dose is preferred to daily steroids.

Precautions

Precautions to be employed when using chronic steroid medications include the following:

1. Because most of the steroid related side effects are dose and duration dependent, always use the minimal effective dose with frequent attempts to decrease the dose.
2. Consider the patient to have hypothalamic-pituitary-adrenal (HPA) axis suppression unless proved otherwise and treat with adequate steroids, 200 to 400 mg/day of hydrocortisone or the equivalent, during the time of acute physical stress.
3. Perform a slit lamp examination for posterior subcapsular cataracts initially and every 6 months as long as steroids are required.
4. Measure height, weight, and blood pressure regularly, and keep a growth chart for children in order to identify growth abnormalities early in the course of the treatment.
5. Check the patient periodically for glycosuria and hypokalemia. Fasting early morning cortisol levels (prior to steroid administration) should be drawn every 6 months to monitor the level of adrenal suppression. A level of less than 5 μg/dl is evidence for clearly abnormal adrenal function. Levels between 5 and 15 μg/dl may indicate partial adrenal suppression. These patients should be protected during stress (see 2).
6. Ensure adequate dietary intake of calcium and vitamin D and encourage regular exercise to avoid or minimize steroid-induced osteoporosis.
7. Check the patient's tuberculin (PPD) sensitivity before starting long-term therapy. A positive control with tetanus or *Candida* should also be placed. Recent converters, or those never adequately treated, should have a full course of antituberculosis therapy. There is no contraindication to the use of steroids for those patients adequately treated or under current therapy.
8. Steroids, if required, may be continued during pregnancy. Severe, uncontrolled asthma with hypoxemia presents a greater risk to both mother and fetus than does the use of corticosteroids. Supplemental steroids should be used during labor and delivery.
9. Try to prevent oral candidiasis in patients taking beclomethasone by having the patients rinse their mouth after use of the inhaler. Candidiasis, if it appears, can be cleared with mycostatin and usually the beclomethasone can be continued.

Ackerman, G. L., and Nolan, C. M.   Adrenocorticol responsiveness after alternate-day corticosteroid therapy. *N. Engl. J. Med.* 278:405–409, 1968.
  Adults on high-dose alternate-day therapy had a normal adrenal response to insulin-induced hypoglycemia and few cushingoid features.
Adinoff, A. D., Hollister, J. R.   Steroid-induced fractures and bone loss in patients with asthma. *J. Int. Med.* 309:265–268, 1983.
  The authors demonstrated that long-term steroid therapy in asthmatic patients is associated with decreased trabecular bone density and an increased prevalence of rib and vertebral fractures.
Bacal, E., and Patterson, R.   Long-term effects of beclomethasone dipropionate on prednisone dosage in the corticosteroid-dependent asthmatic. *J. Allergy Clin. Immunol.* 62:72–75, 1978.
  As expected, the addition of inhaled beclomethasone allowed for significant decrease in prednisone requirements in most patients.
Blodgett, F. M., et al.   Effects of prolonged cortisone therapy on the statural growth, skeletal maturation and metabolic status of children. *N. Engl. J. Med.* 254:636–641, 1956.
  Growth suppression is accompanied by inhibition of skeletal maturation, which should allow catch-up growth if the steroids can be discontinued.

British Thoracic and Tuberculosis Association.   Inhaled corticosteroids compared with oral prednisone in patients starting long-term corticosteroid therapy for asthma. *Lancet* 2:469–473, 1975.
Inhaled steroids were compared to low-dose daily steroids. Equal benefits but fewer side effects were found in the inhalation group.

Bunnag, C., Vipulakom, P., Pacharee, P., and Siriyananda, C.   Intranasal inhalation of beclomethasone dipropionate in the treatment of perennial rhinitis in adults. *Ann. Allergy* 44:100–105, 1980.
This study found good clinical response in 35 of 48 patients, expecially in those with allergic rhinitis.

Clayton, D. E., et al.   Short-term efficacy trial and twenty-four month follow up of flunisolide nasal spray in the treatment of perennial rhinitis. *J. Allergy Clin. Immunol.* 67:2–7, 1981.
In a double-blind, placebo-controlled study flunisolide was significantly more effective than placebo. There was no evidence of adrenal suppression after 2 years of continuous therapy.

Ellul-Micallef, R., and Fenech, F. F.   Intravenous prednisolone in chronic bronchial asthma. *Thorax* 30:312–315, 1975.
Peak improvement occurred 8 hours after a single IV dose, with some improvement apparent at 1 hour.

Fauci, A. S., Dale, D. C., and Balow, J. E.   Glucocorticosteroid therapy: Mechanisms of action and clinical considerations. *Ann. Intern. Med.* 84:304–315, 1976.
A panel discussion reviewed the effects of corticosteroids on various types of white blood cells.

Godfrey, S., Balfour-Lynn, L., and Tooley, M.   A three-to-five year follow-up of the use of the aerosol steroid, beclomethasone dipropionate, in childhood asthma. *J. Allergy Clin. Immunol.* 62:335–339, 1978.
Most of the children were well controlled with beclomethasone. Their growth rate was normal and no serious side effects were found.

Graber, A. L., et al.   Natural history of pituitary-adrenal recovery following long-term suppression with corticosteroids. *J. Clin. Endocrinol. Metab.* 25:11–16, 1965.
In 14 adults the HPA axis recovered in stages with high levels of ACTH appearing first and cortisol level normalizing last; 9 months were required for complete normalization.

Hahn, T. H.   Corticosteroid-induced osteopenia. *Arch. Intern. Med.* 138:882–885, 1978.
A discussion of the mechanisms of inhibition of new bone formation and stimulation of bone resorption, as well as possible therapy with vitamin D and calcium.

Harrison, B. D. W., Rees, L. H., Cayton, R. M., and Nabarro, J. D. N.   Recovery of hypothalamo-pituitary-adrenal function in asthmatics whose oral steroids have been stopped or reduced. *Clin. Endocrinol.* 17:109–20, 1982.
Excellent study on the recovery of adrenal function in 11 asthmatics in whom oral steroid treatment was reduced or stopped. Full recovery may take as long as 5 years. The authors recommend that these patients carry Medic Alert tags and receive supplemental steroids during stressful periods for as long as 5 years after stopping or significantly reducing chronic oral steroids.

Harter, J. G., Reddy, W. J., and Thorn, G. W.   Studies on an intermittent corticosteroid dosage regimen. *N. Engl. J. Med.* 269:591–596, 1963.
This study is the original description of intermittent steroid regimens. The authors found that an every-48-hour, single morning dose, was the most effective regimen with the fewest side effects.

Heimann, W. G., and Freiberger, R. H.   Avascular necrosis of the femoral and humeral heads after high dosage corticosteroid therapy. *N. Engl. J. Med.* 263:672–675, 1960.
The authors present four case reports of avascular necrosis in patients who had been on high-dose daily steroids from 3 months to 1 year. The clinical presentation was joint pain followed by limitation of mobility.

Kerrebijn, K. F.   Beclomethasone dipropionate in long-term treatment of asthma in children. *J. Pediatr.* 89:821–826, 1976.
Significant clinical improvement with minimal side effects was noted in 30 children treated for 18 months with 300 μg/day of beclomethasone.

Kershnar, H., et al.   Treatment of chronic childhood asthma with beclomethasone dipropionate aerosols. II. Effect on pituitary-adrenal function after substitution for oral corticosteroids. *Pediatrics* 62:189–197, 1978.

The authors successfully weaned 30 of 34 asthmatic children off their prednisone by using beclomethasone with excellent clinical control but only partial recovery of adrenal function.

Klinefelter, H. F., Winkenwerder, W. L., and Bledsoe, T.   Single daily dose prednisone therapy. *J.A.M.A.* 241:2721–2723, 1979.
Low-dose daily prednisone in 76 adults resulted in adequate control with partial, dose-related adrenal suppression.

Maberly, D. J., Gibson, G. J., and Butler, A. G.   Recovery of adrenal function after substitution of beclomethasone dipropionate for oral corticosteroids. *Br. Med. J.* 1:778–782, 1973.
The authors demonstrated progressive adrenal recovery over several months in patients whose oral corticosteroids were replaced by inhaled beclomethasone.

Mellis, C. M., and Phelan, P. D.   Asthma deaths in children—a continuing problem. *Thorax* 32:29–34, 1977.
A disturbing report of 5 cases which demonstrates the inadequacy of the ACTH stimulation test in diagnosing adrenal suppression.

Morris, H. G.   Benefits vs risks of corticosteroid therapy in patients with asthma. *Advances in Asthma and Allergy* 5:19–27, 1978.
The author presents a well-written review article that lives up to its title.

Morris, H. G.   Growth and skeletal maturation in asthmatic children: Effect of corticosteroid treatment. *Pediatr. Res.* 9:579–583, 1975.
Severe asthma alone may cause delayed growth, but delayed growth occurs more frequently if long-term daily steroids are taken. The bone age was delayed proportionately to the height age.

Morris, H. G., Neuman, I., and Ellis, E. F.   Plasma steroid concentration during alternate-day treatment with prednisone. *J. Allergy Clin. Immunol.* 54:350–358, 1974.
The authors found a slight but significantly decreased mean fasting cortisol level 48 hours after alternate-day prednisone dose that was not dose dependent.

Norman, P. S., Winkenwerder, W. L., Agbayani, B. F., and Migeon, C. J.   Adrenal function during the use of dexamethasone aerosols in the treatment of ragweed hay fever. *J. Allergy* 40:57–61, 1967.
Intranasal dexamethasone has sufficient systemic steroid activity to suppress adrenal function.

Oh, S. H., and Patterson, R.   Surgery in corticosteroid-dependent asthmatics. *J. Allergy Clin. Immunol.* 53:345, 1974.
With adequate preparation and steroid "coverage" these patients tolerated surgery well.

Peake, M. D., Cayton, R. M., and Howard, P.   Triamcinolone in corticosteroid-resistant asthma. *Br. J. Dis. Chest* 73:39–44, 1979.
Monthly intramuscular triamcinolone resulted in clinical and physiologic improvement in 71% of these steroid-resistant asthmatic patients, with some loss of cushingoid features.

Perlman, K., and Ehlich, R. M.   Steroid diabetes in childhood. *Am. J. Dis. Child.* 136:64–68, 1982.
Significant hyperglycemia requiring insulin may develop during high-dose steroid therapy. It is usually transient but these patients may develop diabetes, especially if there is a family history of diabetes.

Rees, H. A., and Williams, D. A.   Long-term steroid therapy in chronic intractible asthma. A study of 317 adult asthmatics on consecutive steroid therapy for an average period of 2½ years. *Br. Med. J.* 1:1575–1579, 1962.
Dramatic long-term benefits were obtained on low-dose maintenance steroids, however, side effects did develop.

Reimer, L. G., Morris, H. G., and Ellis, E. F.   Growth of asthmatic children during treatment with alternate-day steroids. *J. Allergy Clin. Immunol.* 55:224–231, 1975.
Successful low-dose (less than 15 mg q.o.d.), alternate-day prednisone allowed catch-up growth, while high-dose therapy (greater than 20 mg q.o.d.) caused further growth suppression.

Rooklin, A. R., et al.   Posterior subcapsular cataracts in steroid-requiring asthmatic children. *J. Allergy Clin. Immunol.* 63:383–386, 1979.
Risk of cataracts correlated with dose and presence of growth suppression. Two cases reversed when inhaled beclomethasone was substituted for oral steroids.

Toogood, J. H., Jennings, B., Greenway, R. W., and Chuang, L.   Candidiasis and dysphonia complicating beclomethasone treatment of asthma. *J. Allergy Clin. Immunol.* 65:145–153, 1980.

In 34 patients the risk of thrush and dysphonia was related to dosage and voice stress; however, there was no need to discontinue therapy.

Vogt, F. C.   The incidence of oral candidiasis with the use of inhaled corticosteroids. *Ann. Allergy* 43:205–210, 1979.
Vogt reviewed the literature and found that the incidence of thrush ranged from 4.5 to 13%, and was observed less often in children than in adults.

Wyatt, R., Waschek, J., Weinberger, M., and Sherman, B.   Effects of inhaled beclomethasone dipropionate and alternate-day prednisone on pituitary-adrenal function in children with chronic asthma. *N. Engl. J. Med.* 299:1387–1392, 1978.
Both dosage regimens caused similar partial adrenal suppression. When used together the adrenal suppression effect was additive.

36. MACROLIDE ANTIBIOTICS
Manon Brenner

Macrolide antibiotics, represented by erythromycin base and its various salts (ethyl-succinate, stearate, and estolate), have been used for many years in the treatment of gram-positive infections. With new epidemiologic data concerning *Mycoplasma, Legionella, Campylobacter,* and *Chlamydia* infections, erythromycin, which has been shown to be effective against these organisms, has been used increasingly in both adult and pediatric practice.

Erythromycin is now the drug of choice for clinically suspected *Chlamydia* or *Mycoplasma* infection of the respiratory tract. The asthmatic child in status asthmaticus thought to be secondary to a lower respiratory tract infection is frequently treated empirically with erythromycin when *Chlamydia, Mycoplasma,* or an unrelated bacterial illness is suspected. Because children with wheezing associated with respiratory illnesses are occasionally given a theophylline preparation during their acute illness, and children with asthma are frequently taking maintenance theophylline, clinicians should be aware of the effect of erythromycin on theophylline metabolism (described later in the chapter).

Troleandomycin (TAO) is another macrolide antibiotic that was developed originally in 1957 to treat gram-positive infections. Although not often used as an antibiotic because of its hepatic toxicity, TAO has been used occasionally for a number of years in the treatment of severe adult and adolescent asthmatic patients. TAO has a similar effect on theophylline metabolism as erythromycin, and, as shown recently, interacts with methylprednisolone as well.

The first report of **theophylline toxicity** associated with erythromycin therapy appeared in 1977. Investigators measured theophylline levels prospectively in children taking round-the-clock theophylline who were then placed on various erythromycin preparations for respiratory infections. Four of eleven patients showed significant elevations in theophylline levels while taking erythromycin: two with the stearate, one with the ethyl-succinate, and one with the estolate salt.

Since 1977, three other groups of investigators have performed formal pharmacokinetic studies measuring plasma clearance of theophylline before and after a 7- to 10-day course of erythromycin ethyl-succinate or base. All three groups found a 12 to 26% decrease in theophylline clearance, associated with a concomitant increase in serum theophylline concentration, after a standard course of erythromycin. These studies were performed in persons who were not ill at the time of investigation, excluding the possibility that infection or fever was the cause of decreased theophylline clearance.

Theophylline is primarily metabolized by the liver by 1-demethylation to 3-methylxanthine. Decreased theophylline clearance has been demonstrated in other conditions that affect the liver, such as hepatitis, cirrhosis, and congestive heart failure. Erythromycin may affect the liver's capacity to metabolize theophylline by altering or competing with hepatic enzyme systems.

These studies suggest that patients whose theophylline levels are maintained above 15 μg/ml may be more susceptible to theophylline toxicity when erythromycin therapy is instituted for 7 to 10 days. It also appears that interference with theophylline clearance does not depend on the type of erythromycin preparation, nor on the presence or type of infection.

The efficacy of TAO in treating "infectious" asthma was noted in the early 1960s, and corroborated in two double-blind studies at National Jewish Hospital performed sequentially between 1967 and 1974. In the second of these studies, and the largest one to date, Spector and his co-workers (1974) showed that 85% of 74 severe adult asthmatic patients had moderate to marked improvement in their asthma when TAO was added to their regimen. This effect was shown to be independent of the antibacterial properties of TAO and thought to be caused by an unusual "steroid-sparing" effect, because clinical improvement was achieved despite a marked reduction in maintenance steroid dose.

A recent study by Zeiger and colleagues (1980) in San Diego reported a similarly positive experience in 16 steroid-dependent, severely asthmatic patients, aged 13 to 71. Fifty percent of the patients had at least a 20% improvement in forced expiratory volume in 1 second (FEV$_1$) within 2 weeks of adding TAO, and their maintenance methylprednisolone dose was decreased from a mean of 29 mg/day to 11 mg every other day. Concomitant clinical improvement was observed.

Both of these studies used methylprednisolone (Medrol) because of Spector's early observation that a few of his patients appeared to improve when TAO was added to methylprednisolone therapy, but not when it was added to prednisolone or prednisone therapy. Recent evidence has confirmed that the beneficial synergistic effect observed with TAO is specific to Medrol, and does not occur with other commonly used oral steroids. In most patients with asthma not requiring TAO, Medrol may be used almost interchangeably with prednisone on a dose-equivalent basis.

Reports in the early 1960s indicated that the use of TAO at the recommended antibiotic dosage of 250 mg four times daily resulted in marked elevations in liver enzymes, and in some cases clinical jaundice. Recent studies have shown that the use of much lower amounts of TAO—even 250 mg every other day—can cause mild, transient elevations in serum glutamic-oxaloacetic transaminase (SGOT), serum glutamic-pyruvic transaminase elevations (SGPT), and in some cases elevation of alkaline phosphatase. It appears that the hepatic enzyme elevation is dose related, does not occur at all in some patients, and is not related to clinical improvement of the asthma.

As mentioned, another side effect of TAO therapy is the reduction in theophylline elimination. Patients taking round-the-clock theophylline are in danger of theophylline toxicity if their regular theophylline dose is not reduced at the time TAO is initiated. Depending on their pre-TAO theophylline levels, the theophylline dose should probably be reduced 25 to 30%.

Recent studies by Szefler and colleagues (1980) have investigated the pharmacokinetic parameters of the TAO-Medrol interaction. These studies have shown that TAO significantly inhibits methylprednisolone elimination, with correspondingly prolonged elevated methylprednisolone levels 1 week after TAO is started. Follow-up evaluation in three patients after 1 month on TAO showed continued reduced methylprednisolone elimination even at reduced doses of TAO and Medrol. It appears then that inhibition of methylprednisolone clearance might at least partially explain the beneficial effects of TAO-Medrol therapy.

Szefler and co-workers (1982) have also recently reported that TAO has the capacity to affect other drugs metabolized by the liver, such as anticonvulsants.

The clinical implication of these pharmacokinetic studies is that the marked reduction in steroid dosage achieved with TAO may not be as dramatic as it seems. Rather, the biologic action of TAO-Medrol even at reduced dosages may result in a heightened steroid effect caused by prolongation of steroid interaction with tissues. The increased cushingoid appearance in patients treated with relatively high doses of TAO and their usual maintenance dose of Medrol can be explained by such a heightened or prolonged steroid action. On the other hand, although long-term follow-up is not yet available for many patients, cushingoid features reportedly disappear and clinical improvement remains when patients are tapered to low doses of Medrol and TAO. In addition, the studies of Itkin and Menzel (1970) and Spector and colleagues (1980) indicated that the addition of TAO produced much greater improvement than had been seen with extremely high doses of daily steroids, and they believed that adding TAO was not simply equivalent to adding more steroid.

For the present, TAO should be reserved for only those severely disabled asthmatic patients in whom all other standard pharmacotherapy combinations including high-dose steroids have failed. *Disability* as used here includes daily wheezing that precludes a normal life-style in spite of all conventional medical and psychological therapy. Patients who are still disabled on an oral prednisone dose of 20 mg daily or greater (defined here as high-dose steroid), and who have not been controlled by the addition of inhaled beclomethasone would be considered potential candidates for TAO therapy at our institution.

Before placing a patient on TAO, the as yet unknown risks of TAO and Medrol should be weighed against the known risks of high-dose steroids alone, and should be explained to the patient or parent. Because of the lack of experience with children, it has been routine on our pediatric service to obtain informed consent for use of TAO. In addition, we recommend that TAO therapy be instituted only by physicians familiar with use of steroids and where close monitoring of theophylline levels, liver enzymes, and other potential side effects are available. The potential for interactions with other drugs the patient is taking should be considered.

Given all these considerations, if TAO is to be used, we offer the following guidelines based on Zeiger's recommendations and our own experience:

1. The patient on prednisone or prednisolone should be changed to and stabilized on an equivalent dose of methylprednisolone at least 1 week prior to starting TAO
2. Maintenance theophylline dosage should be reduced 25 to 50% the day TAO is started, and a theophylline level should be obtained within 48 hours after beginning TAO. If the patient is stable, Medrol dosage might also be reduced by 20 to 25% the day TAO therapy is started, and at weekly intervals if the patients maintain their stability.
3. Baseline spirometry and SGPT levels should be obtained prior to starting TAO, with daily spirometry or peak flows and weekly SGPT obtained during the "induction of remission."
4. TAO should be started in a dosage of 14 mg/kg/day or 250 mg two to four times a day for the first week, and, based on response or elevation of SGPT, reduced to 250 mg daily in the morning (given along with the steroid dose) as soon as possible.
5. Medrol dosage may be reduced by 4 mg/week if the patient remains stable until a dose of 4 to 8 mg/day is reached. At this time, the patient should be switched to alternate-day therapy, by tripling the dose (e.g., from 4 mg/day to 12 mg every other day).

6. Once stable on alternate-day Medrol, the patient should be switched to alternate-day TAO as well; the Medrol dose should then be slowly tapered. We have not found any patient who has remained stable on less than 4 mg of Medrol and 250 mg of TAO each taken four times a day (on the same day).
7. During periods of viral infection, increased steroids have to be given as usual for several days, although if TAO is continued during this time the steroid requirements seems to be less.

These recommendations are only guidelines as long-term follow-up, especially with children, is very limited.

Both erythromycin and troleandomycin are useful macrolide antibiotics in asthmatic patients for different reasons, but should be used with caution. Any patient taking erythromycin along with theophylline preparations should be monitored carefully for signs of theophylline toxicity (i.e., nausea, headache, tachycardia, jitterness) or, preferably, have a theophylline level measured 24 to 48 hours after erythromycin therapy is instituted. Patients on maintenance theophylline, particularly those with steady-state concentrations in the upper therapeutic range of 10 to 20 μg/ml, should be particularly closely monitored, and if theophylline levels cannot be monitored, the daily dosage should be decreased by 25% during treatment with erythromycin. If these precautions are observed it is not necessary to avoid this otherwise benign and useful antibiotic.

Daily dosage of theophylline should be reduced 25 to 30% at the onset of TAO therapy. TAO should be used with great caution because of its marked effect on liver functions and its as yet unknown synergistic effect on adverse effects as well as beneficial effects of corticosteroids.

Cummins, L. H., Kozak, P. P., and Gilman, S. A.   Erythromycin's effect on theophylline blood level. *Pediatrics* 59:144–145, 1977.
  Elevated theophylline levels were found in five pediatric patients on stable theophylline doses who developed nausea and vomiting on erythromycin therapy.
Itkin, I. H., and Menzel, M. L.   The use of macrolide antibiotic substances in the treatment of asthma. *J. Allergy* 45:146–162, 1970.
  This is the earliest study comparing TAO with other antibiotics in the treatment of asthma.
Jusko, W. J., et al.   Factors affecting theophylline clearance: Age, tobacco, marijuana, cirrhosis, congestive heart failure, obesity, oral contraceptives, benzodiazepines, barbiturates, and ethanol. *J. Pharm. Sci.* 68:1358–1366, 1979.
  Presents a study of the pathologic conditions and drugs affecting theophylline metabolism.
Kozak, P. P., Cummins, L. H., and Gilman, S. A.   Administration of erythromycin to patients on theophylline. *J. Allergy Clin. Immunol.* 60:149–151, 1977.
  Four of eleven pediatric patients showed significant elevation in theophylline levels when placed on various erythromycin salts for respiratory infections.
LaForce, C. F., Miller, M. F., and Chai, H.   Effect of erythromycin on theophylline clearance in asthmatic children. *J. Pediatr.* 99:153–156, 1981.
  The authors found a 26% decrease in theophylline clearance after 7 days of erythromycin ethyl-succinate in asymptomatic asthmatic patients.
Ogilvie, R. I.   Clinical pharmacokinetics of theophylline. *Clin. Pharmacokinet.* 3:267–293, 1978.
  Ogilvie discusses theophylline pharmacokinetics.
Prince, R. A., et al.   Effect of erythromycin on theophylline kinetics. *J. Allergy Clin. Immunol.* 68:427–432, 1981.
  A 26% decrease in theophylline clearance was observed after a 7-day course of erythromycin base. The subjects were healthy adult males.
Spector, S. L., Katz, F. H., and Farr, R. S.   Troleandomycin: Effectiveness in steroid-dependent asthma and bronchitis. *J. Allergy Clin. Immunol.* 56:367–379, 1974.
  Represents the largest clinical study to date and should be read by anyone interested in using TAO both for a historical perspective and for clinical observations.
Szefler, S. J., et al.   Steroid-specific and anticonvulsant interaction aspects of troleandomycin-steroid therapy. *J. Allergy Clin. Immunol.* 69:455–462, 1982.

The effect of TAO was found to be steroid-specific, and TAO decreased the effect of certain drugs on the induction of steroid metabolism.
Szefler, S. J., et al.   The effect of troleandomycin on methylprednisolone elimination. *J. Allergy Clin. Immunol.* 66:447–451, 1980.
This is the first specific pharmacokinetic study of the effect of TAO on methylprednisolone.
Weinberger, M.   Theophylline for treatment of asthma. *J. Pediatr.* 92:1–7, 1978.
This article reviews guidelines for theophylline use.
Weinberger, M., Hudgel, D., Spector, S., and Chidsey, C.   Inhibition of theophylline clearance by troleandomycin. *J. Allergy Clin. Immunol.* 59:228–231, 1977.
This article documents the effect of TAO on inhibition of theophylline clearance.
Zarowitz, B. J., Szefler, S. J., and Lasezkay, G. M.   Effect of erythromycin base on theophylline kinetics. *Clin. Pharmacol. Ther.* 29:601–606, 1981.
A 20% decrease in theophylline clearance while on erythromycin base was observed in healthy adult men.
Zeiger, R. S., et al.   Efficacy of troleandomycin in outpatients with severe, corticosteroid-dependent asthma. *J. Allergy Clin. Immunol.* 66:438–446, 1980.
This article gives specific recommendations for management based on clinical experience with 16 severe asthmatic patients.

37. ANTIHISTAMINES
Ray S. Davis

The group of drugs most commonly prescribed in the management of allergic disorders are the antihistamines. These drugs act by binding directly to histamine receptors, thereby, blocking the actions of circulating histamine. As competitive antagonists of histamine, antihistamines are mainly "preventive" drugs and are most effective when used in anticipation of symptoms. Antihistamines can only be expected to be partially effective because many mediators besides histamine are involved in allergic disorders. In addition, antagonists, such as antihistamines, are not as potent as the more physiologic agonists such as epinephrine, which is why epinephrine is the drug of choice in allergic emergencies.

Two distinct receptors, H_1 and H_2, are now recognized as the sites on cells where histamine reacts. Manifestations of histamine interaction with H_1 receptors include vasodilatation, increased vascular permeability, and the itch and flare reaction, and are partly responsible for the clinical symptoms of allergic rhinitis, conjunctivitis, and urticaria. Major clinical manifestations of histamine interaction with H_2 receptors are stimulation of gastric acid secretions and vasodilatation. The classic antiallergy drugs are the H_1 antihistamines, which block the various H_1 receptor manifestations. H_2 antihistamines, recognized only over the last decade, act primarily by inhibiting histamine-induced gastric acid secretion, and are currently used primarily to treat peptic ulcer disease. Several research studies have demonstrated beneficial effects of the combined use of H_1 and H_2 antagonists in patients with chronic urticaria.

H_1 and H_2 antagonists often exert undesirable side effects on the central nervous system (CNS), exocrine glands, and cardiovascular system. Common CNS side effects of H_1 antagonists include somnolence and sedation; with higher doses, hyperirritability, ataxia, and even convulsions can occur. H_1 antagonists may potentiate the depressant effects of alcohol or barbiturates. Anticholinergic effects of some H_1 antagonists include drying of salivary and watery nasal secretions, antiemetic properties, antiparkinson effects, and prevention of motion sickness. Cardiovascular effects of H_1 antagonists are generally not noted when the drugs are given orally, but parenteral administration can lead to hypotension, probably from peripheral vasodilation. There is also some evidence of quinidinelike side effects from these drugs. Side effects of H_2 antagonists include headache, fatigue, dizziness, mental confusion, fever, rash, gynecomastia, leukopenia, and neutropenia.

There are five classes of H_1 antihistamines based upon chemical structures. They are the (1) ethanolamines, (2) alkylamines, (3) ethylenediamines, (4) piperazines, and (5) phenothiazines. Each category has slightly different antihistaminic potency and side effects. Keeping in mind the multitude of adverse effects, the physician must choose a drug from the appropriate antihistamine class that will be the most efficacious but have the least side effects.

Ethanolamines include diphenhydramine, which is prescribed for allergic rhinitis and for urticaria, as well as for local anesthesia. Unfortunately, the degree of sedation and atropinelike side effects predominate and are often intolerable. In fact, diphenhydramine is often used as a sedative.

Alkylamines include chlorpheniramine, brompheniramine, and triprolidine. These drugs are probably the most commonly prescribed group and often appear in over-the-counter antiallergy preparations. They appear to be well tolerated by most patients, as they have less sedative and atropinelike side effects.

Ethylenediamines include pyrilamine, mepyramine, clemizole, and antazoline. Although their sedative and atropinelike side effects are low, gastrointestinal intolerance predominates.

Piperazines include cyclizine, meclizine, cyproheptadine, and hydroxyzine. Hydroxyzine is probably the most effective drug for treatment of acute urticaria and other dermatoses such as eczema and contact dermatitis, because of its excellent antipruritic and anti-anxiety effects. Hydroxyzine has also been beneficial as a preoperative medication for surgery because of its antianxiety effects.

Phenothiazines, including promethazine and methdilazine, are also known to have predominantly soporific effects which limit their utility in the treatment of allergic disorders.

Choice of Antihistamine

Antihistamines are the most commonly prescribed drugs in the treatment of allergic rhinitis and conjunctivitis. They are generally more effective with seasonal than with perennial symptoms. Perennial rhinitis frequently responds better to combination preparations of antihistamines and decongestants. Antihistamines are also used in the treatment of nonallergic vasomotor rhinitis.

The alkylamine class is the most commonly prescribed class of antihistamines for allergic rhinitis and conjunctivitis. Drugs like chlorpheniramine and brompheniramine have minimal sedative and atropinelike side effects, and these minimal side effects are generally well tolerated after several days' use. If the soporific effects are predominant, larger doses in the evening and smaller doses during the day will often reduce somnolence.

Antihistamines are valuable in the treatment of **urticaria**. Hydroxyzine and diphenhydramine are the two most commonly prescribed drugs for the acute urticarias. Both of these drugs have also been used in the treatment of chronic urticaria but with less success. Several research studies have demonstrated that addition of H_2 antagonists to the H_1 antagonists has markedly improved the symptoms of chronic urticaria, which have been refractory to H_1 antihistamines alone. Although the research results are encouraging, H_2 antagonists are not approved for clinical use in urticaria at this time. Cyproheptadine appears to be the drug of choice in many cases of cold urticaria, possibly because of its antiserotonin and antikinin activity.

Antihistamines have not been shown to have any substantial beneficial effect on the treatment of **asthma**. They do not appear to objectively worsen asthma by the theoretical drying effect on bronchial secretions mentioned in package inserts in most patients. However, Schuller (1983) was able to demonstrate that a subset of asthmatic children did have a decrease in pulmonary function when challenged orally with antihistamines. Thus, antihistamines are generally not contraindicated in asthma. Nevertheless, a small percentage of patients with asthma do seem to worsen when they take antihistamines and the clinical course of asthma should be monitored closely when an antihistamine is added to the therapeutic regimen.

Hydroxyzine and diphenhydramine are the two most commonly used antihistamines in the treatment of **pruritic skin disorders**. In conditions such as atopic dermatitis, dermatographism, and contact dermatitis the antipruritic as well as the sedative effects of antihistamines may be beneficial.

Although epinephrine is the drug of first choice in the treatment of **anaphylaxis**, antihistamines are useful in the treatment of urticaria, angioedema, and pruritus—all three of which occur in anaphylaxis. Their effectiveness in ameliorating the cardiovascular effects, however, is disappointing. Antihistamines, both H_1 and H_2 have been used alone or in combination with corticosteroids in the prevention of allergic reactions to intravenously administered contrast media (see Chap. 52), as well as in allergic transfusion reactions to blood. Antihistamines are not beneficial in the treatment of hereditary angioedema.

Various textbooks describe a multitude of **other uses** for antihistamines, including the use of piperazines and phenothiazines in the prevention of motion sickness, the use of diphenhydramine as a local anesthetic (e.g., in teething infants) and in the treatment of parkinsonism.

Relative resistance to the beneficial effects of antihistamines is referred to as tachyphylaxis. Tachyphylaxis is often noted by patients especially during periods when their symptoms are generally worse (e.g., during the peak of hay fever season). Patients note that the amount of antihistamine that previously controlled lesser symptoms is no longer successful. Many physicians will alter the medical regimen either by increasing the daily dose of antihistamine until side effects are noted or by doubling the dose of a long-acting antihistamine taken just before bedtime so that the major side effect—somnolence—is not noted as the patient is asleep. Other physicians will try prescribing a drug from a different antihistamine class. This alternative is generally not very beneficial, but occasionally can be rewarding. When tachyphylaxis is truly present and difficult to treat, it makes more sense to withdraw antihistamines completely for 10 to 14 days, use nasal sprays or nasal steroids temporarily, and then restart antihistamines.

In general, antihistamines are safe drugs and fairly effective in allergic disorders mediated by histamine. It should be emphasized, however, that antihistamines are much more effective at preventing the actions of histamine than reversing the manifestations of histamine once they have occurred.

Carpenter, G. B., Bunker-Soler, A. L., and Nelson, H. S.   Evaluation of combined H_1- and H_2-receptor blocking agents in the treatment of seasonal allergic rhinitis. *J. Allergy Clin. Immunol.* 71:412–7, 1983.
In this study of allergic rhinitis there appeared to be a small but statistically significant additive effect of anti-H_2 to the clinical response to anti-H_1. No additional side effects were noted.
Chai, H.   Antihistamines and asthma—Do they have a role in therapy (editorial)? *Chest* 78:420–422, 1980.
This editorial is a review of the literature.
Cook, T. J., et al.   Degree and duration of skin test suppression and side effects with antihistamines. *J. Allergy Clin. Immunol.* 51:71–77, 1973.
A double-blind, controlled study comparing the efficacy of several antihistamines. Hydroxyzine suppressed skin reactivity for the longest duration (4 days) while diphenhydramine was the shortest acting (2 days).
Douglas, W. W.   Histamine and 5-Hydroxytryptamine (Serotonin) and Their Antagonists.

In L. S. Goodman, and A. Gilman (Eds.), *The Pharmacological Basis of Therapeutics* (6th ed.). New York: MacMillian, 1980. Pp. 608–646.
The author presents another classic and thorough discussion of this subject.

Feldman, M., and Richardson, C. T.   Histamine H_2-receptor antagonists. *Adv. Intern. Med.* 23:1–24, 1978.
This article is a nice review of H_2 blockers.

Fisher, A. A.   The antihistamines. *J. Am. Acad. Dermatol.* 3:303–306, 1980.
This article tells how to treat ethylenediamine- and tartrazine-sensitive persons who require antihistamines.

Galant, S. P., Bullock, J., Wong, D., and Maibach, H. I.   The inhibitory effect of antiallergy drugs on allergen and histamine induced wheal and flare response. *J. Allergy Clin. Immunol.* 51:11–21, 1973.
This article showed that hydroxyzine was very effective at inhibiting allergen and histamine-induced wheal-and-flare responses. Aminophylline, ephedrine, and prednisone were not effective.

Goth, A.   Antihistamines. In E. Middleton, C. E. Reed, and E. F. Ellis (Eds.), *Allergy: Principles and Practice.* St. Louis: Mosby, 1978. Pp. 454–463.
This chapter thoroughly reviews the topic.

Harvey, R. P., Wegs, J., and Schocket, A. L.   A controlled trial of therapy in chronic urticaria. *J. Allergy Clin. Immunol.* 68:262–266, 1981.
Nineteen patients with refractory chronic urticaria were treated with a random double-blind regimen including five drug combinations. The combination of hydroxyzine and cimetidine worked the best and improved 58% of these patients.

Howard, J. C., et al.   Effectiveness of antihistamines in the symptomatic management of the common cold. *J.A.M.A.* 242:2414–2417, 1979.
In 271 patients with the common cold, chlorpheniramine was superior to placebo.

Krausen, A. S.   Antihistamines—guidelines and implications. *Ann. Otol. Rhinol. Laryngol.* 85:686–691, 1976.
Presents an ENT specialist's viewpoint of antihistamines.

Pearlman, D. S.   Antihistamines: Pharmacology and clinical use. *Drugs* 12:258–273, 1976.
This article is a nice, concise summary with good references. The "Therapeutic Uses" section discusses the best antihistamines for clinical conditions.

Phanuphak, P., Schocket, A. L., and Kohler, P. F.   Treatment of chronic idiopathic urticaria with combined H_1 and H_2 blockers. *Clin. Allergy* 8:429–433, 1978.
Some patients with chronic urticaria may benefit from the addition of an H_2 antagonist to the regimen.

Rhoades, R. B., Leifer, K. N., Cohan, R., and Wittig, H. J.   Suppression of histamine-induced pruritus by three antihistamine drugs. *J. Allergy Clin. Immunol.* 55:180–185, 1975.
In a double-blind crossover study of diphenhydramine, cyproheptadine, and hydroxyzine, hydroxyzine performed much better than the other two.

Schuller, D. E.   Adverse effects of brompheniramine on pulmonary function in a subset of asthmatic children. *J. Allergy Clin. Immunol.* 72:175–9, 1983.
This article discusses a subset of asthmatic children in whom the use of antihistamines may be harmful.

Weinberger, M., and Hendeles, L.   Pharmacologic Management. In C. W. Bierman and D. S. Pearlman (Eds.), *Allergic Diseases of Infancy, Childhood, and Adolescence.* Philadelphia: Saunders, 1980. Pp. 311–332.
Presents a brief summary with a good table of various groups of antihistamines and their duration of action.

38. IMMUNOTHERAPY
Robert Berkowitz

Immunotherapy, injection therapy, or hyposensitization (also referred to as desensitization or "shots") has gained widespread acceptance in the therapy of allergic disorders. These terms are used to describe the method of decreasing clinical sensitivity to offending allergens by administering injections of increasing dosages of certain selected allergens to which a patient is clinically sensitive for diseases that involve IgE-mediated mechanisms. Since it was introduced by Noon as "prophylactic inoculation" against hay fever in 1911, immunotherapy has been a part of the therapeutic approach to many allergic diseases. Anecdotal experience as well as clinical trials have shown immunotherapy to be effective in modifying some disease entities (Table 28), while it is ineffective in others (Table 29).

That allergic disease can be treated immunologically was postulated as early as 1903 when Dunbar in Germany attempted to passively immunize patients suffering from grass-sensitive allergic rhinitis and conjunctivitis with specific horse antiserum directed against pollen. In 1911, Noon suggested that active immunization with grass pollen vaccine should be attempted in certain allergic patients. Working with his sister, Dorothy Noon, a botanist, who was able to collect grass pollen, he began an active immunization program for grass-sensitive allergic rhinitis subjects. Because Dr. Noon considered allergic rhinitis to be the result of a "toxin" in the pollen, his scientific rationale was predicated on the concept that the successful induction of an antitoxin might be therapeutic. Of Noon's 18 original patients, the hay fever was completely "cured" in 30%, "greatly diminished" in 35%, "diminished to a slight extent" in 24%, and brought no improvement in 12%. He also demonstrated that higher concentrations of grass pollen extract were needed to induce positive provocative conjunctival tests after immunization than before the grass pollen injections were given. Dr. Robert A. Cooke was the chief American proponent of the newly developing field of allergy

Table 28. Reactions in which immunotherapy is effective as an adjunct to avoidance and medical therapy

Type I hypersensitivity reactions
Hypersensitivity to Hymenoptera stinging insects
Seasonal allergic rhinitis
Perennial allergic rhinitis and its complications such as serous otitis media and sinusitis
Allergic component of asthma
Biting insect antigens
Desensitization of drug reactions (e.g., penicillin, insulin)

Table 29. Conditions for which immunotherapy is not indicated

Vasomotor rhinitis
Eosinophilic nonallergic rhinitis
Nonallergic asthma
Chronic urticaria
Angioedema
Atopic dermatitis
Migraine headache
Food allergy
Bacterial vaccines for "infectious asthma"
Allergic bronchopulmonary aspergillosis
Extrinsic allergic alveolitis (e.g., pigeon breeder's disease, Bagassosis, and so on)
Chronic sinusitis

at that time, and he developed the method of allergy injections that is still used by most practitioners.

As immunotherapy gained popularity, further attempts were made to clarify its mechanism of action. Perhaps the most significant contribution in this regard was again made by Cooke. In 1935 he discovered a substance in the blood of patients treated with immunotherapy that inhibited the allergic reaction as manifested by the Prausnitz-Küstner reaction. This substance was absent in the sera of untreated patients and was specific for the allergen in question. Cooke reasoned that this substance was an antibody and suggested the term *blocking antibody* to describe it.

Investigations in subsequent years have shown that specific nonreaginic, or IgG, blocking antibody is formed after repeated injections of allergen. Several investigations have demonstrated that immunotherapy is associated with other measurable immunologic changes. These include (1) blunting of the seasonal rise in allergen-specific serum IgE concentrations; (2) after an initial rise in IgE, a gradual decline over several months to years of allergen-specific IgE serum concentrations; (3) a decrease in basophilic leukocyte sensitivity to the specific allergen; and (4) development of suppressor T-lymphocytes that actively decrease the synthesis of allergen-specific IgE. No single immunologic change explains why immunotherapy induces a clinical state of relative tolerance to a specific allergen, and this remains an area of active research.

Although immunotherapy has been in use since early in the 20th century, the first double-blind controlled studies were not done until the 1950s. Most investigators have studied seasonal allergic rhinitis, although there have been some studies in patients with allergic asthma and Hymenoptera hypersensitivity. Trials to evaluate the efficacy of immunotherapy are difficult because they depend on the patient's subjective evaluation of his or her symptomatology. Other problems include lack of applicable objective physiologic measurements for some of the diseases studied, chronicity of the diseases, geographic variability, the multifactorial nature of the disease states, and the fact that allergic diseases may spontaneously remit. In addition, immunotherapy usually only modifies the disease and rarely abolishes it, making the end point of the studies imprecise.

The criteria to determine justification and initiation of immunotherapy are reviewed in Tables 30 and 31. The documentation of specific sensitivity is usually satisfied with an extensive history along with selective skin tests. Radio allergosorbent tests (RAST) or bronchial provocation challenges may help to quantify the reactions, but are often unnecessary. Assessment of allergic diseases by their severity and duration by subjective and objective criteria is done both during the initial evaluation and on careful follow-up. Prior to initiating immunotherapy, different forms of therapy including avoidance, pharmacologic therapy, and physiotherapy should be utilized to their fullest. It is also essential to consider how associated concurrent diseases may be affected by drugs that would be used prior to the initiation of immunotherapy; if adverse effects to the use of these drugs are likely, it may be necessary to use immunotherapy earlier in the treatment plan than it would be in the absence of complicating illness. After defining the disease, the pros and cons of immunotherapy, such as the expense and discomfort of years of weekly injections, should be considered prior to initiating immunotherapy (see Table 30).

Indications for beginning immunotherapy depend on the disease being treated (see Table 30). As an example, let us take the current recommendation for IgE-mediated rhinitis and asthma. Both of these diseases can result in significant morbidity. The patient should have unavoidable exposure to common inhaled allergens of clinical significance to be considered for immunotherapy. Therefore, immunotherapy should not be initiated for allergies to foods or nonoccupationally related household pets. Immunotherapy should be considered as treatment for a

Table 30. Considerations for immunotherapy of atopic disorders

Documentation of specific sensitivity
  History–temporal relation between exposure to putative antigen and appearance of symptoms
  Presence of specific IgE antibody by skin testing (puncture, dilutional ID), in vitro assay (RAST, histamine release), or provocative challenge
  Severity and duration of symptoms
    Subjective symptoms
    Objective correlates (i.e., time lost from school or work, emergency room visits, spirometry, medication usage, and so on)
    Response to conventional medication
  Coexisting illnesses (e.g., cystic fibrosis, nasal polyps, bronchiectasis, chronic serous otitis media or sinusitis, diabetes, cardiac disease)
Potential risks
  Anaphylaxis (accompanied by urticaria, asthma, shock, death)
  Symptom exacerbation, immediate or delayed
  Local reactions (i.e., immediate or delayed swellings)
  Precipitation of immunologic disorders (e.g., serum sickness ?, eosinophilic pneumonia ?, polyarteritis nodosa ?)
  Aggravation of other coexisting immunologic disorder (e.g., systemic lupus erythematosus, rheumatoid arthritis, dermatomyositis ?)
Present-day shortcomings
  Relative cost (expensive)
  Inconvenience (time and duration of therapy)
  Lack of standardized allergens
  Inability to predict favorable responders
  Determination of objective responses often difficult
    Variations in allergen exposure
    Noncompliance in recording diary cards
  Inability to establish objective parameters for discontinuation
  Not curative for respiratory allergies
  Potential of adverse reactions

Source: From R. S. Zeiger and M. Schatz, Immunotherapy of atopic disorders: Present state of the art and future prospectives. *Med. Clin. North Am.* 65:987–1012, 1981.

Table 31. Immunotherapy: current recommendations

Clinical situation	Immunotherapy indicated	
	No	Yes
IgE-induced rhinitis or asthma		
Controlled by environmental avoidance	X	
Controlled with tolerated low-risk medications	X	
Controlled with medication but intolerable side effects (e.g., urinary disturbance, hypertension, and so on)		X
Uncontrolled by environmental avoidance and medication		X
Progressively more severe and requiring more medications		X
Need for medications, that may complicate management of coexisting severe diseases (e.g., hypertension, diabetes)		X
Secondary to occupational dander (in a veterinarian, laboratory worker, and so on)		X
Secondary to foods	X	
IgE disease only in part (e.g., allergic bronchopulmonary aspergillosis)	X	
IgE-induced Hymenoptera (venom) sensitivity		
Large local reactions	X	
Mild hives	X	
Life-threatening reactions (e.g., shock, laryngeal edema, wheezing, and so on)		X
IgE-induced drug hypersensitivity		
Clinically effective alternative drug available	X	
Clinically effective alternative drug unavailable		
Non-life-threatening illness	X	
Life-threatening illness		X
Non-IgE induced disease		
Extrinsic allergic alveolitis (e.g., pigeon breeder's disease, bagassosis, and so on)	X	
Intrinsic asthma, infectious asthma, exercise-induced asthma, infectious nasopharyngitis-sinusitis, frequent URIs, eosinophilic nonallergic rhinitis, vasomotor rhinitis	X	
Rhus dermatitis	X	

Source: Modified from R. S. Zeiger and M. Schatz, Immunotherapy of atopic disorders: Present state of the art and future prospectives. *Med. Clin. North Am.* 65:987–1012, 1981.

patient's persistent respiratory tract symptoms only after there has been an inadequate response to environmental manipulation and to a trial of ordinary doses of drugs that are generally known to be safe and effective. Requirement for the more potent agents (e.g., corticosteroids) that are frequently associated with harmful side effects is further justification to begin immunotherapy. Recommended considerations for asthma, rhinitis, and other diseases are detailed in Table 31.

Methods of Immunotherapy

In practice, immunotherapy is the administration of offending allergens in increasing concentrations in an attempt to ameliorate the symptoms associated with exposure to those allergens. Immunotherapy for allergic disease consists of a series of increasing doses of allergen administered subcutaneously at progressively longer intervals for a variable duration, depending on the disease being treated. Generally treatment lasts for at least 3 to 5 years at which time a reevaluation is indicated, whether or not the symptoms have been ameliorated. The duration of benefit that patients receive after successful immunotherapy when injections are stopped is variable and unpredictable, ranging from a rapid increase in symptoms requiring reinstitution of immunotherapy, to long-term relief of symptoms. Therefore, it is advisable to stop immunotherapy to determine if the patient will remain improved without continued therapy.

The selection of allergens for immunotherapy is based on a history of allergen exposure-symptom relationships with confirmation of specific sensitivity by skin tests with appropriate allergens. In formulating a mixture of allergens to be used in treatment, the patient's sensitivity to the specific allergens to be used must be considered. Allergens to which the patient is most sensitive may limit the amount of the other allergens injected because of adverse reactions to that allergen. If the allergen to which the patient is most sensitive is injected separately from the others, this problem can be eliminated. Mold allergen extracts are notorious for causing adverse reactions in many patients and these extracts usually should be given as separate injections. High-dose immunotherapy (differing from the low dose, or Rinkel method) has been shown to be essential for obtaining an optimal response to injections. With this in mind, the dose of extracts administered should be pushed to the highest tolerated levels, the potency of extracts should be maintained by keeping them refrigerated at 4°C, and the number of constituents in an extract bottle should be limited so that each individual allergen has adequate concentration. Ten allergens, each with adequate individual concentrations, should be the largest number allowed in any mixture. To prevent loss of potency, some physicians add preservatives such as 10% glycerin or 0.03% human serum albumin or both to the most dilute extracts. Because there is no standardization of extracts, and most dilute extracts are unstable and quickly lose their potency, the initial dosages of each new bottle of extract (e.g., a new bottle of maintenance extract) are decreased by half to avoid reactions that may occur when the more potent extracts are administered. For example, consider the patient on maintenance immunotherapy who needs a new batch of extract. For ongoing therapy the patient receives 0.5 ml of 1:100 weight/volume of the aqueous extract every 3 to 4 weeks. When the new bottle is started, the patient should be given 0.25 ml of the new 1:100 bottle. The dose is then built back to 0.5 cc in 5 weekly or biweekly intervals.

Specific injection schedules differ, but two general approaches have been used: preseasonal and perennial. Preseasonal therapy consists of a treatment period of 3- to 6-months' duration immediately before the symptomatic season. Perennial treatment is given at regular intervals throughout the year. With currently available extracts, perennial treatment is usually recommended because this method allows a patient on maintenance immunotherapy to receive monthly injections throughout the year rather than requiring a patient to have more frequent injections each year during the asymptomatic time of year (preseason). In most practices compliance seems to be better with perennial therapy. Also, perennial therapy allows more total antigen to be given than the preseasonal method, enhancing the possibility that the therapy will be effective.

There are many reasons why immunotherapy may fail to be effective or may cause adverse reactions. Stock allergen extracts theoretically are extracts of single allergen sources, but standardization of commercial allergen extracts is presently based on parameters unrelated to specific antigen content. Extracting crude allergens with present technology often results in a mixture of proteins with the major antigens often being only a small fraction of the total protein extracted. Also many of the proteins may be unrelated to those causing the atopic symptoms. Other reasons for failure of immunotherapy are an incorrect diagnosis, improper environmental control, inappropriate or incomplete choice of allergens, inappropriate dose of allergens, or use of immunotherapy for conditions for which it is of little or no value.

Immunotherapy must be given under the supervision of a physician. Before an injection is given, reactions to previous dosages as well as current symptoms of the disease for which the patient is being treated should be reviewed. A disposable tuberculin syringe with 0.01-ml graduations and a 25- or 27-gauge needle is usually used for injection. After carefully checking for the correct extract and the correct dilution, the injections are given subcutaneously in the outer aspects of the upper arm. Injections are usually administered weekly during the time course in which the allergen dose is being increased. This is the standard frequency of injections but some patients are given "rush" immunotherapy with injections every few hours to once every day, or "cluster" immunotherapy technique consisting of several injections given at 30-minute intervals every 2 to 3 weeks. Once maintenance dosages are reached the interval between injections is usually lengthened. The recommended maximum interval for aqueous extracts is one injection every 3 to 4 weeks.

Although immunotherapy is relatively safe, adverse reactions are not uncommon. The most serious reaction is anaphylaxis. Because of this danger of anaphylaxis from injection of allergen and the fact that most immediate adverse reactions occur within 20 to 30 minutes of injections, patients are requested to wait in the physician's office for 20 to 30 minutes after injections. Less serious but more frequent reactions include local painful erythema and swelling and immediate or delayed exacerbation of symptoms (including rhinitis, conjunctivitis, urticaria, angioedema, and mild wheezing) within several hours of allergen administration. Once the problem is diagnosed, the adverse reactions are appropriately treated. Table 32 lists adverse reactions to immunotherapy. A common reason for an adverse reaction occurring is technical error, such as using the wrong dilution of antigen for the injection. For this reason the nurse or technician administering the injections must not be interrupted and must work in surroundings that allow for concentration. Changes in dosing schedules after adverse reactions or missed dosages are outlined in Table 33.

Because conventional immunotherapy treatment has some serious potential adverse reactions and requires repeated weekly injections of aqueous extracts of allergens, there have been many efforts to modify the extracts in order to reduce the incidence of adverse reactions as well as increase their duration of action. Polymerization of the allergens with gluteraldehyde offers the most promise; however, allergens in this form are not currently available.

This is a list of *some* of the many good reviews on immunotherapy in allergic diseases. Major differences between reviews occur because of varied interpretations of the available data.

General Reviews of Immunotherapy

Johnstone, D. E.   Immunotherapy in children: Past, present and future. *Ann. Allergy* 46:1–7, 59–66, 1981.

Lockey, R. F., and Bukantz, S. C.   Diagnostic Tests and Hyposensitization Therapy in Asthma. In E. B. Weiss and M. S. Segal (Eds.), *Bronchial Asthma: Mechanisms and Therapeutics*. Boston: Little Brown, 1976, Pp. 613–637.

Normal, P. S.   An overview of immunotherapy: Implications for the future. *J. Allergy Clin. Immunol.* 65:87–96, 1980.

Norman, P. S., and Rose, B.   Specific therapy in allergy—pro (with reservations) and immunotherapy—areas of doubt. *Med. Clin. North Am.* 58:111–133, 1974.

Patterson, R.   Clinical efficacy of allergen immunotherapy. *J. Allergy Clin. Immunol.* 64:155–158, 1979.

Table 32. Adverse reactions to injections

Type of reaction	Treatment
Local reactions Reaction associated with great discomfort Reactions that do not disappear completely within a few hours	Oral antihistamine Local application of cold
Systemic reactions Mild systemic reactions—symptoms include mild asthma, mild rhinitis Generalized reactions—symptoms include those of the disorder for which allergy treatment is being given, and can also include generalized itching, urticaria, faintness, flushing, perspiration, nausea, vomiting, pallor, cyanosis, a "thick" throat, tightness of the chest, and frank cardiovascular collapse.	Treat as a medical emergency (1) Apply a tourniquet proximal to the site of allergen injection (2) Immediately inject 0.01 ml/kg to a maximum of 0.3 ml aqueous epinephrine 1 : 1000 sc into the arm that was not used for allergen injection. This dose may be repeated at 20-minute intervals as needed. (3) Give an additional 0.01 ml/kg to a maximum of 0.2 ml epinephrine 1 : 1000 into the site of allergen injection to retard the antigen absorption (4) Inject diphenhydramine (1–2 mg/kg) IV *slowly* to a maximum of 50 mg
Specific reactions Bronchospasm Laryngeal edema Hypotension Cardiac arrest	Treatment needed to supplement the general measures Intravenous aminophylline may be given after checking serum theophylline level (if patient is on theophylline) or a dose of 5 mg/kg IV over 15–20 minutes (if the patient is not on theophylline); aqueous hydrocortisone 5 mgm/kg to a maximum of 200 mgm; oxygen. Oxygen, intubation IV fluids, vasopressors, corticosteroids Resuscitation, appropriate medications

Table 33. Alteration in dosing schedule after adverse reactions or missed doses

Local reactions (sustained for longer than a few hours)
  Negative (swelling up to 15 mm; i.e., dime size): progress according to
    schedule
  A (swelling 15–20 mm; i.e., dime to nickel size): repeat the same dosage
  B (swelling 20–25 mm; i.e., nickel to quarter size): return to the last dosage that
    caused no reaction
  C (swelling persisting more than 12 hours or over 25 mm; i.e., quarter size or larger):
    according to the schedule, reduce to ½ the dose that caused the reaction and
    increase dosage cautiously to the highest concentration unassociated with a
    significant reaction.
Systemic reactions
  Mild systemic reaction: reduce dosage to ¼ the dose that produced symptoms. If the
    lower dose is well tolerated, increase dosage cautiously by standard increments to
    tolerance.
  Generalized reactions: generally the dosage is reduced to ¼ the *last dosage that caused
    no reaction* and repeated 3 times before increasing dose according to schedule.
If the patient misses the scheduled injection by:
  1 or 2 scheduled doses: increase according to schedule.
  3 or 4 scheduled doses: repeat the last dose.
  5 to 7 scheduled doses: reduce the dose by ¼ for each missed dose over 4.

Patterson, R.   Allergen immunotherapy with modified allergen. *J. Allergy Clin. Immunol.* 68:85–90, 1981.
Patterson, R., et al.   Immunotherapy. In E. Middleton, C. E. Reed, and E. F. Ellis (Eds.), *Allergy: Principles and Practice.* St. Louis: Mosby, 1978. Pp. 877–898.
Rocklin, R. E.   Clinical and immunologic aspects of allergen-specific immunotherapy in patients with seasonal allergic rhinitis and/or allergic asthma. J. Allergy Clin. Immunol. 72:323–334, 1983.
Tipton, W. R., and Nelson, H. S.   Experience with daily immunotherapy in 59 adult allergic patients. *J. Allergy Clin. Immunol.* 69:194–199, 1982.
Zeiger, R. S., and Schatz, M.   Immunotherapy of atopic disorders: Present state of the art and future perspectives. *Med. Clin. North Am.* 65:987–1012, 1981.

Immunology of Immunotherapy Reviews
Irons, J. S., Pruzansky, J. J., Patterson, R., and Zeiss, C. R.   Studies of perennial ragweed immunotherapy. *J. Allergy Clin. Immunol.* 59:190–199, 1977.
Rocklin, R. E., Sheffer, A. L., Greineder, D. K., and Melmon, K. L.   Generation of antigen specific suppressor cells during allergy desensitization. *N. Engl. J. Med.* 302:1212–1219, 1980.

Other Reviews
Grieco, M. H.   Controversial practices in allergy. *J.A.M.A.* 247:3106–3111, 1982.
Levinson, A. I., et al.   Evaluation of adverse effects of long-term hyposensitization. *J. Allergy Clin. Immunol.* 62:109–114, 1978.
Metzger, W. J., Turner, E. and Patterson, R.   The safety of immunotherapy during pregnancy. *J. Allergy Clin. Immunol.* 61:268–272, 1978.

HYPERSENSITIVITY DISEASES

Jeffrey H. Hill

During the last half of the 19th century many physicians noted the systemic symptoms of fever, urticaria, lymphadenopathy, proteinuria, arthritis, and even sudden death that occurred in humans after the injection of antitoxin antisera from other species. During the first decade of this century, von Pirquet termed this symptom complex *serum sickness* and postulated that it was the result of the combination of patient antibodies with foreign proteins and the subsequent release of "toxic" materials. He also suggested that similar symptoms associated with infectious diseases such as scarlet fever, tuberculosis, and syphilis might be the result of the same mechanism. During the 1950s, elegant studies by several groups confirmed the hypothesis of von Pirquet and demonstrated the pivotal role of immune complexes (IC) in the development of serum sickness in animals. As a result, many clinical investigators renewed their efforts to define "immune complex diseases" in humans. Immune complexes have now been demonstrated to be of clinical significance in many autoimmune diseases, such as systemic lupus erythematosus (SLE) and rheumatoid arthritis, and in symptom complexes associated with bacterial infections (e.g., poststreptococcal glomerulonephritis, endocarditis), viral infections (e.g., glomerulonephritis associated with hepatitis B), and parasitic infections (e.g., glomerulonephritis, nephrosis associated with malaria).

Properties of Immune Complexes
The formation and pathogenicity of IC are dependent on the properties of both the antigen and antibody (immunoglobulin, or Ig) molecules involved. The IC that mediate disease are formed when polyvalent antigen and at least divalent antibody are present in similar concentrations. These IC can be formed in the circulation, in the extravascular fluid space, or in the subendothelial and subepithelial ground substance. There are also three major types of IC that do not mediate immune complex disease. (1) The IC that consist of one antigen molecule and two or fewer immunoglobulin molecules are relatively inactive biologically. Thus, monovalent antigens or monovalent immunoglobulins that do not allow cross-linking between multiple antigen and antibody molecules do not mediate immune complex disease. (2) The IC that are formed in more than five times antigen excess do not favor antigen-antibody lattice formation. (3) IC that are formed in specific antibody excess with polyvalent antigen molecules are rapidly cleared by the reticuloendothelial system and do not mediate immune complex disease.

Complement Activation
The majority of biologic activities associated with IC are initiated through the activation of complement. Pathologic IC usually consist of antigen associated with specific IgG1, IgG2, IgG3, or IgM, which activates the classical complement pathway. Aggregated IgA and IgG4, and possibly aggregated IgE, will also activate complement through the properdin pathway; however, these are special cases that will not be dealt with further in this chapter.

When antigen is bound in the antigen binding sites (Fab portion) of IgG1, IgG2, IgG3, or IgM, alterations in the configuration of the opposite end of the antibody molecule (Fc portion) occur that result in binding of C1, the initial component of the classical complement pathway, and in complement activation. Complement and Fc receptors on phagocytic cells facilitate binding and ingestion of IC by fixed macrophages in the liver, spleen, and lungs, as well as by free macrophages and granulocytes, a process that results in the release of many mediators of the inflammatory process. Complement can also directly mediate cell lysis when the IC are bound to cell surfaces, releasing more mediators. Soluble complement fragments that result from the activation of complement through the classical pathway and its amplification through the properdin pathway, mediate increased vascular permeability and chemotaxis of leukocytes. The phagocytes that respond to those complement-derived chemotactic factors also release mediators during phagocytosis of the IC. These mediators cause local damage of host tissues and are responsible for the majority of the pathologic findings associated with immune complex disease.

Detection of Immune Complexes

IC are conventionally detected in tissues by demonstrating closely associated immunoglobulin and complement with immunofluorescent staining. The distribution of immunoglobulin and complement can be regular or irregular. The regular pattern is usually associated with antibody to that tissue (e.g., the anti-glomerular–basement membrane antibody seen in Goodpasture's syndrome), whereas the irregular pattern is more likely to be associated with circulating immune complexes that have been deposited in the tissue.

Many methods for detecting circulating IC have been described. The most sensitive and reproducible depend on the presence of products of complement that have been activated by the IC (e.g., C1q assays), on binding of the Fc portions of immunoglobulin in the IC to receptors of cells added to test plasma (e.g., platelet aggregation assays), or on binding of the IC to test cells via the C3 fragments bound to the IC during activation of complement (e.g., Raji cell assay, conglutinin assay). These assays and many others are discussed in detail in the chapter references; however, a general description of the two most commonly used techniques may be helpful.

The most commonly used techniques for detecting IC are the Raji cell assay and variations of the C1q assay. The Raji cell assay uses a human B-lymphocyte cell line that originated from a Burkitt's lymphoma and is now maintained in continuous cultures. Normal B-lymphocytes have receptors for Fc and complement on their surfaces, in addition to their membrane immunoglobulinlike antigen. In contrast, Raji cells have high affinity receptors for complement but have fewer, or lower affinity, receptors for Fc than normal B-lymphocytes, and completely lack the immunoglobulinlike antigen seen on normal B-lymphocytes. Therefore, Raji cells preferentially bind immune complex–complement aggregates via the complement receptor, but have little binding affinity for native immunoglobulin. After incubation of Raji cells with the test plasma, the amount of immune complex on Raji cells is quantitated by the addition of an anti-human immunoglobulin antibody that is bound to a radioactive molecule of iodine. The radiolabelled antibody attaches to the immunoglobulin in the IC bound to the Raji cells. The amount of immune complex is then related to the amount of radioactivity detected after the Raji cells are washed. A standard curve is developed with known amounts of IC.

C1q assays take advantage of the activation of the classical complement pathway by the IC. The first protein of the classical complement sequence that binds to IC is C1q, which is the largest subunit of the C1 molecule. C1q assays can be done in several ways. The one most commonly used quantitates the amount of immune complex by testing its capacity to bind to C1q. A standard amount of purified, radiolabelled C1q is added to the test serum. After an incubation period to allow the C1q to bind, IC are selectively precipitated from the serum, leaving C1q that has not reacted in the supernatant. Similar to the Raji cell assay, the amount of immune complex is related to the amount of radioactivity detected in precipitate. A standard curve is developed with known amounts of IC.

Neither of these assays is perfect for they depend on the presence of IC that

Table 34. Diseases with immune complexes of clinical significance

Endogenous antigens
  Systemic lupus erythematosus
  Rheumatoid arthritis

Exogenous antigens
  Poststreptococcal glomerulonephritis
  Erythema nodosum leprosum
  Lepromatous leprosy
  Syphilis-associated glomerulonephritis
  Dengue hemorrhagic fever
  Hepatitis B–associated polyarthritis and nephritis
  Malaria-associated nephritis and nephrosis
  Schistosomiasis-associated nephritis
  Toxoplasmosis-associated nephritis

contain C3 fragments or IC that can bind to C1q. Using both of these assays, as well as other assays available in research labs, provides more information than using any single test, which may give false-negative results depending on the nature of the IC present in that disease. Therefore, a negative result with any single test does not mean that IC are not present in the test serum.

Clinical Significance
Many diseases are associated with the presence of circulating IC, but the pathologic significance of these IC is not always clear. Table 34 lists some of the diseases in which the clinical significance of IC is established by the following criteria: (1) circulating IC are present, (2) immunoglobulin and complement can be consistently demonstrated in diseased tissues, and (3) specific antigen or antibody or both can be isolated from circulating IC or IC deposits in diseased tissue.

SLE is probably the best and most widely studied example of human immune complex disease. The etiology of SLE is unknown, but the major pathologic findings of nephritis, vasculitis, and arthritis seem to be caused by the deposition of IC in these tissues. The antigens consist primarily of native DNA, single-stranded DNA, and DNA fragments. DNA, DNA fragments, various anti-DNA antibodies, rheumatoid factor (antibody of the IgG or IgM class that bind native IgG), and complement are all commonly detected in circulating IC, and at sites of tissue damage in SLE (e.g., kidneys, dermoepidermal junction, blood vessel walls, lungs, and so on). The activity of SLE correlates with increased levels of anti-DNA antibody and IC, and with decreased complement levels. Circulating IC frequently disappear with remission, and reappear as the first sign of relapse. It has been suggested that the most reliable assessment of disease activity can be obtained by following circulating immune complex levels, complement levels, and DNA binding.

Altenburger, K. M., and Johnston, R. B., Jr.   The Complement System and its Disorders in Man. In R. K. Chandra (Ed.), *Primary and Secondary Immunodeficiency Disorders*. London: Churchill Livingstone, 1983. Pp. 113–132.
  Presents a very helpful review of the complement system. This reference article will provide essentially "all you need to know" about complement to the student of medicine and the practicing physician.
Davis, P., Cumming, R. H., and Verrier-Jones, J.   Relationship between anti-DNA antibodies, complement consumption and circulating immune complexes in SLE. *Clin. Exp. Immunol.* 28:226–232, 1977.
  Presents evidence to support use of anti-DNA antibody titers and complement assays to monitor SLE disease activity.

Koffler, D., Agnello, V., Thoburn, R., and Kunkel, H. G.   SLE: Prototype of immune complex nephritis in man. *J. Exp. Med.* 134:169s–179s, 1971.
This article is a classic presentation of SLE nephritis and its correlation with the presence of IC, and was taken from a symposium on immune complexes and glomerulonephritis in man chaired by Dr. Koffler.

Mannik, M.   Physicochemical and functional relationships of immune complexes. *J. Invest. Dermatol.* 74:333–338, 1980.
This article is an excellent in-depth discussion of the physicochemical and functional properties of immune complexes.

Nydegger, U. E., and Davis, J. S.   Soluble immune complexes in human diseases. *C.R.C. Crit. Rev. Clin. Lab. Sci.* 12:123–170, 1980.
Exhaustive, though excellent, review of IC disease with a more basic science approach, which contains a brief review of antibody structure and characteristics important for formation of pathogenic IC, as well as an exhaustive discussion of IC detection procedures including advantages, disadvantages, and limitations of each. It also contains a comprehensive but more superficial discussion of immune complex–associated diseases.

Pussell, B. A., et al.   Value of immune complex assays in diagnosis and management. *Lancet* 2:359–364, 1978.
This articles supports the use of IC assays in the management of SLE.

Theofilopoulos, A. N.   Evaluation and clinical significance of circulating immune complexes. *Prog. Clin. Immunol.* 4:63–106, 1980.
Presents an excellent review with a clinical orientation. It contains a brief review of various IC assay techniques, characteristics, and biologic activities as well as a comprehensive discussion of immune complex– associated diseases

Winfield, J B., Koffler, D., and Kunkle, H. G.   Specific concentration of polynucleotide immune complexes in the cryoprecipitates of patients with SLE. *J. Clin. Invest.* 56:563–570, 1975
This research paper presents evidence on the nature of immune complexes in SLE.

40. INSECT STING REACTIONS
Don A. Bukstein

Honeybees, wasps (*Polistes*), yellow jackets, bald- and yellow-faced hornets, and fire ants all belong to the order Hymenoptera. The sting of these insects can produce local reactions, anaphylaxis, and more unusual vascular and neurologic reactions. Retrospective studies suggest that 0.4 to 0.8% of the population has a history of a systemic reaction. Actual statistics indicate that at least 40 deaths occur each year in the United States as a result of Hymenoptera sensitivity. Many more deaths probably go unreported. Severe reactions may occur in persons with no atopic background, although 30 to 40% of persons do have an atopic history. In two studies, 18 to 47% of patients with fatal anaphylactic reactions had a prior history of insect sting reactions.

The usual reaction to a Hymenoptera sting lasts for several hours, and consists of intense stinging, pain, swelling, and redness at the site. Swelling that extends from the sting site over a large area and lasts for several days is not always predictive of future severe reactions.

A person with multiple stings may suffer a generalized toxic reaction to the venom. Symptoms of toxic reaction are gastrointestinal upset, faintness, edema, headache, fever, muscle spasms and, rarely, convulsions and renal failure.

Anaphylactic reactions generally begin within several minutes to 15 minutes, and include generalized urticaria, angioedema, laryngeal stridor, wheezing, and manifestations of shock.

Treatment
Local reactions are treated by applying ice or a paste of meat tenderizer, which contains enzyme of papaya, or both to the site of the sting. Oral antihistamines, analgesics, and oral corticosteroids are administered in cases of extensive large, local reaction.

Anaphylaxis is treated with the following measures:

1. Aqueous epinephrine (1:1000) subcutaneously. Dosage for children is 0.01 ml/kg up to 0.4 ml for adults.
2. Careful attention to maintenance of airway patency
3. Antihistamines: diphenhydramine 25 to 50 mg orally or parenterally (never to be used as a substitute for epinephrine)
4. Oxygen
5. IV fluids and vasopressors to maintain blood pressure
6. Aminophylline IV, 3 to 5 mg/kg over 15 minutes if bronchospasm occurs
7. Corticosteroids. Corticosteroids may be helpful if one anticipates the symptoms may continue for a number of hours, even though they are not helpful in the acute situation (e.g., hydrocortisone, 100–200 mg IV every 4–6 hours or methylprednisolone, 20–40 mg every 4–6 hours).

Identification of the insect that caused the sting can be difficult; the patient's identification of the insect may be incorrect. Only one insect, the honey bee, leaves a stinger at the wound site, which can aid in identification. The stinging apparatus, complete with venom sac, remains in the victim's skin and should be scraped or flicked off with a knife blade or fingernail. The place where the sting occurred may provide valuable information. The yellow jacket is a scavenger and is often found near the ground and encountered while gardening. The hornet and the wasp are nest builders frequenting the sides of barns and houses.

Pathogenesis
Generalized allergic reactions appear to be mediated by IgE antibodies against insect venom antigens. This is supported by the following observations:

1. Skin sensitivity is passively transferred to insensitive patients with serum from Hymenoptera-sensitive patients.
2. Absorption of IgE from sensitized serum prevents the passive transfer of the cutaneous response.
3. Venom-specific IgE to a variety of venom proteins is present in sera of patients who have been stung.
4. Patients with a history of reactions to insect stings have basophils that release histamine when stimulated with the appropriate Hymenoptera venom.

Until recently it was believed that patients with Hymenoptera sensitivity reacted to allergens in the body of the insect, as well as in the venom. In the past, treatment with whole-body extracts from the insect was regarded as the only effective mode of therapy. Recently it has been established that skin tests with whole-body extracts do not discriminate between normal persons and patients allergic to insect stings. In addition, treatment with whole-body extracts do not provide any greater protection than placebo. The apparent benefit from whole-body extracts seen in the past was probably the result of the natural loss of sensitivity, which occurs in as many as 40% of people with a history of systemic reactions to insect stings.

Recent studies using specific venoms have confirmed that the venoms alone induce the allergic response. Specific venoms given as immunotherapy are 95% protective against future stings. These results led to the FDA's 1979 release of Hymenoptera venoms for diagnosis and treatment of insect sensitivity. Although proved protective, venom immunotherapy has several drawbacks, including patient inconvenience, high cost, potential toxicity, undetermined duration of effectiveness, and treatment of a disease with an unknown natural history (especially in children).

While it is still difficult to determine which patients should be recommended for Hymenoptera venom immunotherapy, the following six categories of possible candidates for evaluation for venom immunotherapy have been described in the literature:

1. Patients without a history of systemic or large local reaction, but with a positive skin test
2. Patients with a history of a large local reaction, with a negative skin test
3. Patients with a history of large local reactions, with a positive skin test
4. Patients with a history of systemic reactions, with a negative skin test (Most patients with clinical anaphylaxis do not have specific IgE detected by either skin testing or RAST.)
5. Patients with a history of non-life-threatening systemic reaction (e.g., erythema or urticaria), with a positive skin test.
6. Patients with a history of a life-threatening systemic reaction (e.g., anaphylaxis, respiratory distress, hypotension), with a positive skin test.

It appears that adults and possibly children who have had previous life-threatening reactions (category 6) are the ones at greatest risk for future life-threatening reactions and should receive immunotherapy. Investigators at Johns Hopkins University have studied children who fall into category 5 and are not being treated with venom. Preliminary data showed that patients with non-life-threatening reactions (urticaria or angioedema only) after one sting will continue to have non-life-threatening reactions (urticaria or angioedema) after subsequent stings. However, some investigators feel that a person's previous reaction to an insect sting is not a reliable indicator of severity of future reactions. Not enough data is available to give definitive recommendations on categories 1, 2, 3, or 4. It appears that patients who have had large local reactions might be more at risk to have a worse reaction in the future. Category 4 is quite worrisome and long-term follow-up of these patients is underway.

Evaluation and Treatment

The FDA recommends evaluation and treatment for only those patients who have had systemic reactions to Hymenoptera stings. Although useful data may be collected through leukocyte histamine release and RAST testing, skin testing has been found to be the most sensitive and specific method of evaluation. Although skin tests detect current sensitization (i.e., the presence of specific IgE sensitization) they *do not* predict risk or severity of future reactions.

Nevertheless, all patients with a history of systemic reactions probably should be skin tested, keeping in mind that the use of venom skin tests presents unique problems. Although some *sensitive* persons react to venom concentrations of 1 ng/ml, approximately 80% have positive skin tests at concentrations of 10 to 1000 ng/ml. Nonspecific positive responses can be induced in very sensitive normal skin at concentrations of 1000 ng/ml. There is, therefore, a narrow range between diagnostic reactions and reactions from irritant effects. Further, 35 to 40% of patients with histories of anaphylaxis and positive skin tests may not be at risk of anaphylaxis with future stings. Although rare, systemic allergic reactions during skin testing have occurred, and full precautions to treat anaphylaxis should always be immediately available.

All persons with a history of systemic reactions and positive skin test to a venom at 1000 ng/ml or less are potential candidates for treatment. Patients and family must be fully informed of treatment alternatives. They must understand that venom treatment could confine the outcome of future stings to only a local reaction. The following general considerations should be kept in mind:

1. Because treatment is greater than 95% effective in preventing reactions to single stings, there is substantial reason to treat.
2. Treatment is generally well tolerated, particularly if administered in a careful manner. Risk of systemic reactions during therapy is approximately 2 per 100 injections and can be reduced if dosage is cut one-third to one-half when large local reactions are noted during previous injections.
3. A consent to treatment commits a patient to life-long therapy. Studies underway may allow shortening of the total period. A decision to treat might be made for a young child incapable of self-administering epinephrine, but might not be made for an older child or adult who prefers to be prepared with an anaphylaxis kit during possible exposure.
4. A life-threatening systemic reaction would weigh in favor of treatment.
5. Cost and possible future unavailability of certain venoms weighs against treatment.
6. The risk of sensitization of venom protein constituents to which a patient is not already sensitive weigh against treatment.
7. If the morbidity of treatment in children proves to be as high as the morbidity of the disease, this, of course, would weigh against treatment of children.
8. Venom skin tests and RAST detect prior sensitization, but do not predict risk or severity of future reactions.

Immunotherapy causes a rise in venom-specific IgE, followed several weeks later by a rise in IgG. Some patients are protected without an IgG rise. There are a few patients who have a rise in IgG antibody, but are not protected to resting challenge. These occurrences are exceedingly rare. Passive immunization of venom-specific IgG will protect against sting reactions and leukocyte histamine release. During the first few weeks of therapy, however, until a rise in antivenom IgG occurs, patients are at greater risk than before therapy. Most studies have shown that IgE remains high throughout the period of treatment, and that discontinuation of therapy leads to a precipitous fall in protective IgG and slow fall in IgE. IgE levels during therapy are much higher than before therapy.

Although rush regimens have been advocated by some, the venom suppliers' recommendations for therapy include a 16-week schedule to reach maintenance of 100 µg/month. This maintenance dose was chosen because an average sting injects 50 µg of venom. Each venom to which a person is sensitive should be administered during treatment. A mixed vespid venom containing 300 µg/ml of yellow jacket, yellow- and bald-faced hornet venoms should be used to treat only those patients with positive skin tests to all three venoms.

Prevention and Further Treatment

All patients should be instructed in the use of epinephrine (0.01 ml/kg) whether or not they are treated with venom. When patients reach maintenance of 100 µg of venom per month, they are theoreteically protected and should not require epinephrine; however, if they are stung by an insect for which they are not receiving treatment, they still could have a serious reaction.

The prevention of stings is of paramount importance for the allergic person. The patient must avoid not only the insects, but also the habitats and items that might attract the insects, such as bright colored clothing, flowers, perfume, over-ripe fruit, and clover fields. The patient (especially the young child) should never go barefoot outdoors, and should have his or her home inspected for Hymenoptera nests. In addition, the allergic person should wear an identification tag indicating his or her hypersensitivity, and should always carry one of the commercially available insect-sting treatment kits.

The efficacy of venom therapy has been widely publicized in the lay literature, and because some allergists may be less practiced in using venom therapy for patients with *systemic* reactions and *positive* skin tests, one should refer patients to competent local practitioners if immunotherapy is requested by the patient or the patient's family. By no means, however, should a sensitive patient be left without an adequate source of care.

The fire ant, also in the order Hymenoptera, is spread over 13 southern states. It attaches to its victim by biting with its mandible, and then it stings many times with a stinger that protudes from the abdomen. Within 24 hours of a sting, a sterile pustule, which is diagnostic of the fire ant sting, appears. A significant number of systemic hypersensitivity reactions to fire ant stings occur each year. Skin tests with fire ant extracts prepared from both the whole body and venoms appear to be reliable in identifying allergic individuals. Immunotherapy with fire ant whole body extracts is apparently effective, in contrast to immunotherapy with whole body extracts with other Hymenoptera.

Numerous studies continue to evaluate problems such as required length of treatment, cross-reactivity of venom protein constituents, and diagnostic criteria (particularly for non-life-threatening and nonsystemic reactions). Close attention must be paid to changes in recommendations based upon these studies.

Benson, R. L., and Semenov, H.   Allergy in its relation to bee sting. *J. Allergy* 1:105–115, 1930.
  Presents the first evidence that skin sensitivity can be passively transferred with serum from Hymenoptera sensitive to insensitive persons; and includes the hypothesis that severe reactions to bee stings were on "allergic" basis.

Chipps, B. E., et al.   Diagnosis and treatment of anaphylactic reactions to Hymenoptera stings in children. *J. Pediatr.* 97:177–184, 1980.
  Venom therapy in 13 children was safe and effective, but long-term studies suggest that many children with preceding mild systemic reactions to insect stings are at low risk for subsequent, more serious reactions and may not require venom immunotherapy.

Green, A. W., Reisman, R. E., and Arbesman, C. E.   Clinical and immunologic studies of patients with large reactions following insect stings. *J. Allergy Clin. Immunol.* 66:186–189, 1980.
  The article assesses the potential need for specific immunotherapy in patients with large local reactions following insect stings; patients must be assessed individually.

Hunt, K. J., et al.   A controlled trial of immunotherapy in insect hypersensitivity. *N. Engl. J. Med.* 229:157–161, 1978.
  A classic study demonstrating that venom therapy was effective but that therapy with whole-body extracts was no better than placebo. After treatment with pure venom 58 patients with insect hypersensitivity could be challenged by a sting without any adverse reactions.

Lichenstein, L. M., Valentine, M. D., and Sobotka, A. K.   Insect allergy: The state of the art. *J. Allergy Clin. Immunol.* 64:5–12, 1979.
  The article is a recent review of the scientific background for the use of venom in the diagnosis and therapy of insect allergy. It reviews the extensive experience of the Johns Hopkins investigators with these venoms, outlining indications on classification and diagnosis of sting reactions, immediate and long-term management of Hymenoptera sensitivity, and some unresolved problems.

Medical Letter   22:37–38, 1980.
  Outlines the use of venom extracts in skin testing and immunotherapy to insect allergy.

Parrish, H. M.   Analysis of 460 fatalities from venomous animals in the United States. *Am. J. Med. Sci.* 245:129–141, 1963.
  Presents an epidemiologic statistical estimate of the morbidity and mortality of insect stings.

Paull, B. R., Coghlan, T. H., and Vinson, S. B.   Fire ant hypersensitivity. I. Comparison of fire ant venom and whole body extract in the diagnosis of fire ant allergy. *J. Allergy Clin. Immunol.* 71:448–451, 1983.
  The authors demonstrated that fire ant venom and fire ant whole body extract both contain relevant allergens important in fire ant-allergic individuals and that skin tests and

radioallergosorbent tests with both preparations are valid diagnostic tests for fire ant allergy.

Ramirez, D. A., and Evans, R.   Adverse reactions to venom immunotherapy (abstr.). *J. Allergy Clin. Immunol.* 65:200, 1980.
Systemic and large local reactions during immunotherapy with pure venom extracts were greatly decreased by adjustment of venom dose.

Schuberth, K. C., et al.   An epidemiologic study of insect allergy in children (abstr.). *J. Allergy Clin. Immunol.* 65:198, 1980
Many children with preceding mild systemic reactions to insect stings are at low risk for subsequent, more serious reactions and may not require immunotherapy.

Yunginger, J. W.   Advances in the diagnosis and treatment of stinging insect allergy. *Pediatrics* 67:325–328, 1981.
An excellent update that summarizes advances and new thoughts on classification and diagnosis of sting reactions, immediate and long-term management of Hymenoptera sensitivity, and some unresolved problems.

41. FOOD HYPERSENSITIVITY
Michael E. Martin

The area of food allergy is very confusing to many physicians because of the numerous anecdotal reports and unscientific observations contained in the literature. The term *food allergy* itself has become so imprecise that the term *food hypersensitivity* is preferred for those adverse reactions to foods involving immunologic mechanisms. The application of basic scientific principles, using controlled observations to obtain objective, unbiased results is critically important to the proper evaluation of suspected food hypersensitivity reactions. Only by these methods can we avoid confusion about the relationship of food to many psychophysiologic symptoms or other unrelated physical complaints. This approach can be used in clinical practice and need not be considered solely a research procedure.

Basic Principles
A brief review of immunologic principles is germane to a basic grasp of the pathophysiology of immune injury and to an adequate understanding and interpretation of immunologic tests. Sensitization occurs when antigenic materials penetrate protective barriers (e.g., skin, respiratory mucosa, or gastrointestinal mucosa) and come into contact with immunocompetent cells. In the gut these cells are present in nodules of lymphatic tissue (Peyer's patches), which lie in close apposition to a specialized epithelium at the gut lumen. In addition, the lamina propria has numerous lymphocytes (both T and B cells) and plasma cells, as well as mast cells and eosinophils. When intact antigenic material penetrates the intestinal barrier, it stimulates the production of antibody-producing plasma cells and lymphocytic memory cells. Subsequent contact with antigen in the sensitized person can lead to a variety of immunologic events including the formation of antigen-antibody complexes, complement activation, lymphocyte proliferation, direct cytotoxicity, and the release of numerous mediators from various cells involved in the inflammatory response. Ordinarily the physical and immunologic barriers at the mucosa prevent the penetration of sufficient amounts of antigen to induce any clinical response. If the barrier is weakened by disease or immunodeficiency, larger amounts of antigen can penetrate and lead to a symptomatic response. In addition, allergens absorbed may reach the circulation in sufficient quantities to stimulate clinically apparent reactions at distant sites.

Two essential concepts for the understanding of food hypersensitivity evolve from the foregoing considerations. These are the stimulus-response relationship and the concept of symptomatic versus asymptomatic sensitivity. When considering the stimulus-response relationship, it is important to enumerate the sequence of events occurring after the ingestion of a food. This sequence begins with penetration of the intestinal mucosa by antigenically intact food proteins. These antigens then come in contact with immunoreactive cells, which results in mediator release, lymphocyte stimulation, or cell damage. Finally, the effect of these responses is to produce clinically recognizable end-organ symptoms. If the quantity of antigen or the degree of sensitivity is not sufficient, this sequence of events can be broken at any point and no clinical symptoms will be observed. It should not be surprising then, that some patients may tolerate a small amount of food, but have symptoms upon exposure to a larger amount.

The second important concept, symptomatic versus asymptomatic sensitivity, is a corollary of the stimulus-response relationship. An apparent dilemma may exist between *sensitization* and the presence of symptoms. The terms *symptomatic sensitivity* and *asymptomatic sensitivity* are used to describe immunologically mediated reactions to foods that are clinically significant (symptomatic) or clinically insignificant (asymptomatic). Symptomatic sensitivity means that sensitization has been demonstrated, and that the adverse reaction has been objectively confirmed and other causes of the reaction ruled out. Asymptomatic sensitivity means that sensitization has been demonstrated, but that no reaction is observed when the food is consumed. In other words, sensitization to a food has been demonstrated by immunologic methods (e.g., skin testing, RAST, or circulating nonreaginic antibodies), but that this sensitization is of too low a degree to result in symptoms, or that too small an amount of antigen has penetrated the mucosa, so that there has been too little effect on end organs to result in a clinically apparent reaction.

Clinical Evaluation

The clinical evaluation of a patient suspected of having an adverse reaction to a food consists of a thorough history and physical examination, objective confirmation of the adverse reaction that was reported in the history, differentiation of hypersensitivity from other forms of adverse reactions to foods, evidence of specific immunologic sensitization with identification of an immunologic mechanism, and observation of the effects of elimination of the food from the diet.

A differential diagnosis is important from the onset in evaluating patients with a history of an adverse reaction to foods. In patients presenting with chronic or recurrent symptom complexes, such as rhinitis, wheezing, dermatitis, or diarrhea, a differential diagnosis may exist, with an adverse reaction to foods being only one of the possible explanations. Other patients may present with complaints of specific symptoms following ingestion of a particular food. Here, it is helpful to consider the principle categories of adverse reactions to foods: (1) deficiency of intestinal enzymes, (2) poisonous natural constituents, (3) contaminants (e.g., microorganisms, chemicals, and toxins), (4) psychological, and (5) immunologic or hypersensitivity reactions. Psychological factors, including beliefs, dislikes, or attendant feeding stresses, can greatly influence interpretation of an adverse reaction to foods and be confused with hypersensitivity reactions. These reactions may be convincingly described by good historians but are not confirmed by objective double-blind challenge.

Immunologically mediated reactions to foods are divided currently into two categories. First, **reagin-mediated** sensitivity is caused by antibodies of the IgE or IgG4 isotypes. Symptoms occur within minutes to less than 2 hours with the following manifestations: anaphylaxis, abdominal pain, vomiting, diarrhea, angioedema, urticaria, rhinitis, or asthma. Second, **nonreaginic** sensitivity reactions are mediated by antibodies of the IgG, IgM, and (possibly) IgA isotypes

Generally the time between ingestion of the food and onset of symptoms is longer than 4 hours and may be up to 48 hours or more. Clinical manifestations include vomiting, diarrhea, enteropathies, pneumonitis, asthma, urticaria, and contact dermatitis. Although the reaction may take days to become evident, the immunologic process begins as soon as the antigen comes into contact with the antibody or sensitized cells within the lamina propria.

Clinical syndromes of nonreaginic sensitivity generally take the form of enteropathies. Gluten-sensitive enteropathy (GSE) is the disease for which the most data are available supporting the process of nonreagin-mediated immunological events resulting in mucosal injury. Other syndromes include acute gastroenteropathy associated with sensitivity to cow's milk protein or soy protein, which may commonly occur in the first several months of life as intractable diarrhea of infancy. Chronic gastroenteropathy associated with cow's milk protein sensitivity can also occur. Both of these are transient problems that resolve spontaneously by 2 to 3 years of age, but serious failure to thrive may result if the diagnosis is not made. GSE and the acute and chronic forms of cow's milk gastroenteropathy have characteristic changes in small bowel morphology consisting of flattened intestinal mucosal villae with infiltration of the lamina propria with lymphocytes, plasma cells, and eosinophils. The lesions are frequently patchy in nature in the gastroenteropathy syndromes, and may even be absent in the chronic form. The literature also describes several infants with chronic pneumonitis and pulmonary infiltrates associated with ingestion of cow's milk. This disorder generally begins within the first 6 months of life and is associated with anemia and abnormally high titers of milk antibodies in serum. Elimination of cow's milk from the diet results in the disappearance of symptoms.

Diagnostic Tests

At present there are relatively few diagnostic procedures that are helpful in evaluating patients with suspected food sensitivity. The first and most fundamental step in evaluating a potential food sensitivity problem is to objectively confirm or refute the suspicion that ingestion of the food is associated with the reported symptoms. The double-blind challenge is a necessary technique to eliminate the influence of bias or imagination on the part of the subject or the observers. Also, sound observations of reactions to foods cannot be made unless the patient is free of symptoms or brought to a steady state at the time of challenge. Opaque capsules containing placebo or known amounts of a dried food can be used for children old enough to swallow the capsules. In younger children, the food is disguised in another food normally tolerated in that child's diet. Based on the child's history, the challenge food is given every 2 to 4 hours in increasing dosages, up to a maximum of 8 gm. At this point the food is added openly to the child's diet and administered in the customary manner. Generally, the use of placebo is not necessary, but if questionable results are obtained, a repeat challenge with placebo capsules is performed.

Briefly summarized, the technique of clinical double-blind testing consists of the following: (1) Eliminate suspected food from the diet for at least 1 week. (2) Provide a diet of foods rarely causing reactions. (3) Challenge with food in opaque capsules or hidden in a food known not to cause a reaction. (4) Arrange to have the subject and observers blinded to the materials being used. (5) Administer the food in increasing amounts. (6) Record the manifestations systematically. Even if the symptoms are shown objectively and unequivocally to be associated with the ingestion of a certain food, further evaluation is necessary to determine if immunologic mechanisms are responsible.

Reaginic sensitization may be detected by allergy skin testing with food extracts or by RAST. Food skin testing has been repeatedly said to be unreliable because of too many false-positive and false-negative reactions. However, several recently published studies have shown that skin testing with food extracts is clinically relevant, but requires the same verification and interpretation as skin testing for inhalant antigens. These studies have demonstrated that food extracts do not produce nonspecific irritant reactions in nonatopic control populations and that they do detect specific antibodies in the food-sensitive person. A clinically significant positive reaction is one with a net wheal of 3 mm or more in diameter by the puncture test, using 1 : 20 wt/vol concentration extracts. In a reported series of more than 200 children evaluated for suspected food sensitivity, no child older than 3 years of age with a skin-test wheal less than 3 mm in diameter had a positive food challenge. In children younger than 3 years of age, the immediate skin test may be somewhat less reliable in predicting symptomatic food sensitivity because reactions in this younger group are often nonreagin mediated. It must be remembered that a reliable and verified extract preparation must be used for proper interpretation of skin test results. Also, as previously mentioned, the presence of a positive skin test indicating sensitization does not necessarily mean that clinical symptoms will occur with ingestion (asymptomatic sensitivity).

The RAST is a radioimmunoassay that is used to measure circulating levels of IgE antibody to a specific antigen. While the RAST does detect specific IgE antibodies to food in patients who have symptomatic food sensitivity, it offers no more sensitivity or reliability than skin testing. Other considerations and limitations, such as cost and time factors, suggest that the RAST is not appropriate for routine clinical use.

Biopsies of the gastrointestinal tract offer another method for making the diagnosis of protein sensitive enteropathies. Certain limitations exist, as similar lesions of the bowel are produced by different food proteins, and some enteropathies (cow's milk and soy proteins) produce a patchy mucosal lesion that can be missed if only a single biopsy is obtained. To increase the probability of obtaining a biopsy specimen of abnormal bowel, the patient should be on a diet containing the suspected food and should be having symptoms at the time of the biopsy.

Other potentially useful clinical tests include the quantitation of circulating nonreaginic antibodies to food proteins, and tests of cell-mediated immunity to food through assay of the production of lymphokines after specific antigen stimulation of the patient's lymphocytes. Laboratory tests of investigational interest include measurements of serum complement and circulating immune complexes.

Management and Prevention

The mainstay of management in the food-sensitive patient is avoidance of the confirmed offending food or foods. It is essential in all cases to ensure that a nutritionally adequate diet is maintained. The use of an elimination diet consisting of foods rarely documented to cause sensitivity is occasionally helpful in the evaluation of a patient in whom food sensitivity may be causing a chronic problem when no specific food has been implicated. Several drugs including antihistamines, cromolyn, and corticosteroids have been used to treat food sensitivity. The usefulness of these medications is not well substantiated in the literature—except for the use of corticosteroids in some cases of intractible diarrhea in infancy. No scientific support for the effectiveness of oral or parenteral hyposensitization for food sensitivity can be found in the literature; therefore, this form of therapy is not recommended.

Another interesting and controversial area involves the prevention of atopic disease by delaying the introduction of common offending foods into the diet until later in infancy. There are a number of studies to both refute and support the hypothesis that prolonged breast feeding will decrease the incidence of allergic symptoms in children with a family history of allergy. At present, a recommendation to have mothers breast-feed exclusively for the first 6 months of life seems appropriate when there is an immediate family history of atopy. Even if symptoms of allergic disease are only delayed, they may be less detrimental to growth and development, and easier to manage when the child is older. The mother also should probably avoid excessive intake of highly allergenic foods such as cow's milk, eggs, and peanuts, because sensitization and occurrence of symptoms have been reported after exposure to food antigens through the breast milk. Two studies suggest that serum IgE measured at birth or in the first year of life can be used to predict which infant may be particularly at risk for the development of atopic diseases. Further well-designed studies are needed to determine what beneficial effect, if any, would be attained by strict antigen-avoidance diets in the early months of life.

Aas, K. The diagnosis of hypersensitivity to ingested foods. Reliability of skin prick testing and radioallergosorbent test with different materials. *Clin. Allergy* 8:39–50, 1978.
RAST was not more reliable than skin testing.

Ament, M. E., and Rubin, C. E. Soy protein: Another cause of the flat intestinal lesion. *Gastroenterology* 62:227–234, 1972.
Reviews a case of soy protein enteropathy with biopsy evidence of mucosal villous damage.

Ashkenazi, A., et al. In vitro cell mediated immunologic assay for cow's milk allergy. *Pediatrics* 66:399–402, 1980.
Cell-mediated immune assay to B lactoglobulin was shown to be a reliable test for the diagnosis and management of cow's milk protein sensitivity.

Bock, S. A. Food sensitivity. A critical review and practical approach. *Am. J. Dis. Child.* 134:973–982, 1980.
This article is a comprehensive review with detailed description of clinical evaluation including practical application of the double-blind challenge.

Bock S. A., Lee, W.-Y., Remigio, L., Holst, A., and May, C. D. Appraisal of skin tests with food extracts for the diagnosis of food hypersensitivity. *Clin. Allergy* 8:559–564, 1978.
The reliability of skin testing was established. The interpretation and verification of extracts are discussed.

Buisseret, P. Drug treatment of allergic gastroenteritis. *Am. J. Clin. Nutr.* 33:865–871, 1980.
Report of a fascinating new concept of involvement of prostaglandins in GI symptoms and use of prostaglandin inhibitors in treatment.

Chandra, R. K. Prospective study of the effects of breast feeding on incidence of infection and allergy. *Acta Paediatr. Scand.* 68:691–694, 1979.
Significantly less atopic disease was noted in group of infants with family history of atopy who were breast-fed compared with a similar group fed cow's milk formula.

Cunningham-Rundles, C., Brandeis, W. E., Good, R. A. and Day, N. K. Bovine antigens and the formation of circulating immune complexes in selective IgA deficiency. *J. Clin. Invest.* 64:272–279, 1979.
Characterizes immune complexes, with a discussion of possible pathophysiologic consequences.

Dannaeus, A., Foucard, T., and Johansson, S. G. O. The effect of orally administered sodium cromoglycate on symptoms of food allergy. *Clin. Allergy* 7:109–115, 1977.
In this double-blind cross-over study 5 of 20 patients had remarkable relief of skin symptoms while on cromolyn but overall there was no significant difference in symptom scores on and off cromolyn.

Eastham, E. J., Lichauco, T., Grady, M. I. and Walker, W. A. Antigenicity of infant formulas: Role of immature intestine on protein permeability. *J. Pediatr.* 93:561–564, 1978.
Soy protein was shown to be as antigenic as cow's milk protein; therefore, it may have limitations in the use of prophylaxis of allergic disease.

Ferguson, A., McClune, J. P., MacDonald, T. T., and Holden, R. J. Cell-mediated immunity to gliadin within the small-intestinal mucosa in coeliac disease. *Lancet* 1:895–897, 1975.
This article proposes a role for cell-mediated immunity in mucosal injury by measuring macrophage inhibitory factor production after gliadin exposure in organ culture of small bowel biopsy from a patient with GSE.

Galant, S. P. Common Food Allergens. In C. W. Bierman and D. S. Pearlman (Eds.),

Allergic Diseases of Infancy and Childhood. Philadelphia: Saunders, 1980. Pp. 211–218.
This article is a brief general review of traditional considerations in food sensitivity.

Goldbert, T. M.　A review of controversial diagnostic and therapeutic techniques in allergy. *Allergy Clin. Immunol.* 56:170–190, 1975.
The lack of reliability of leukocytotoxic test for food allergy and lack of efficacy of oral desensitization was reviewed.

Halsey, J. F., Johnson, B. H., and Cebra, J. J.　Transport of immunoglobulins from serum to colostrum. *J. Exp. Med.* 151:767–772, 1980.
The mechanism by which secretory IgA reaches mammary secretions was explored in an animal model. The findings suggest that serum IgA may be secreted in colostrum.

Heiner, D. C., Sears, J. W. and Kniker, W. T.　Multiple precipitins to cow's milk in chronic respiratory disease. A syndrome including poor growth, gastrointestinal symptoms, evidence of allergy, iron deficiency anemia, and pulmonary hemosiderosis. *Am. J. Dis. Child.* 103:634–654, 1962.
The earliest description of patients with GI and respiratory symptoms associated with multiple precipitins to cow's milk, positive skin tests, and relief of symptoms upon removal of milk from diet.

Jakobsson, I., and Lindberg, T.　Cow's milk as a cause of infantile colic in breast fed infants. *Lancet* 2:437–439, 1978.
Intriguing report of colic in breast-fed infants whose symptoms related to the mother's intake of cow's milk. Immunologic studies on jejunal mucosa biopsy specimens from infants with similar histories are reported in Austr. Paediatr. J. *13:276, 1977.*

Kjellman, N-I. M., and Johansson, S. G. O.　IgE and atopic allergy in newborns and infants with a family history of atopic disease. *Acta Paediatr. Scand.* 65:601–607, 1976.
Determinations of serum IgE in infants predicted atopic allergy.

Kjellman, N-I. M., and Johansson, S. G. O.　Soy versus cow's milk in infants with a biparental history of atopic disease: Development of atopic disease and immunoglobulins from birth to 4 years of age. *Clin. Allergy* 9:347–358, 1979.
No apparent benefit was noted by use of soy formula to decrease atopic symptoms after 5 year follow-up.

Kocoshis, S., and Grybowski, J. D.　Use of cromolyn in gastrointestinal allergy. *J.A.M.A.* 242:1169–1173, 1979.
Cromolyn afforded significant protection and may be useful in the multiple food-sensitive patients. Presents a good review of previous studies also.

Kuitunen, P., Visakorpi, J. K., Savilahti, E., and Pelkonen, P.　Malabsorption syndrome with cow's milk intolerance. Clinical findings and course in 54 cases. *Arch. Dis. Child.* 50:351–356, 1975.
Fifty-four cases reported with laboratory data and clinical course. Symptoms generally resolve by the age of 2 years but sensitivity to other food proteins are not uncommon.

Lloyd-Still, J. D., Schwachman, H., and Filler, R. M.　Protracted diarrhea of infancy treated with intravenous alimentation. I. Clinical studies of 16 infants. *Am. J. Dis. Child.* 125:358–364, 1973.
The roles of cow's milk sensitivity and the use of corticosteroids in treatment is discussed.

Matthews, T. S., and Soothill, J. F.　Complement activation after milk feeding in children with cow's milk allergy. *Lancet* 2:893–895, 1970.
Eight patients were reported with positive skin test to milk and reaction to cow's milk on challenge. All patients had a decrease in serum complement after challenge; however, results have not been reliably reproduced by others since.

May, C. D., and Bock, S. A.　A modern clinical approach to food hypersensitivity. *Allergy* 33:166–188, 1978.
This article develops a rational, scientific method for study of food sensitivity. The importance of the double-blind challenge is emphasized as only one-third of children and one-half of infants had their history confirmed upon challenge.

May, C. D., Remigio, L., and Bock, S. A.　Usefulness of measurement of antibodies in serum in the diagnosis of sensitivity to cow milk and soy proteins in early childhood. *Allergy* 35:301–310, 1980.
Quantitative measurement of antibodies to milk proteins showed a clearly higher level in children with a confirmed adverse reaction to milk.

Minor, J. D., Tolber, S. G., and Frick, O. L.　Leukocyte inhibition factor in delayed-onset food allergy. *J. Allergy Clin. Immunol.* 66:314–321, 1980.

A cellular immune component was suggested in the pathogenesis of delayed-onset food sensitivity.

Orgel, H. A., et al.   Development of IgE and allergy in infancy. *J. Allergy Clin. Immunol.* 56:296–307, 1975.
Elevated serum IgE levels correlated with atopic disease in the first 2 years of life. The limitations of clinical application are discussed.

Saarinen, U. M., Backman, A., Kajosaari, M., and Siimes, M. A.   Prolonged breast feeding as prophylaxis for atopic disease. *Lancet* 2:163–166, 1979.
This article studied 256 newborns and reached the conclusion that prolonged breast-feeding for 6 months resulted in a lower incidence of atopic disease.

Savilahti, E.   Immunochemical study of the malabsorption syndrome with cow's milk intolerance. *Gut* 14:491–501, 1973.
An analysis of immunologic processes in the serum and small bowel biopsies is presented.

Shiner, M., Brook, C. G. D., Ballard J., and Herman, S.   Intestinal biopsy in the diagnosis of cow's milk protein intolerance without acute symptoms. *Lancet* 2:1060–1063, 1975.
Pre- and postchallenge biopsies are reported to be the most helpful in establishing the diagnosis of cow's milk sensitivity.

Strober, W., et al.   The pathogeneses of gluten-sensitive enteropathy. *Ann. Intern. Med.* 83:242–256, 1975.
Describes the elegant studies of the mucosal immune response in GSE, and the association of GSE with histocompatibility antigens.

Thomas, H. C., and Jewell, D. P.   *Clinical Gastrointestinal Immunology.* Oxford: Blackwell, 1979.
This book provides comprehensive, informative chapters on immune defense of the GI tract, celiac disease, and gastrointestinal allergy.

Tomasi, T. B. Jr., Larson, L., Challacombe, S., and McNabb, P.   Mucosal immunity: The origin and migration pattern of cells. *J. Allergy Clin. Immunol.* 65:12–19, 1980.
This article is an excellent review of developmental and functional aspects of the secretory immune system.

Walker-Smith, J., Harrison, M., Kilby, A., Phillips, A., and France, N.   Cow's milk sensitive enteropathy. *Arch. Dis. Child.* 53:375–380, 1978.
Serial biopsies after milk challenge may provide definitive information for the diagnosis.

42. HYPERSENSITIVITY PNEUMONITIS
Allen D. Adinoff

The hypersensitivity pneumonitides represent a group of diffuse inflammatory diseases involving alveoli, bronchioles, and interstitium. They are caused by sensitization and subsequent exposure to inhaled organic dusts, animal or plant proteins, microorganisms, and, rarely, low-molecular-weight chemicals. Acute episodes usually resolve without residua; however, repeated exposure may progress to a noncaseating granulomatous lesion or intestinal fibrosis, leading to irreversible lung damage. The pathophysiology involves an incompletely understood interplay of various immunologic mechanisms, including humoral, cellular, and local immunity.

Hypersensitivity pneumonitis (HP) secondary to occupational exposure was first recognized by Ramazzini in 1713. In 1932, Campbell reported an acute pneumonitis in British farmers with repeated exposure to moldy hay (farmer's lung). Since then, a multitude of HP syndromes have been identified, each type labeled according to the particular exposure, condition, or etiologic agent (see Table 35).

The **pathogenesis** of HP is incompletely understood. The development of HP seems to be related to certain characteristics of the antigen, the conditions of exposure, and host susceptibility. Antigens involved in production of this disease

Table 35. Etiology of hypersensitivity pneumonitis

Antigen	Antigen source	Name of disorder
Thermophilic actinomycetes		
Micropolyspora faeni	Moldy hay	Farmer's lung
Thermoactinomyces vulgaria	Moldy sugarcane	Bagassosis
Thermoactinomyces sacchari	Moldy compost	Mushroom worker's disease
Thermoactinomyces candidus	Contaminated home humidifier and air-conditioning ducts	Humdifier lung
Thermoactinomyces viridis	Cattle	Fog fever
	Moldy cork	Suberosis
	Vineyards	Vineyard sprayer's lung
	Ventilation system	—
True fungi		
Aspergillus clavatus	Moldy barley	Malt worker's lung
	Moldy cheese	Cheese washer's lung
Cryptostroma corticale	Moldy maple logs	Maple bark disease
	Maple bark	Maple bark stripper's lung
Graphium sp.	Moldy wood dust	Sequoiosis
Pullularia sp.	Moldy wood dust	Sequoiosis
Alternaria sp.	Moldy wood pulp	Wood pulp worker's disease
Mucor stolonifer	Moldy paprika pods	Paprika slicer's lung
Penicillium casei	Cheese mold	Cheese worker's lung
Animal products		
Pigeon serum proteins	Pigeon droppings	Pigeon breeder's disease
Duck proteins	Feathers	Duck fever
Turkey proteins	Turkey products	Turkey handler's disease
Parrot serum proteins	Parrot droppings	Budgerigar fancier's disease
Chicken proteins	Chicken products	Feather plucker's disease
Bovine and porcine proteins	Pituitary snuff	Pituitary snuff taker's lung
Rat serum protein	Rat urine	—
Bat serum protein	Bat droppings	Bat lung
Insect products		
Ascaris siro (mite)	Dust	—
Sitophilus granarius (wheat weevil)	Contaminated grain	Miller's lung
Amebae		
Naegleria gruberi	Contaminated water	—
Acanthamoeba polyphaga		
Acanthamoeba castellani		
Vegetable products	Sawdust (redwood, maple, red cedar)	Sequoiosis
Unknown	Cereal grain	Grain measurer's lung
	Dried grass and leaves	Thatched roof disease
	Tobacco plants	Tobacco grower's disease
	Tea plants	Tea grower's disease
	Cloth wrappings of mummies	Coptic disease
Chemicals, drugs		
Toluene diisocyanate	Urethane foam	—
Nitrofurantoin	Iatrogenic	—
Sodium cromolyn	Iatrogenic	—
Hydrochlorothiazide	Iatrogenic	—

exert several important biologic effects, including specific humoral and cellular immune responses, nonspecific activation of complement, immune response enhancement, and tissue destruction. Apart from their antigenic properties, certain agents can also be nonspecifically irritating and may serve as adjuvants for induction of specific cell-mediated immunity. Factors that modulate host susceptibility clearly exist, as only a minority of exposed subjects contract the disease. The prevalence of atopic diseases or reactivity to common aeroallergens is not increased in patients with HP. Total eosinophil counts and IgE are typically normal. Certain HLA types appear to occur with increased frequency in patients with farmer's lung and pigeon breeder's disease.

Specific immune responses have been interpreted largely in terms of the Gell and Coombs classification. Little evidence supports the involvement of type I (anaphylactic) or type II (cytotoxic) hypersensitivity mechanisms. Much emphasis has been placed on the type III or immune complex mechanism. The presence of late clinical reactivity, complement-fixing antibodies, Arthus-type skin reactivity, and acute pulmonary vasculitis in patients biopsied early in their disease course all support the involvement of this mechanism. A type IV cell-mediated reaction is believed by some investigators to be necessary for the development of HP. Support of the involvement of this mechanism includes delayed skin tests in some patients, sensitization of lymphocytes to the antigens, lung histology showing lymphocytic infiltration with granulomas, and passive transfer of sensitivity in animal models of the disease via lymph node cells, but not serum. Local immune factors are probably important in HP, and may not parallel systemic sensitization. "Activated" alveolar macrophages are believed to act as the pathogenic focal point, serving as a functional link between inhaled antigen and production of the pulmonary lesion.

The **clinical features** of HP are similar for all varieties. The acute form usually occurs within several hours of a brief, intensive antigen exposure. Cough, fever, chills, malaise, and dyspnea, most often without wheezing, are seen, and these symptoms are often misdiagnosed as infectious pneumonia. Symptoms usually resolve within several hours to weeks unless the patient is reexposed to the offending antigen. The subacute form of HP is more common and occurs after low-dose, long-term exposure. Symptoms are insidious and resemble chronic bronchitis, with anorexia, weight loss, productive cough, and dyspnea on exertion. It is important to suspect the diagnosis at this stage, as continued exposure can lead to chronic irreversible lung damage (i.e., interstitial fibrosis and pulmonary insufficiency). The diagnosis of HP is based on the connection between antigen exposure and disease. If the exposure is occupational, for example, symptoms may begin toward the beginning of the work week or abate during the weekend. Recurrence of symptoms after returning to work from a prolonged absence may be helpful. Often, the antigen or antigen source is obscure, requiring a detailed history and careful search of the patient's home, car, workplace, school, and so on. It should also be emphasized that Table 35 lists only the known HP antigens. New offenders are discovered every year, and the astute clinician should always suspect the possibility that a previously undescribed agent may be causing the patient's symptoms. Physical findings are nonspecific and typical of a pneumonitis, often with cor pulmonale. Wheezing is occasionally found.

Laboratory studies may be a useful aid in diagnosis. Serum-precipitating antibodies directed against the antigen are found in the vast majority of patients with HP using commercially available Ouchterlony double-diffusion plates. However, a significant number of asymptomatic exposed persons will also have serum antibodies, limiting the usefulness of this test. In addition, the antigens tend to be poorly standardized. Skin testing will produce immediate wheal-and -flare reactions in most exposed patients, although specific IgE is usually not found. Late-onset (4–6 hours) skin reactions are also seen in most symptomatic, exposed patients. Skin biopsies of these reactions reveal findings typical of the Arthus reaction, with a perivascular neutrophil infiltrate, and IgG and C3 in blood vessels walls. Delayed type hypersensitivity reactions in the skin are less common. Changes in total hemolytic complement (CH50) are seen following bronchial provocation testing with the offending agent. Perhaps paradoxically, values of CH50 are increased in symptomatic patients following bronchial provocation testing, whereas the opposite is seen in asymptomatic exposed persons. Lymphocytes can be stimulated with antigen to undergo blast transformation or to produce lymphokines, such as macrophage inhibitory factor. Pulmonary function testing generally shows restriction with diffusion defects. Mild obstruction may also be seen. Chest roentgenographic findings are typical of an interstitial abnormality. Bronchial provocation testing is occasionally helpful in making the diagnosis, although false-positive reactions can occur because of impurities in the extracts. The histopathology shows alveolar and interstitial inflammation, with infiltrates of lymphocytes, plasma cells, and alveolar macrophages. Often bronchiolar involvement characteristic of bronchiolitis obliterans is seen. If patients are biopsied soon after antigen exposure, acute vasculitis may be seen with infiltrates around alveolar capillaries, and IgG and C3 within vessel walls. While most of these acute processes resolve, continued exposure can lead to the development of noncaseating granulomas and interstitial fibrosis.

The **diagnosis** of IIP rests mainly upon the clinician's awareness that the syndrome exists and that offending agents may be difficult to identify. A careful history and search for the antigen are the basis for the diagnosis. Laboratory tests may be helpful. Antigen avoidance is the most effective treatment. Treatment of HP rests mainly on identification and avoidance of the offending antigen. Protective masks are usually of little benefit in filtering the 1 to 6 μ particles. Corticosteroids are probably helpful during acute attacks. Bronchodilators are indicated if airway hyperreactivity is a component.

Barrowcliff, D. F., and Arblaster, P. G. Farmer's lung: A study of an early acute fatal case. *Thorax* 23:490–500, 1968.
Lung histology in this study suggests a type III (Arthus) reaction.
Edwards, J. H., Baker, J. T., and Davies, B. H. Precipitin test negative farmer's lung—activation of the alternative pathway of complement by mouldy hay dusts. *Clin. Allergy* 4:379–388, 1974.
In vitro conversion of C3 proactivator (factor B) to C3 activator (Bb) was shown.
Freedman, P. M., and Ault, B. Bronchial hyperreactivity to methacholine in farmer's lung disease. *J. Allergy Clin. Immunol.* 67:59–63, 1981.
In this study, symptomatic patients had greater methacholine sensitivity than exposed asymptomatic farmers, but less sensitivity than asthmatic patients.
Freedman, P. M., et al. Skin testing in farmer's lung disease. *J. Allergy Clin. Immunol.* 67:51–63, 1981.
This study is an excellent review.
Kagen, S. L., et al. *Streptomyces albus:* A new cause of hypersensitivity pneumonitis. *J. Allergy Clin. Immunol.* 68:295–299, 1981.
Presents a biopsy proved case of hypersensitivity pneumonitis from a spore-producing bacteria uniformly present in processed dirt.
Karr, R. M., and Salvaggio, J. E. Infiltrative Hypersensitivity Diseases of the Lung. In C. W. Parker (Ed.) *Clinical Immunology.* Philadelphia: Saunders, 1980. Pp. 1336–1350.
The book gives an overview of hypersensitivity pneumonitis with an extensive reference list.
Moore, V. L., Hensley, G. T., and Fink, G. An animal model of hypersensitivity pneumonitis in the rabbit. *J. Clin. Invest.* 56:937–944, 1975.
In a study of artificially induced HP in rabbits, changes in humoral and cellular immune responses were demonstrated.
Schatz, M., Patterson, R., and Fink, J. Immunologic lung disease. *N. Engl. J. Med.* 300:1310–1320, 1979.

Presents an excellent review of various types of immunologically mediated pulmonary diseases.

Schatz, M., Patterson, R., and Fink, J. Immunopathogenesis of hypersensitivity pneumonitis. *J. Allergy Clin. Immunol.* 60:27–37, 1977.
Reviews recent evidence and theories of immunopathogenesis. Clinical aspects are included.

Unger, J. S., and Fink, J. N. Pigeon breeder's disease: A review of the roentgenographic pulmonary findings. *Radiology* 90:683, 1968.
This article is an excellent discussion of the radiologic findings in pigeon breeder's disease.

Wenzel, F. J., Emanuel, D. A., and Gray, R. L. Immunoflourescent studies in patients with farmer's lung. *J. Allergy Clin. Immunol.* 48:224–229, 1971.
Lung histology in this article suggests a type II (cytotoxic) reaction.

43. ALLERGIC BRONCHOPULMONARY ASPERGILLOSIS
Don A. Bukstein

Allergic bronchopulmonary aspergillosis (ABPA) is a disease characterized by reversible airways obstruction (i.e., asthma), transient pulmonary infiltrates, eosinophilia, and fever caused by hypersensitivity response to *Aspergillus* antigens. It was first described in 1952, and hundreds of cases were reported in England within the next few years. The first cases in the United States were not published until 1968. Initially the condition was thought to be rare in the United States. Recent evidence, however, has demonstrated that the disease occurs more frequently than previously suspected, especially in patients receiving corticosteroids to control their asthma.

ABPA can occur at any age in both males and females, although most patients with clinically evident ABPA are less than 35 years of age. The incidence of new cases as well as the frequency of symptoms is increased in fall and winter months—September through March—when *Aspergillus* spore counts are high. Although the prevalence of ABPA in the United States is unknown, the disease has been estimated to occur in the United Kingdom in more than 20% of asthmatic patients admitted to a hospital for chronic chest disease. Accurate incidence figures are difficult to obtain and probably underestimate the true incidence of this disorder.

The most common species of *Aspergillus* associated with ABPA is *A. fumigatus,* though other species have been implicated. The spores of these *Aspergillus* organisms are ubiquitous in soil and decaying organic material and are present in the air in all but the coldest periods of the year. In the atopic host, *Aspergillus* colonization (not actual tissue invasion) of the airways provides a potent source of hyphal antigens. These antigens initiate an immediate IgE-mediated reaction that accounts for the acute bronchospastic symptoms of this disorder. IgE antibody must be present for this disease to occur. The reaction of the anitgen with the IgE antibody and the associated release of mediators may also act by allowing the absorption and further trapping of *Aspergillus* antigen into the tissues surrounding the airways.

Once it is absorbed, the antigen reacts with IgG-precipitating antibody that also must be present for the disease to be expressed. The antigen-IgG precipitating antibody reaction is responsible for the tissue damage that is manifested in the roentgenographic features of ABPA, as well as in the peribronchial inflammation that can lead to the destructive changes seen in ABPA (e.g., bronchiectasis).

The exact pathophysiology of this disorder is complex and far from completely understood. Long-standing inflammation from these immunologic processes probably leads to the chronic sequelae of ABPA such as fibrosis, bronchiectasis, lung contraction, and lobar shrinkage. Although specific stages of ABPA have been described, the degree of pulmonary involvement depends on a multiplicity of host factors, not yet well defined. The ultimate clinical manifestations of ABPA cannot be reliably predicted in a given patient.

Clinical Features

ABPA is an episodic, recurrent disorder that has a wide range of clinical presentations depending upon the severity of the disease. Hallmarks of the disease include reversible airways obstruction with wheezing (i.e., asthma), transient pulmonary infiltrates, peripheral blood eosinophilia, fever, elevated IgE levels, and the expectoration with cough of "brown sputum plugs." Milder cases may be mistaken for "extrinsic" asthma, while chronic cases can have symptoms more compatible with bronchiectasis and irreversible lung disease. These patients also have a high incidence of rhinitis, conjunctivitis, eczema, urticaria, and food and drug hypersensitivity.

Pulmonary function tests will reflect the current status of the disease, and can have a spectrum from pure bronchospasm to irreversible lung disease (as in ABPA-induced bronchiectasis and fibrosis). In more chronic cases, reversibility with bronchodilators is usually minimal although some reversibility is usually seen even in severe cases. Impairment of the diffusion capacity is common and usually correlates with the duration and severity of the disease.

Radiographically, there are transient pulmonary infiltrates during an acute attack. These take the form of homogeneous ill-defined densities ranging in size from patchy infiltrates to lobar consolidation with an upper lobe predilection. They are often bilateral and may recur in different areas of the lung. Transient pulmonary infiltrates may also occur in some patients without significant clinical symptoms of asthma. Chronic radiographic changes include parallel tram-line shadows representing mucoid impactions in areas of branching bronchi. Proximal saccular bronchiectasis, in contrast to the changes seen in asthma and infectious bronchiectasis, is considered by some to be unique to ABPA. Bronchography and bronchoscopy can aid in the diagnosis of saccular proximal bronchiectasis; however, these procedures must be approached with caution because of the bronchospastic potential of the agents used in such procedures.

Aspergillus obtained from bronchoscopy in multiple cultures suggests the diagnosis of ABPA. Routine sputum cultures cannot be considered diagnostic as *Aspergillus* may be found in persons with no evidence of disease.

Total IgE is always elevated during an acute attack, and may remain elevated for weeks to months. It is also helpful in monitoring the activity of disease. IgE levels often rise prior to clinical exacerbations, and will decrease with remission, whether or not steroid therapy has been used. Chronic corticosteroids may also suppress total IgE levels to below those normally seen in ABPA. But as a general rule, if the total IgE levels are normal during an actue attack the diagnosis of ABPA should be reconsidered. Specific IGE directed against *Aspergillus* antigen is usually elevated during an acute attack, but may be only 5% of the total IgE. In contrast to total IgE levels, the specific IgE falls rapidly after an acute attack. Thus, the specific IgE may aid in diagnosis when it is elevated in the more chronic corticosteroid-dependent asthmatic patient or in the fibrotic stage of ABPA when total IgE has returned to nearly normal levels.

Puncture skin testing using *Aspergillus* antigens demonstrates a positive immediate wheal-and flare reaction in all patients. Many patients will also have a positive late-phase response approximately 6 to 8 hours after skin testing. The percentage of patients with a late-phase response increases when an intradermal skin test is performed but is still not positive in all patients. There are problems in screening of suspected ABPA patients using *Aspergillus* skin tests. Antigenic

Table 36. Criteria for the diagnosis of ABPA

Primary
    Episodic bronchial obstruction
    Peripheral blood eosinophilia
    Immediate skin reactivity to *Aspergillus* antigens
    Precipitating antibodies against *Aspergillus* antigens
    Elevated serum IgE
    History of infiltrates
    Central bronchiectasis
Secondary
    Aspergillus in sputum
    History of mucous plug expectoration
    Late skin (Arthus) reactivity to *Aspergillus* antigens

Source: Modified from Rosenberg et al., Clinical and immunologic criteria for the diagnosis of allergic bronchopulmonary aspergillosis. *Ann. Intern. Med.* 86:404–414, 1977.

extracts for testing have not been standardized, and most commercial preparations are a mixture of *Aspergillus* species; thus, the *A. fumigatus* antigen is diluted by irrelevant antigens. The test also lacks specificity because as many as 40% of asthmatic patients without other evidence of ABPA have immediate positive skin tests. When it occurs, the late reaction may be more helpful in supporting the diagnosis of ABPA.

Serum precipitating antibody (precipitins) to *Aspergillus* antigen can be demonstrated in 80 to 90% of patients with ABPA by using several different methods, such as double-gel immunodiffusion, complement fixation, or counterimmunoelectrophoresis. The precipitating antibody is an IgG antibody. Because the precipitin tests also rely on unstandardized *Aspergillus* antigenic extracts, many of the same problems mentioned in skin testing also exist with these assays. There is a rough correlation with ABPA disease activity and the level of the precipitin reaction, although steroid therapy will inhibit the precipitin reaction.

Diagnosis
ABPA is a syndrome-complex with few unique pathologic or roentgenographic features. Diagnosis is often a problem because findings such as asthma, eosinophilia, positive skin tests to *Apergillus,* elevated serum IgE, pulmonary infiltrates, and precipitins are seen in other diseases often associated with ABPA. Criteria for diagnosis have varied among investigators and have been revised to accommodate new immunologic discoveries (Table 36). The first six primary signs should be present to establish the diagnosis of ABPA. In addition, bronchial challenge tests may be helpful. A suggested approach to the diagnosis of ABPA is presented in Fig. 15.

Treatment and Course
The mainstay of therapy for ABPA is corticosteroids. Steroids hasten the resolution of pulmonary infiltrates and clinical symptoms; steroids also decrease serum precipitin and IgE levels. Current recommendations for treatment include prednisone, 0.5 mg/kg daily, until the chest roentgenogram is clear, and then a tapering of the dose over several months while following total serum IgE levels to monitor disease activity. There is some evidence that the chronic sequelae of ABPA can be prevented by early diagnosis and prednisone therapy.

As in other forms of reactive airways disease, the most useful drugs to treat the bronchospasm that occurs in this disease are theophylline and inhaled beta$_2$ sympathomimetics. Cromolyn may also be useful in preventing acute bronchospasm. None of these drugs, however, including cromolyn, will prevent the

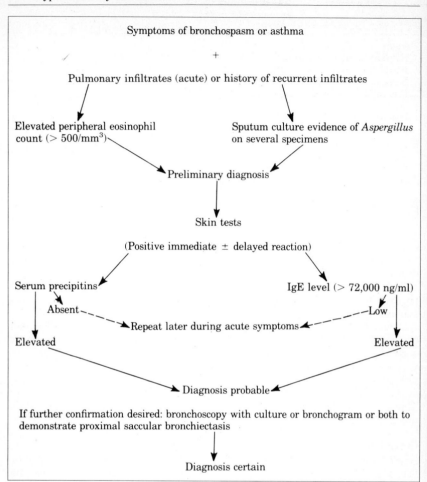

Fig. 15. A suggested approach to the diagnosis of allergic bronchopulmonary aspergillosis.

chronic sequelae of ABPA, and they should never be used instead of steroid therapy. Treatment with antifungal drugs, either oral or inhaled, and hyposensitization, have been disappointing; use of these agents probably should be avoided.

Basich, J. E., et al.   Allergic bronchopulmonary aspergillosis in corticosteroid-dependent asthmatics. *J. Allergy Clin. Immunol.* 68:98–102, 1981.
   This study suggests previously undiagnosed ABPA can be detected in populations of corticosteroid-dependent asthmatic patients. Corticosteroid therapy may mask ABPA.
Glimp, R. A., and Bayer, A. S.   Fungal pneumonias. Part 3: Allergic bronchopulmonary aspergillosis. *Chest* 80:85–94, 1981.
   This article is an excellent, brief overview of allergic bronchopulmonary aspergillosis.
Greenberger, P. A., et al.   Late sequelae of allergic bronchopulmonary aspergillosis. *J. Allergy Clin. Immunol.* 66:327–335, 1980.
   Reviews the late fibrotic sequelae of ABPA, which remain undiagnosed for years.
Henderson, A. H., English, M. P., and Vecht, R. J.   Pulmonary aspergillosis: A survey of its occurrence in patients with chronic lung disease of the significance of diagnostic tests. *Thorax* 23:513–518, 1968.

The article provides an excellent discussion of the value of various diagnostic tests in the diagnosis of ABPA.

Patterson, R., Greenberger, P. A., Radin, R. C., and Roberts, M.   Allergic bronchopulmonary aspergillosis: Staging as an aid to management. *Ann. Intern. Med.* 96:286–291, 1982.
Five stages of ABPA were identified on the basis of clinical parameters and measurements of IgE and IgG antibodies against Aspergillus fumigatus.

Pepys, J., et al.   Clinical and immunologic significance of *Apergillus fumigatus* in the sputum. *Am. Rev. Respir. Dis.* 80:167–180, 1959.
This study is one of the original descriptions of this syndrome. Skin-prick tests for A. fumigatus *were positive in all patients with* A. fumigatus *in sputum and pulmonary eosinophilia.*

Ricketti, A. J., Greenburger, P. A., and Patterson, R.   Immediate-type reactions in patients with allergic bronchopulmonary aspergillosis. *J. Allergy Clin. Immunol.* 71:54–5, 1983.
The authors showed that ABPA patients are a subset of atopic individuals with a greater predisposition for the development of a wide spectrum of allergic diseases, despite the lack of manifestations of other major immunologic disease patterns.

Ricketti, A. J., Greenberger, P. A., Mintzer, R. A., and Patterson, R.   Allergic bronchopulmonary aspergillosis. *Arch. Int. Med.* 143:1553–7, 1983.
This is an excellent review on the diagnosis and treatment of ABPA.

Rosenberg, M., et al.   Clinical and immunologic criteria for the diagnosis of allergic bronchopulmonary aspergillosis. *Ann. Intern. Med.* 86:405–414, 1977.
Clinical and immunologic characteristics are reported in 20 patients with ABPA, using the most recently revised list of criteria for diagnosis.

Wang, J. L. F., et al.   Allergic bronchopulmonary aspergillosis in pediatric practice. *J. Pediatr.* 94:376–381, 1979.
Twelve cases of ABPA in pediatric patients (aged 6–18 yr) are reported.

Wang, J. L. F., Patterson, R., Roberts, M., and Ghory, A. C.   The management of allergic bronchopulmonary aspergillosis. *Am. Rev. Respir. Dis.* 120:87–92, 1979.
Reviews the use of steroids in the management of ABPA.

ADVERSE REACTIONS TO DRUGS

44. PENICILLIN
Allen D. Adinoff

Penicillin has been remarkable for its lack of toxicity during its approximately 40 years of usage; however, the penicillins are the most common pharmacologic cause of allergic reactions, occurring in 1 to 10% of therapeutic courses. Anaphylaxis occurs with the frequency of 1 to 15 per 10,000 courses, with fatal reactions seen in 1.5 to 2 per 100,000 courses. It has been estimated that penicillin may be responsible for as many as 75% of anaphylactic deaths in the United States and may cause 400 to 800 deaths per year. Anaphylactic reactions to penicillin occur most commonly in adults 20 to 49 years of age, although anaphylaxis has occurred in both infants and the elderly. Fatal anaphylaxis has been reported in infants as young as 3 months of age.

The route of administration probably affects the incidence of penicillin reactions. Topical application will most frequently cause contact-hypersensitivity reactions, while systemic allergic reactions are more commonly seen with parenteral rather than oral administration. Certain diseases may predispose individuals to an adverse penicillin reaction. These diseases include infectious mononucleosis, cytomegalovirus infection, the chronic lymphocytic leukemias, and hyperuricemia, especially when it is treated with allopurinol. Sex, race, and human leukocyte antigen (HLA) phenotype do not appear to affect the incidence of penicillin allergy. Early investigations found that anaphylaxis to penicillin was more common in atopic individuals; however, recent evidence has not confirmed this observation. There appears to be no correlation between penicillin reactivity and a personal or family history of allergy; nor does a relationship exist between positive skin tests to penicillin in nonatopic persons versus atopic persons. Most deaths from penicillin anaphylaxis have occurred in persons with no history of allergy.

Penicillin as an Antigen
Penicillins all share the molecular nucleus, 6-aminopenicillanic acid. Its major components are a beta-lactam ring and a thiazolidine ring (Fig. 16). The side chain determines the penicillin type and whether it will be resistant to beta-lactamase. It is primarily the metabolic products of penicillin rather than penicillin itself that form the immunogenic moieties. Of the penicillin that ultimately becomes conjugated to proteins, perhaps 95% is in the penicilloyl configuration (see Fig. 16). Because penicilloyl is the major conjugated product, it is referred to as the "major determinant." A small amount of protein-bound penicillin, probably 5% or less, is metabolized by several other pathways in vivo, or in vitro by alkaline hydrolysis (see Fig. 16). The fact that these metabolites are formed in such small quantities has led to their designation as "minor determinants." Their structures are not fully known. The primary minor determinants identified to date are crystalline penicillin, sodium penicilloate, benzyl penicilloate, and sodium alpha-benzyl penicilloyl-amine.

Drugs of low molecular weight are not intrinsically immunogenic. Penicillin (molecular weight 333) and its by-products induce an immune response only after covalent binding to serum and tissue proteins to form a hapten-protein complex. To elicit symptoms of hypersensitivity, the haptenic antigen must be multivalent—to form a "bridge" between antibody molecules. Univalent haptens not only fail to elicit allergic responses, but may compete with multivalent antigens for antibody. Penicillin, unlike most drugs, has the property to form multivalent antigens. It will produce an immune response in nearly every person who receives the drug. Antibodies of all the major classes—IgE, IgG, IgM, IgA, IgD—

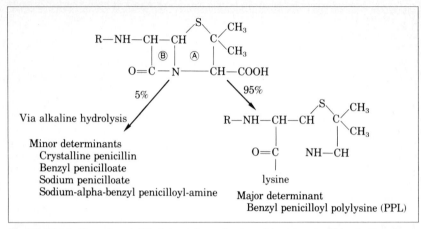

Fig. 16. Metabolism of penicillin into major and minor determinants. Thiazoladine ring (A) and beta-lactam ring (B) are the major components of the 6-aminopenicillanic acid nucleus, which is the structure basic to all penicillins. When R = phenyl-CH_2-CO, the molecule is benzyl penicillin G.

are formed. Antibody formation, however, does not necessarily mean that clinical reactions will occur.

Clinical Manifestations and Pathophysiologic Correlation

Patients with adverse reactions to penicillin present in a variety of ways. In addition, not all forms of reactions are immunologically mediated. Other possible reactions such as a vasovagal episode or a "pseudopenicillin anaphylaxis" from the procaine in the penicillin preparation need to be considered. It is therefore crucial that a detailed account of the reaction be obtained, both to authenticate the history and to attempt to categorize the type of reaction. Significant aspects of the history include the following: (1) the exact drug preparation used, (2) the nature of the illness for which the penicillin was given, (3) the time elapsed between drug administration and onset of reaction, (4) the nature and extent of the response, and (5) whether the patient has received penicillin since the reaction and if so, whether a second reaction has occurred.

Clearly, **anaphylaxis**, or immediate hypersensitivity reaction, is the most serious adverse reaction to penicillins. Usually within 20 minutes of administration, patients complain of a sensation of "impending doom." This complaint may be followed by diffuse urticaria and hypotension and, less commonly, by wheezing, rhinitis, laryngeal edema, cardiac arrythmias, and hyperperistalsis. These reactions are mediated by IgE and possibly IgG4. Minor determinant–specific IgE is the most frequent mediator despite the more common occurrence of specific IgE to penicilloyl. Specific IgE on mast cells or basophils reacts with the multivalent penicillin hapten-protein complex leading to release of the chemical mediators of anaphylaxis.

Because of their similar immunologic mechanisms, **accelerated reactions and late urticaria reactions** have been grouped together. Accelerated reactions usually begin 2 to 48 hours after drug administration and consist of generalized or local urticaria. Laryngeal edema may also develop. Late reactions begin 3 days after initiating treatment. These reactions are associated with antibody to the penicilloyl group. Studies indicate the reaction is mediated by IgE and modulated by IgG. Clinically, it is observed that patients with these reactions often lose their rash as treatment is continued, corresponding with the rise in specific IgG (interfering or blocking antibody). The difference between accelerated and late reactions is that the former have specific antibody (IgE) prior to treatment, whereas the latter develop it during the course of treatment. If penicillin treatment is continued, the risk of serious allergic reactions is rare and no fatalities have been reported. Patients should be closely observed for hypotension, laryngeal edema, hematologic manifestations (explained in a later section), and exfoliative dermatitis.

Maculopapular rashes pose a dilemma for the clinician because these rashes probably constitute the majority of penicillin "allergic reactions" by history. The lesions usually occur over the trunk and proximal extremities and may be pruritic, lasting 3 to 21 days. Symptoms of generalized immunoreactivity such as fever, lymphadenopathy, or arthritis do not occur. While the precise etiology of these rashes is not known, IgE mediation does not appear to play a role in most cases. Up to 40% of patients with maculopapular rashes may have positive skin tests to penicillin, especially when pruritus is present. Many patients have elevated IgM antibodies of penicilloyl specificity suggesting that the reaction is mediated by antigen-antibody complexes. Ampicillin therapy is associated with a higher incidence of maculopapular rash (5–10%) compared with other penicillins (approximately 2%).

Penicillin is now probably the most common cause of drug-related **serum sickness–like** reactions. Symptoms occur approximately 6 days into treatment although they may begin after the drug has been discontinued. Most of the classic clinical manifestations (i.e., fever, rash, lymphadenopathy, arthritis, nephritis) are believed to be initiated by drug-antibody complexes (IgG or IgM). Local deposition of immune complexes may be facilitated by IgE-mediated release of vasoactive substances. Patients with serum sickness reactions probably should not receive penicillin in the future. A syndrome similar to the more classic serum sickness has also been described, which consists of recurrent urticaria and arthralgias that begin 3 to 21 days after withdrawal of penicillin therapy. Symptoms may persist for 2 to 15 weeks. Unlike true serum sickness, no evidence of joint inflammation is found, and no fever, lymphadenopathy, or renal or cardiac involvement has been noted. IgE of minor determinant specificity without IgG or IgM has been described, but the mechanism of the syndrome is not known.

Penicillin-induced hemolytic anemia is not common although it is probably second in incidence only to that caused by methyldopa. Penicillin or penicilloyl groups combine with red blood cell membranes and stimulate production of IgG antibody (and probably IgM and IgA in some cases) directed against the drug–cell membrane complex. These antibodies can be detected by direct antiglobulin (Coombs') tests in approximately 3% of patients receiving large doses (10–20 million units/day) of IV penicillin. If the antibodies are present in high enough concentration, they can cause hemolysis. This hemolysis generally occurs extravascularly in the macrophages in the liver, spleen, and lungs by cellular recognition of the Fc portion of IgG. Intravascular hemolysis may also occur if complement is activated. Hemolysis is usually of gradual onset and is mild, although it may become life-threatening if unrecognized. Immune hemolysis usually occurs in the absence of other allergic symptoms. It is interesting that penicillin-specific IgG appears toxic in one situation (hemolysis) and protective in another (accelerated and late urticaria). Neutropenia, thrombocytopenia, and inhibition of factor VIII have been reported in association with penicillin treatment.

In addition to the **nephritis** occurring in serum sickness–like reactions, acute interstitial nephritis can also be seen rarely, especially with methicillin therapy. Fever, rash, urinary abnormalities, eosinophilia, and azotemia are seen in patients on prolonged courses of penicillin for serious infections. Recovery is usually good if the penicillin is discontinued. Recurrence or exacerbation of the disease has been noted in patients reexposed to these drugs. The pathogenesis is unclear although humoral and cell-mediated mechanisms may play a role.

It is well known that penicillin is a potent topical sensitizing agent and is capable of causing immune **contact dermatitis** via cell-mediated delayed hypersensitivity. **Other cutaneous reactions** from systemic administration, such as erythema multiforme, Stevens–Johnson syndrome, exfoliative dermatitis, and erythema nodosum, have been associated with penicillin therapy. The specific immune mechanisms involved in these reactions are unknown and risk upon reexposure has not been defined.

Pulmonary disease is probably the least common manifestation of penicillin related adverse reactions. Pulmonary infiltrates with associated peripheral eosinophilia have been reported. Acute airways obstruction may occur as a result of inhaled penicillin.

Approach to the Patient with Penicillin Allergy

Patients with suspected penicillin allergy present an interesting and challenging set of problems. The author's opinion is that no patient need seriously be evaluated for an adverse reaction to penicillin unless the situation arises in which a penicillin (or cephalosporin) is the only antibiotic indicated for the patient's infection. If an alternate drug can be administered without risk of major toxicity, and the history of penicillin is convincing, then no further evaluation is indicated. Routine testing of patients for penicillin allergy is probably not useful.

If a patient clearly requires a penicillin for a serious infection and the risk of a serious immediate reaction seems likely by history, skin testing should be performed. It is the most valuable and convenient method to evaluate the risks of subsequent penicillin therapy. A variety of other tests, including Prausnitz-Küstner (passive transfer) reaction, passive cutaneous anaphylaxis, direct and indirect basophil degranulation, and the enzyme-linked immunosorbent assay (ELISA), are available, but have not been found clinically useful. The radioallergosorbent test (RAST) correlates well with skin tests to penicilloyl major determinants, but there is a slightly greater risk for a false-negative test. In addition, there is no suitable RAST for the minor determinants.

Skin testing must include both the major and minor determinants, since many patients with the most severe immediate reactions are sensitive only to the minor determinant. Multivalent penicilloyl haptens such as penicilloyl polylysine (PPL) are available commercially as Pre Pen (Kremers Urban Company, Milwaukee, Wisconsin) in a single skin-test strength. Minor determinant mixtures (MDM) are not available commercially although benzyl penicillin (penicillin G) potassium or sodium (1 million U/vial supplied by E. R. Squibb and Son), which has been reconstituted and allowed to sit at room temperature for 2 weeks may be an acceptable substitute. Other researchers recommend the use of a mildly alkaline solution of penicillin, which has been allowed to stand at room temperature for several days (see Sullivan et al., 1981). Freshly prepared penicillin should also be used. The penicillin study group of the American Academy of Allergy recommends the skin-testing procedure presented in Table 37.

Various studies in both children and adults have clearly demonstrated the safety and reliability of penicillin skin testing to predict which patients are at increased risk of developing an immediate allergic reaction if given penicillin. The combined use of PPL and penicillin G will detect 90 to 95% of potential anaphylactic reactors. The 5 to 10% of reactors that are not detected probably are sensitive to minor determinants not present in the skin-testing mixtures commonly used. Skin testing is not without its limitations or dangers. Some false-negative reactions do occur. Skin reactions are of no value in predicting the occurrence of non-IgE-mediated reactions to penicillin such as a delayed exanthem or hemolytic anemia. Most serious is that both nonfatal and fatal anaphy-

Table 37. Penicillin skin test

Skin test[a]	Concentration	Volume	Dose
Penicillin G[b]			
Prick or scratch	10,000 U/ml	1 drop	
Intradermal	100 U/ml	0.02 ml	2 U
	1000 U/ml	0.02 ml	20 U
	10,000 U/ml	0.02 ml	200 U
Penicilloyl polylysine[c]			
Prick or scratch	6×10^{-5} M	1 drop	
Intradermal	6×10^{-5} M	0.02 ml	

[a]Skin tests are read at 10-minute intervals.
[b]Penicillin G obtained from Squibb and Company and prepared fresh weekly.
[c]Penicilloyl polylysube obtained from Kremers Urban Company, supplied in skin-test strength.

lactic reactions have occurred as a result of skin testing with penicillin. In each instance, however, either the volume of antigen injected was large or the concentration used was excessively high. Despite these risks, skin testing is generally an extremely safe procedure, especially when used appropriately by those experienced in the technique.

Because the 6-aminopenicillenic acid nucleus is common to all semisynthetic penicillins, it is not surprising that **cross-allerginicity** exists. Although exceptions may occur, if a person reports a history of an allergic response to one penicillin, the assumption must be made that the person is allergic to all penicillins, at least until skin testing can be done. Major determinants for the semisynthetic penicillins are not commercially available. Suitable concentrations of cephalosporins for skin testing are 0.025 mg/ml, 0.25 mg/ml, and 2.5 mg/ml.

Treatment
Patients who have immediate reactions to penicillins represent a medical emergency. Treatment of anaphylaxis is discussed in Chapter 1.

Desensitization is necessary in patients hypersensitive to penicillin who must be given the drug. The process involves the administration of increasing amounts of drug over a short period of time. The rationale is that small incremental doses allow a gradual binding of penicillin to IgE antibody fixed to mast cells or basophils, allowing gradual rather than massive release of histamine and other mediators. When all the antibody is bound, penicillin can be given with impunity. After a lag period of 3 to 4 days, antibody binding is followed by production of IgG antibodies that are believed to be protective. Various methods of desensitization have been proposed; Tables 38 and 39 outline examples of a subcutaneous and intravenous program. Recently oral desensitization to penicillin was successfully accomplished in 30 penicillin allergic patients by Sullivan and colleagues (1982). The vast majority of patients can be desensitized with little or no difficulty although fatal anaphylactic reactions have occurred. Once the gradual administration procedure has been completed, full therapeutic doses of penicillin should be started immediately. At the conclusion of therapy the patient should be informed that once the penicillin has been stopped, he or she may once again become clinically sensitive to penicillin.

Administration of univalent haptens capable of reacting with the antigen-combining site on the IgE molecule, thus preventing the binding of IgE by the complete antigen, have given mixed results. Induction of immunologic tolerance to penicillin is at the level of experimental research in animals.

Table 38. Subcutaneous penicillin G desensitization program

Drug concentration (units/ml)	Volume given (ml)	Dose given (units)	Cumulative dose given (units)
100	0.05	5	5
	0.01	10	15
	0.2	20	35
	0.4	40	75
	0.8	80	155
1,000	0.15	150	305
	0.3	300	605
	0.6	600	1,205
	1.0	1,000	2,205
10,000	0.2	2,000	4,205
	0.4	4,000	8,205
	0.8	8,000	16,205
100,000	0.15	15,000	31,205
	0.3	30,000	61,205
	0.6	60,000	121,205
	1.0	100,000	221,205
1,000,000	0.2	200,000	421,205
	0.4	400,000	621,205

Table 39. Intravenous penicillin G desensitization program

Drug concentration (units/ml)	Volume given (ml)	Dose given (units)	Cumulative dose given (units)
1	50	50	50
10	50	500	550
100	50	5,000	5,500
1,000	50	50,000	55,500
10,000	50	500,000	555,550

The rate of infusion of each drug concentration depends on whether anaphylactic reactions occur. Once the maximum dose has been achieved, regular IV doses may be safely given.

Baldwin, D. S., Levine, B. B., McCluskey, R. T., and Gallo, G. R. Renal failure and interstitial nephritis due to penicillin and methicillin. *N. Engl. J. Med.* 279:1245–1252, 1968.
The clinical, laboratory, histologic, and immunologic findings of seven patients with nephropathy due to penicillin or methicillin are described. Speculation as to the hypersensitivity mechanism for the nephropathy is given.
Bierman, C. W., and Van Arsdel, P. P., Jr. Penicillin allergy in children: The role of immunological tests in its diagnosis. *J. Allergy Clin. Immunol.* 43:267–272, 1969.
Skin testing to penicillin in children was an accurate means of identifying patients who were likely to have positive reactions with penicillins and also of eliminating those with questionable histories.
Chandra, R. K., Joglekar, S. A., and Tomas, E. Penicillin allergy: Antipenicillin IgE antibodies and immediate hypersensitivity skin reactions employing the major and minor determinants of penicillin. *Arch. Dis. Child.* 55:857–860, 1980.
The diagnosis of penicillin hypersensitivity can be reliably confirmed by skin tests in children using major and minor determinants of benzyl penicillin. Correlation with the RAST was good. Such hypersensitivity is not permanent.
Erffmeyer, J. E. Adverse reactions to penicillin. *Ann. Allergy* 47:288–300, 1981.

This article is a recent and thorough review of adverse reactions to penicillins with 234 references.

Green, G. R., Rosenblum, A. H., and Sweet, L. C. Evaluation of penicillin hypersensitivity: Value of clinical history and skin testing with penicilloyl-polylysine and penicillin G. *J. Allergy Clin. Immunol.* 60:339–345, 1977.

A cooperative prospective study of the penicillin study group of the American Academy of Allergy. In a study of almost 3000 patients, the usefulness of skin tests to penicillin G and penicilloyl polylysine was confirmed in the evaluation of penicillin hypersensitivity.

Grieco, M. H. Cross-allergenicity of the penicillins and the cephalosporins. *Arch. Intern. Med.* 119:141–146, 1967.

A cross-allergenicity of these two groups of antibiotics was studied. It is suggested that all cephalosporin derivatives be used with the same caution as are penicillin derivatives in patients with a past history of penicillin allergy.

Levine, B. B. Immunologic mechanisms of penicillin allergy. *N. Engl. J. Med.* 275:1115–1125, 1966.

Levine provides a more clinical approach to the subjects discussed in his article in the Journal of Clinical Investigation.

Levine, B. B., et al. Penicillin allergy and the heterogeneous immune responses of man to benzylpenicillin. *J. Clin. Invest.* 45:1895–1906, 1966.

Correlations with immune responses and clinical manifestations of penicillin hypersensitivity were studied. This is a classic paper upon which the majority of the latter penicillin allergy literature is based.

Levine, B. B., and Zolov, D. M. Prediction of penicillin allergy by immunological tests. *J. Allergy Clin. Immunol.* 43:231–244, 1969.

A prospective study was done to evaluate objective immunologic tests to predict penicillin allergy. Skin tests were found to be a valuable predictive tool for immediate (including anaphylactic) and accelerated urticarial allergic reactions to penicillin.

Parker, C. W. Drug allergy. *N. Engl. J. Med.* 292:511–514, 732–736, 957–960, 1975.

This article is an excellent review of mechanisms of drug hypersensitivity with special emphasis on penicillin allergy.

Solley, G. O., Gleich, G. J., and VanDellen, R. G. Penicillin allergy: Clinical experience with a battery of skin test reagents. *J. Allergy Clin. Immunol.* 69:238–244, 1982.

Skin testing was done to reagents consisting of penicillin G, ampicillin, and methicillin, as well as their major and minor determinant products. Skin testing with semisynthetic penicillins increases the number of skin reactors. The incidence of allergic reactions is low in patients treated with a cephalosporin who are penicillin sensitive.

Sullivan, T. J., et al. Skin testing to detect penicillin allergy. *J. Allergy Clin. Immunol.* 68:171–180, 1981.

This study extends and confirms previous observations that skin testing with major and minor determinants is a rapid, safe, and effective method for identifying patients at risk or not at risk for allergic reactions to penicillin.

Sullivan, T. J., et al. Desensitization of patients allergic to penicillin using orally administered beta-lactam antibiotics. *J. Allergy Clin. Immunol.* 69:275–282, 1982.

This article is a description of a new protocol for desensitization, which is safe and effective.

45. ASPIRIN
Linden Ho

Aspirin idiosyncrasy may be characterized by bronchospasm or urticaria-angioedema or both following ingestion of the drug. In 1902, 3 years after the synthesis of aspirin, the syndrome was first described in a person with facial and laryngeal edema. Subsequent reports have established the association—known as the aspirin triad—of aspirin idiosyncrasy, nasal polyposis, and asthma.

Population surveys, based on patient recall, estimate the prevalence of aspirin idiosyncrasy among asthmatic patients at 2 to 4%. However, significant bronchospasm can be induced in 8 to 28% of asthmatic patients following deliberate oral challenge. The frequency of sensitivity in adult and pediatric populations is comparable, although the full-blown symptomatic syndrome is found much more often in adults.

The profile of the classic aspirin-idiosyncratic person has been best described by Samter (1973). The initial manifestation is a vasomotor rhinitis with intermittent but profuse watery rhinorrhea developing during the second or third decade of life. These symptoms evolve into more chronic nasal congestion resistant to vasoconstrictor therapy. Nasal polyps, usually bilateral, are discovered on physical examination at this stage. By middle age, bronchial asthma develops in a significant number of these persons. The asthma is initially responsive to bronchodilators or low-dose corticosteroid therapy but can then become intractable. Overt intolerance to aspirin, manifested by bronchospasm or urticaria, is frequently delayed for years. Avoidance of aspirin does not clearly halt the progression of the disease. Patient characteristics include a high incidence of sinusitis and eosinophilia of the blood and nasal secretions, and a low incidence of atopy. Females are more at risk.

Although a stereotypic patient clearly exists, aspirin idiosyncrasy is now recognized to be more variable and heterogeneous than previously thought. In fact, the aspirin triad may be an inappropriate concept, as some affected patients do not manifest all three features simultaneously, and the full-blown syndrome may only develop with time. Absence of atopy is not a consistent finding, and although nasal eosinophilia is common in adults with aspirin idiosyncrasy, blood eosinophilia is variable. Neither feature predicts idiosyncrasy in children.

Strong evidence exists for at least two distinct, though overlapping, subtypes of aspirin idiosyncrasy—one characterized by asthma and bronchospasm, the other by rhinitis and urticaria-angioedema. In one study of a selected group of asthmatic patients, 64% reacted with bronchospasm following oral challenge, while only 28% had urticaria or angioedema. Bronchospasm usually occurred within 30 minutes to 3 hours. In contrast, nearly 100% of a selected group of patients with rhinitis but no asthma developed urticaria or angioedema, and the reaction was later in onset, occurring 90 minutes to 12 hours after challenge. The latter was also more frequently associated with hypotension.

Aspirin-idiosyncratic persons are at risk for cross-sensitivity to other agents such as nonsteroidal anti-inflammatory drugs, azo and nonazo dyes, and a variety of food preservatives. The incidence of reactivity to aspirinlike anti-inflammatory drugs such as indomethacin is probably high and may be related to their similar mechanism of action. Reactions to artificial dyes found in foods and medications occur infrequently, although sensitivity to tartrazine (FD&C yellow dye no. 5) has been reported in up to 33% of aspirin-idiosyncratic patients. Food preservatives such as sodium benzoate and sodium salicylate rarely cause symptoms, but have been implicated in some cases of chronic urticaria.

The pathogenesis of aspirin idiosyncrasy is unknown, and a number of unrelated mechanisms have been proposed. One of the most attractive hypotheses relates idiosyncratic reactions to aspirin's inhibition of prostaglandin synthesis. Prostaglandins of the E series cause bronchodilation and inhibit histamine release, whereas those of the F series induce bronchoconstriction. Conceivably, the E prostaglandins may be inhibited preferentially in persons with idiosyncrasy, allowing for actions of the F prostaglandins to be manifested. In addition, in these persons, inhibition of prostaglandin synthesis may tend to drive arachidonic acid metabolism into the alternative lipoxygenase pathway, which leads to formation of leukotrienes—several of which are potent bronchoconstrictors. Support for these hypothesized mechanisms comes primarily from the observations that the aspirinlike anti-inflammatory drugs that inhibit prostaglandin synthesis are also potent inducers of bronchospasm or urticaria in aspirin-idiosyncratic persons.

Attempts to demonstrate specific immunologic mechanisms have been unsuccessful.

Diagnosis of aspirin idiosyncrasy is based on clinical suspicion. A history should be solicited from patients with symptoms occurring after ingestion of aspirin, nonsteroidal anti-inflammatory drugs, yellow-colored foods and medications, or over-the-counter preparations containing salicylates. Physical examination should focus on the presence of underlying asthma or rhinitis, sinusitis, and nasal polyposis. Eosinophilia of nasal secretions may be helpful as well. There are no useful in vitro tests for the diagnosis of aspirin idiosyncrasy, and at present definitive confirmation requires oral challenge in accordance with standard, published protocols. Routine challenge, however, is not recommended and is contraindicated in patients with an unequivocal history of severe reaction. Oral challenge is indicated in the following situations (see also the recommendations for oral challenge by Farr and colleagues, 1970):

1. Asthmatic patients who need aspirin or nonsteroidal anti-inflammatory drugs for another medical condition should be challenged.
2. Persons with a history of asthma or urticaria after ingestion of aspirin or yellow-colored food or drugs should be considered for tartrazine challenge.
3. Persons with intractable asthma or known aspirin idiosyncrasy should probably be tested for tartrazine idiosyncrasy.

Aspirin idiosyncrasy should be managed by avoidance of aspirin-containing medications and aspirinlike anti-inflammatory drugs that inhibit prostaglandin synthesis. In most instances, acetaminophen may be safely substituted. For tartrazine-sensitive patients, medication and foods must be screened for tartrazine. It should be noted that tartrazine may be present even when the medication or food is a color other than yellow or orange. Inhaled cromolyn has been reported to protect against aspirin-induced bronchospasm. Recently it has been demonstrated that oral desensitization to aspirin can be achieved. It is important to warn patients undergoing desensitization that the desensitization will gradually disappear over several days when additional aspirin is withheld. Thus there must be strict compliance with the desensitization protocol to avoid severe reactions from aspirin ingestion after a period of not taking the drug. Such a desensitization program allows the therapeutic use of aspirin or other nonsteroidal anti-inflammatory drugs in aspirin-sensitive patients with coexisting chronic rheumatic, cardiovascular, or neurologic syndromes. Potential therapeutic benefits of producing prolonged aspirin desensitization by daily administration of aspirin to patients with aspirin-sensitive asthma are not yet defined.

Basomba, A., et al.   The effect of sodium cromoglycate in preventing aspirin-induced bronchospasm. *Clin. Allergy* 6:269–275, 1976.
Cromolyn prior to and during oral aspirin challenge was protective against bronchospasm.
Farr, R. S., Spector, S. L., and Wangaard, C. H.   Evaluation of aspirin and tartrazine idiosyncrasy. *J. Allergy Clin. Immunol.* 64:667–668, 1979.
Guidelines for oral challenge are described.
Lumry, W. R., et al.   Aspirin-sensitive rhinosinusitis: The clinical syndrome and effects of aspirin administration. *J. Allergy Clin. Immunol.* 71:580–7, 1983.
Of the 17 patients who were treated with aspirin daily after desensitization, 77% experienced improvement in their nasal symptoms.
Phills, J. A., and Perelmutter, L.   IgE mediated and non-IgE mediated allergic-type reactions to aspirin. *Acta Allergologica* 29:474–490, 1974.
Evidence is presented for an IgE-mediated mechanism in rhinitis-urticaria group of idiosyncratic patients.
Pleskow, W. W., et al.   Aspirin desensitization in aspirin-sensitive asthmatic patients: Clinical manifestations and characterization of the refractory period. *J. Allergy Clin. Immunol.* 69:11–19, 1982.
This presents a follow-up to other Stevenson reference. More patients are reported with

definition of treatment protocol and a demonstration that desensitization will gradually disappear when additional aspirin is withheld.

Samter, M.   Intolerance to aspirin. *Hosp. Pract.* 8(12):85–100, 1973.
Reviews and describes the classic aspirin-idiosyncratic patient.
Settipane, G. A., Chafee, F. H. and Klein, D. E.   Aspirin intolerance. II. A prospective study in an atopic and normal population. *J. Allergy Clin. Immunol.* 53:200–204, 1974.
The ariticle gives the incidence of idiosyncrasy by history, with a discussion of clinical subtypes.
Spector, S., Wangaard, C. H., and Farr, R. S.   Aspirin and concomitant idiosyncrasies in adult asthmatic patients. *J. Allergy Clin. Immunol.* 64:500–506, 1979.
Oral challenges to aspirin, tartrazine, acetaminophen, and sodium salicylate in adult asthmatic patients are reported.
Stevenson, D., Simon, R. A., and Mathison, D. A.   Aspirin-sensitive asthma: Tolerance to aspirin after positive oral aspirin challenges. *J. Allergy Clin. Immunol.* 66:82–88, 1980.
This article provides case reports of two idiosyncratic patients made refractory to aspirin following oral desensitization.
Szczeklik, A., Gryglewski, R. J., and Czerniawska-Mysik, G.   Clinical patterns of hypersensitivity to nonsteroidal anti-inflammatory drugs and their pathogenesis. *J. Allergy Clin. Immunol.* 60:276–284, 1977.
The pathogenesis of aspirin idiosyncrasy was related to prostaglandin synthesis inhibition. Clinical subtypes of asthma-bronchospasm versus rhinitis-urticaria are described.
Vane, J.   The mode of action of aspirin and similar compounds. *J. Allergy Clin. Immunol.* 58:691–712, 1976.
Comprehensively reviews prostaglandin synthesis and its relation to aspirin.
Vedanthan, P. K., Menon, M. M., Bell, T. D., and Bergin D.   Aspirin and tartrazine oral challenge: Incidence of adverse response in chronic childhood asthma. *J. Allergy Clin. Immunol.* 60:8–13, 1977.
Similar study to Spector's but the study group consists of institutionalized asthmatic children.
Weber, R. W., Hoffman, M., Raine, D. A., and Nelson H. S.   Incidence of bronchoconstriction due to aspirin, azo dyes, non-azo dyes, and preservatives in a population of perennial asthmatics. *J. Allergy Clin. Immunol.* 64:32–37, 1979.
The title is self-explanatory title. A very low incidence of reactions to dyes and preservatives is reported.
Weinberger, M. Analgesic sensitivity in children with asthma. *Pediatrics* 62 (Suppl.):910–915, 1978.
This is a good review, with special reference made to the syndrome in children.

46. LOCAL ANESTHETICS
Karl M. Altenburger

Reactions associated with the use of local anesthetics are not uncommon and vary from minor to severe and life-threatening. When presented with a history of a reaction after injection with local anesthetics, most physicians or dentists are understandably reluctant to reexpose their patients until further clarification has been obtained. This is especially true when the history is vague and incomplete, as it often is. Further clarification before any reexposure is especially necessary in those patients who report severe reactions to all "caines." Frequently, referral to an allergist results.

Reactions can be classified as toxic, vasovagal (psychogenic), or immunologic. Toxic reactions are due to the direct effects of these agents on the cardiovascular and central nervous systems, and are caused by rapid absorption of the drug into the systemic circulation. Reactions usually begin with signs of CNS stimulation (i.e., restlessness, rapid slurred speech, euphoria, nausea, vomiting, disorientation), and as the reaction progresses coma, hypotension, and cardiac arrest can

Table 40. Antigenic grouping of local anesthetics

Group I (para-aminobenzoic esters)	Group II (lack p-aminophenyl group)
Procaine (Novocain)	Lidocaine (Xylocaine)
Benzocaine	Mepivacaine (Carbocaine)
Tetracaine (Pontocaine)	Dibucaine (Nupercaine)
Chloroprocaine (Nesacaine)	Phenacaine (Holocaine)
Butethamine (Monocaine)	Piperocaine (Metycaine)
Benoxinate (Dorsacaine)	Amydricaine (Alypin)
Butacaine (Butyn)	Cyclomethycaine (Surfacaine)
Butyl aminobenzoate (Butesin)	Dimethisoquin (Quotane)
Larocaine	Diperodon (Diothane)
Naepaine (Amylsine Hydrochloride)	Dyclonine (Dyclone)
	Hexylcaine (Cyclaine)
	Oxethazine (Oxaine)
	Pramoxine (Tronothane)
	Proparacaine (Ophthaine)
	Pyrrocaine (Endocaine)
	Cocaine

Source: R. D. DeSwarte, Drug Allergy. In R. Patterson (Ed.), *Allergic Diseases: Diagnosis and Management* (2nd ed.). Philadelphia: Lippincott, 1980.

occur. Epinephrine mixed with the anesthetic is used for the purpose of delaying systemic absorption and prolonging the local effects. However, although its use will reduce reactions from the rapid absorption of the anesthetic, the epinephrine can also produce reactions of its own, most notably, anxiety, tachycardia, and hypertension. Many reactions are vasovagal in nature and have more to do with the surgical or dental procedure itself than the agent used. Unfortunately, the local anesthetic is often implicated as the causative agent. Toxic and vasovagal reactions are by far the most common causes of reactions to local anesthetics. Immunologically mediated reactions are less common and the overwhelming majority of these are contact reactions (presumed lymphocyte-mediated, delayed hypersensitivity). Contact reactions can be a special problem for health professionals who are frequently exposed. Use of the topical anesthetic agents that are present in popular over-the-counter medications may cause sensitization to the anesthetic agent and thus predispose a patient to an immunologically mediated reaction. Immediate hypersensitivity (IgE-mediated, allergic) reactions to the local anesthetic agent itself are fortunately very uncommon.

Local anesthetics can be divided into two groups (see Table 40). The first group are para-aminobenzoic esters. Hypersensitivity to members of this group is thought to be especially common and cross-reactivity among individual members occurs. Examples of this group include procaine (Novocain), first introduced into wide use in 1905, and benzocaine, which is commonly used as a surface anesthetic in over-the-counter medications. The agents in the second group—the amide type—are generally not structurally related to each other; therefore, patients sensitive to one agent in this group are generally not sensitive to any other compound in the group. Reactions to members of this group are rare. Lidocaine (Xylocaine) and mepivacaine (Carbocaine) are the most widely used group II agents. If the history suggests sensitivity to a group I agent, then a group II agent is chosen for subsequent challenge. If a group II agent is implicated, then a group I agent or another group II agent should be used.

Table 41. Provocative test dosing procedure

Patient: _____ Date: _____

Drug: _____ Referred by: _____

1. Make dilutions as:
   (a) concentrate _____ without epinephrine or preservatives
   (b) 1:10
   (c) 1:100
2. Have resuscitation equipment ready (i.e., O_2, laryngoscope, endotracheal tubes, epinephrine, benadryl, IVs, steroids, and so on)
3. Patient seated and comfortable
   Pulse _____ RR _____ B/P _____
4. Place histamine and diluent controls on one arm. Do epicutaneous and intracutaneous tests on opposite forearm and give subcutaneous injections in same arm (posterior–lateral)
   Step 1. Histamine and diluent controls
        Time _____ Site _____ Reaction _____
   Step 2. Puncture test with (c) (1:100)
        Time _____ Site _____ Reaction _____
   Step 3. If negative after 20 minutes, perform puncture test with (a) (concentrate)
        Time _____ Site _____ Reaction _____
        Pulse _____ RR _____ B/P _____
   Step 4. If negative after 20 minutes, do intradermal skin test with 0.02 ml (c) (1:100)
        Time _____ Site _____ Reaction _____
   Step 5. If negative after 20 minutes, do intradermal skin test with 0.02 ml (a) (concentrate)
        Time _____ Site _____ Reaction _____
   Step 6. If negative after 20 minutes, give 0.1 ml subcutaneously (b) (1:10)
        Time _____ Site _____ Reaction _____
   Step 7. If negative after 20 minutes, give 0.1 ml subcutaneously (a) (concentrate)
        Time _____ Site _____ Reaction _____
   Step 8. If negative after 20 minutes, give 0.5 ml subcutaneously (a) (concentrate)
        Time _____ Site _____ Reaction _____
   Step 9. If negative after 20 minutes, give 1.0 ml subcutaneously (a) (concentrate)
        Time _____ Site _____ Reaction _____
        Pulse _____ RR _____ B/P _____

Source: Modified from protocols of R. D. DeSwarte, Drug Allergy. In R. Patterson (Ed.), *Allergic Diseases: Diagnosis and Management*. Philadelphia: Lippincott, 1980; R. D. deShazo and H. S. Nelson, An approach to the patient with a history of local anesthetic hypersensitivity: Experience with 90 patients. *J. Allergy Clin. Immunol.* 63:387–394, 1979; and G. Incaudo, et al., Administration of local anesthetics to patients with a history of prior adverse reactions. *J. Allergy Clin. Immunol.* 61:339–345, 1978.

The issue of allergy to these agents is easily clarified by the use of a well-controlled provocative challenge. Before the challenge is designed, the history of all previous reactions should be thoroughly explored in an attempt to identify precisely the etiologic agent (i.e., anesthetic, epinephrine, preservative) responsible for the reaction and the mechanisms involved. The referring physician or dentist is consulted and an appropriate agent is chosen for challenge. After a full and detailed explanation, the patient is scheduled for the challenge as close as possible to the procedure for which exposure is necessary (e.g., the day before). In a relaxed and comfortable environment the challenge is begun using any of a number of established protocols (see Table 41 for an example). After the application of appropriate controls, a low concentration of the agent is introduced using an epicutaneous skin test. The patient is observed closely for at least 20 minutes. In the absence of any adverse reactions, intracutaneous and subcutaneous injections are used to introduce progressively larger amounts of the drug. The protocol may be modified, depending on the history. If an extreme degree of sensitivity is suggested, one may wish to begin with much higher dilutions and progress even more cautiously. If the history suggests the occurence of delayed reactions, appropriately longer intervals between injections should be chosen. Successful completion of the challenge without any adverse reactions indicates that the patient is not at an increased risk of sustaining a serious, immunologically mediated reaction on subsequent exposure to the agent.

Chin, T. M., and Fellner, M. J.   Allergic hypersensitivity to lidocaine hydrochloride. *Int. J. Dermatol.* 19:147–148, 1980.
A 39-year-old man developed acute onset of pruritis and erythema with wheals and flares at sites where lidocaine was injected. He showed marked urticarial dermographism.
deJong, R. H.   Toxic effects of local anesthetics. *J.A.M.A.* 239:1166–1168, 1978.
deJong gives a brief, but good, review of the topic.
deShazo, R. D., and Nelson, H. S.   An approach to the patient with a history of local anesthetic hypersensitivity: Experience with 90 patients. *J. Allergy Clin. Immunol.* 63:387–394, 1979.
The authors used skin testing and progressive challenge and found that both techniques were useful.
DeSwarte, R. D.   Drug Allergy. In R. Patterson (Ed.), *Allergic Diseases: Diagnosis and Management* (2nd ed.). Philadelphia: Lippincott, 1980. Pp. 542–583.
The article is an excellent, general review that includes a specific section on problems with local anesthetics.
Eisenberg, L.   Allergy to procaine and mepivacaine. *J.A.M.A.* 230:613, 1974.
Question-and-answer article that discusses the practical approach to these allergies.
Fregert, S., Tegner, E., and Thelin, I.   Contact allergy to lidocaine. *Contact Dermatitis* 5:185–188, 1979.
Two cases of lidocaine allergy are reported. The patients also reacted to chemically related anesthetics of the amide type.
Hofman, H., Maibach, H. I., and Prout, E.   Presumed generalized exfoliative dermatitis to lidocaine. *Arch. Dermatol.* 111:266, 1975.
This letter to the editor reports a single case of contact allergy. The subject was a 21-year-old man who had received 2% lidocaine as a dental anesthetic. The reaction occurred originally after his first two doses cleared, and then reoccurred after an inadvertent third dose.
Incaudo, G., et al.   Administration of local anesthetics to patients with a history of prior adverse reaction. *J. Allergy Clin. Immunol.* 61:339–345, 1978.
The authors found: a low incidence of reaction compatible with a systemic IgE-mediated reaction, no value from dilutional skin tests, and the safety and usefulness of careful challenge with a local anesthetic with chemical nonsimilarity.
Latronica, R. J., Goldberg, A. F., and Whitman, J. R.   Local anesthetic sensitivity. Report of a case. *Oral Surg.* 28:439–441, 1969.
A 45-year-old man with a history of reactions to local anesthetics had a positive intradermal skin test to a lidocaine solution containing methylparaben, but not to lidocaine without preservative.
Nagal, J., Fusaldo, J. T., and Fireman, P.   Paraben allergy. *J.A.M.A.* 237:1594–1595, 1977.
A hydrocortisone preparation containing methylparaben and propylparaben provoked bronchospasm and pruritus when given IM to an asthmatic patient, whereas another hydrocortisone preparation without paraben preservative did not.
Ritchie, J. M., and Greene, N. M.   Local Anesthetics. In A. G. Gilman, L. S. Goodman, and A. Gilman (Eds.), *The Pharmacological Basis of Therapeutics* (6th ed.). New York: Macmillan, 1980. Pp. 300–320.
This article is an excellent review of pharmacology of these drugs.

47. DRUG-INDUCED LUPUS
Nancy P. Cummings

Systemic lupus erythematosus (SLE) may occur spontaneously or may appear after the ingestion of certain drugs. In 1947, Hoffman described the first patient with possible drug-related lupus and incriminated sulfadiazine. Case reports followed of patients with lupus-like symptoms in association with sulfonamide or penicillin. It was not until 1953, however, that convincing evidence for a true drug-induced lupus syndrome appeared during treatment of hypertension with hydralazine. At least 35 drugs have presently been implicated in causing drug-induced lupus, with the major groups including drugs used in heart disease and hypertension, anticonvulsants, and phenothiazines. Controlled prospective studies and proof of association of drug-induced lupus is present with hydralazine, procainamide, and isoniazid. Drugs with possible associations include certain anticonvulsants, chlorpromazine, methyldopa, penicillamine, quinidine, propylthiouracil, various beta blockers, lithium carbonate, and nitrofurantoin. A third group of drugs has been implicated, but the evidence is even less conclusive; it includes griseofulvin, phenylbutazone, gold salts, and oral contraceptives.

The majority of the patients with drug-induced lupus fulfill the criteria of the American Rheumatism Association for classification of SLE, however, clinical features are usually milder. The age of onset relates to the population at risk for which the drugs are used. Most case reports with drug-induced lupus in childhood are secondary to anticonvulsants, in middle-aged patients isoniazid is implicated most frequently, and in older patients reports of procainamide-induced lupus predominate. Clinical features commonly include fever, constitutional symptoms, arthralgias, myalgias, and true polyarthritis. Rashes, oral ulcers, and alopecia are less common in drug-induced than in spontaneous lupus. Pleuropericarditis has been seen with hydralazine, procainamide, and isoniazid. Renal involvement is unusual but occurs most commonly with hydralazine. When renal histology has been obtained, it has shown mesangial or focal proliferative nephritis.

Laboratory features generally include an elevated erythrocyte sedimentation rate and anemia. Leukopenia and thrombocytopenia occur, but less commonly than in spontaneous lupus. Coombs' test positivity, false-positive serologic test for syphilis (STS), rheumatoid factor, circulating anticoagulants, antilymphocyte antibodies, hypocomplementemia, and immune complexes have all been described in drug-induced lupus. More than 90% of patients will have antinuclear antibodies and lupus erythematosus (LE) cells. Antinuclear antibodies may be present in patients who never develop clinical signs or symptoms. There have been a few reports of antibodies to native DNA and antibodies to Sm antigen, however, these are generally specific for spontaneous lupus. Antibodies to histones are present in almost all patients with procainamide-induced lupus and in only 25% of patients with spontaneous lupus.

Procainamide and hydralazine are the most extensively studied drugs in this illness. Procainamide, introduced in 1951 for the treatment of arrhythmias and myotonic dystrophy, is the most common cause of adult drug-induced lupus. Antinuclear antibodies develop in 50 to 80% of patients taking procainamide for longer than 1 year, whereas only 10 to 15% of patients have clinical symptoms. Fever, adenopathy, skin changes, central nervous system and kidney involvement are rare; however, there is a frequent occurrence of pleuropericarditis with or without effusions and pulmonary infiltrates. Hydralazine, introduced in 1952 for the treatment of hypertension, leads to drug-induced lupus in approximately 10% of patients. Antinuclear antibodies occur in all patients with clinical symptoms. Large initial doses of the drug—400 mg or more a day—as well as initial severe hypertension with good response to hydralazine seem to correlate with the development of lupus. With hydralazine there is a high incidence of arthralgias but skin lesions are infrequent.

Isoniazid has also been reported to cause sporadic drug-induced lupus. Large studies show that antinuclear antibodies occur in 20% of patients on long-term isoniazide therapy after a year of treatment.

Several hypotheses exist for the etiology of drug-induced lupus. The most frequently evoked is that drug-nucleoprotein interactions enhance the autoimmunogenicity of nuclear constituents. There is no direct evidence, however, that drugs interact with nuclear antigens in vivo leading to antinuclear antibody formation. Other hypotheses include cross-reactive antigens at the T and B cell levels and lack of suppressor cells. Genetically, the most important consideration is the acetylator phenotype. A genetically controlled polymorphism of the hepatic acetyltransferase enzyme is responsible for different rates of inactivation of drugs such as hydralazine, procainamide, and isoniazid. In the United States the population is evenly divided between slow and rapid acetylators. The slow acetylators are homozygous for an autosomal recessive gene and rapid acetylators are either homozygous or heterozygous for the dominant gene. With hydralazine, slow acetylators are more prone to develop antinuclear antibodies, and almost all patients who develop clinical symptoms of hydralazine-induced lupus are slow acetylators. Procainamide-induced lupus is seen in both slow and rapid acetylators; however, changes occur sooner in the slow acetylators. There are no definite effects of acetylator phenotype on the development of lupus with isoniazid.

The most important aspect in the management of drug-induced lupus is to discontinue the drug. Salicylates or other nonsteroidal anti-inflammatory agents will usually control milder symptoms of arthralgias and myalgias. With more severe symptoms, corticosteroids in moderate dosage (20–40 mg daily) should be used. In patients with life-threatening disease, high-dose corticosteroids are indicated. After symptoms remit, corticosteroid therapy can gradually be withdrawn. Some patients will have the continued presence of antinuclear antibodies after clinical manifestations of the disease have disappeared. Treatment should not be given for persistence of antinuclear antibodies alone.

Alarcon-Segovia, D.   Drug-induced systemic lupus erythematosus and related syndromes. *Clin. Rheum. Dis.* 1:573–582, 1975.
Reviews drug-induced lupus.

Alarcon-Segovia, D., Wakim, K. G., Worthington, J. W., and Ward, L. E.   Clinical experimental studies on the hydralazine syndrome and its relationship to systemic lupus erythematosus. *Medicine* 46:1–32, 1967.
Reviews hydralazine-induced lupus.

Blomgren, S. E., Condemi, J. J., and Vaughan, J. H.   Procainamide-induced lupus erythematosus. *Am. J. Med.* 52:338–348, 1972.
The clinical symptoms of procainamide-induced lupus are reviewed.

Perry, H. M., Jr.   Possible mechanisms of hydralazine-related lupus-like syndrome. *Arthritis Rheum.* 24:1093–1105, 1982.
The mechanisms of hydralazine-induced lupus are reviewed.

Schoen, R. T., and Trentham, D. E.   Drug-induced lupus: An adjuvant disease? *Am. J. Med.* 71:5–7, 1981.
Proposals regarding pathogenesis of drug-induced lupus are introduced.

Sheikh, T. K., Charron, R. C., and Katz, A.   Renal manifestations of drug-induced systemic lupus erythematosus. *Am. J. Clin. Pathol.* 75:755–762, 1981.
This article provides a review of the renal findings in drug-induced lupus and of the first case of crescentic glomerulonephritis reported.

Tanem, N., and Portanova, J. P.   The role of histones as nuclear autoantigens in drug-related lupus erythematosus. *Arthritis Rheum.* 24:1064–1069, 1981.

Antihistone antibodies are present in patients with procainamide-induced lupus but not hydralazine-induced lupus.

Uetrecht, J. P., and Woosley, R. L.   Acetylator phenotype and lupus erythematosus. *Clin. Pharmacokinet.* 6:118–134, 1981.
The authors provide a review of acetylation.

Walshe, J. M.   Penicillamine and the SLE syndrome. *J. Rheumatol.* 8:155–160, 1981.
In 120 patients with Wilson's disease treated with penicillamine, 8 patients developed the serologic changes of SLE.

Weber, W. W., and Tannen, R. H.   Pharmacogenetic studies on the drug-related lupus syndrome: Differences in antinuclear antibody development and drug-induced DNA damage in rapid and slow acetylator animal models. *Arthritis Rheum.* 24:979–986, 1981.
Mice with a slow acetylator phenotype, when exposed to hydralazine, have greater DNA damage in hepatocytes than do mice with rapid acetylator phenotype.

Weinstein, A.   Drug-induced systemic lupus erythematosus. *Prog. Clin. Immunol.* 4:1–21, 1980.
Weinstein has written an excellent review of drug-induced lupus.

48. DIABETES MELLITUS AND ADVERSE REACTIONS TO INSULIN
Uwe Manthei

Although the recent introduction of purified insulins has decreased the incidence of adverse reactions to insulin, most patients are still using standard, non-purified, commercially available preparations for reasons of cost and availability. Therefore, knowledge of the nature of the reaction to these insulins is still essential in treating diabetic patients and in developing a plan to deal with adverse reactions to insulin. Previous publications report that between 1 and 55% of all patients receiving insulin experience adverse reactions, which can range from mild local manifestations to severe anaphylaxis. Eight to twelve percent of all insulin-dependent diabetic patients require alteration of their therapy because of either local or systemic reactions. One author reported that 25% of all patients with insulin allergy have adverse reactions to other drugs, with penicillin-induced reactions being the most frequent.

The standard, commercially available preparations of insulins are usually beef and pork mixtures made by acid ethanol extraction from animal pancreas. Pure beef extractions and pure pork extractions are also available.

Neutral regular insulin is a crystallized zinc extract of pork and beef pancreas.
Neutral protamine Hagedorn (NPH) is a mixture of protamine zinc and crystalline zinc insulin peaking in its biologic activity between 6 and 12 hours post-subcutaneous injection.
Lente insulins use zinc acetate buffer instead of zinc phosphate buffer. They have a high zinc concentration that allows delayed absorption without the use of protamine.

Adverse reactions to the commercially available insulin preparations may be caused by impurities that are incompletely removed during the purification process, or from additives that are used to stabilize the protein, inhibit bacterial growth, and ensure delayed release. Inappropriate injection technique associated with the introduction of cleansing alcohol into the skin by the hypodermic needle may also cause reactions that can be misjudged as insulin-specific adverse reactions.

Antibodies to the following hormonal impurities present in insulin prepara tions have been found in varying percentages in insulin-dependent diabetic patients:

Glucagon	(6%)
Pancreatic polypeptide (PP)	(63%)
Vasoactive intestinal peptide (VIP)	(6%)
Somatostatin	(0.5%)

Proinsulin (present only as 10 parts per million [ppm] in purified insulins) has been suggested as a cause of adverse reactions, however, no antibodies specific to proinsulin as opposed to insulin itself have been found. Furthermore, proinsulin reacts with antibodies against the insulin molecule. Arginine insulin and desaminoinsulin, both with allergenic properties, have been shown to be present in commercial preparations.

Stabilizing chemicals, such as phenol, metacresol, and parabens (used only in lente), are added and may be irritating or cause reactions similar clinically to the immunologic reactions. Zinc has been found to be antigenic. The protamine moiety of NPH forms a complex with the insulin, which first has to be split by proteolytic enzymes to allow the release of the insulin, thus ensuring delayed absorption. Protamine alone has antigenic properties, and the combination with insulin may increase the antigenic potential of the molecule. Isopropyl alcohol has been shown to be the cause of reactions similar to the immediate type of hypersensitivity; these reactions can be avoided by modifying the methods of disinfection and injection.

Adverse reactions to insulin can be classified into the following categories:

A. Allergy
   1. Local reactions
      a. immediate wheal-and-flare reaction
      b. biphasic reaction
      c. toxic complex disease (Arthus-type reaction)
      d. delayed hypersensitivity ("tuberculin" type reaction)
   2. Systemic reactions
B. Resistance
C. Autoimmune antireceptor disease

The *immediate wheal-and-flare reaction (WFR)* usually is seen within 2 weeks after the introduction of insulin therapy. It is similar to classic immediate skin response, which is seen after injection of an allergen, and is observed within 15 minutes after the injection of the insulin. The reaction peaks during the next 15 minutes, then decreases in size and resolves over the next 1 to 2 hours.

In some patients the immediate WFR is followed by a late-phase reaction (LPR) characterized by a circumscribed area that is pruritic, painful, edematous. This *biphasic reaction* develops 2 to 6 hours postinjection and resolves by 24 hours. A LPR can also be observed without a preceding WFR. Both WFR and LPR can be passively transferred (i.e., Prausnitz-Küstner reaction) and are IgE mediated.

Toxic complex disease, or Arthus-type reaction, will occur 3 to 5 hours postinjection, without a preceding WFR. It peaks at 12 to 24 hours and resolves by approximately 48 hours. The mediating antibodies are probably IgG or IgM, with involvement of the complement system (C3a, C5a) and lysosomal enzymes derived from neutrophils.

Delayed hypersensitivity, or tuberculin type, reaction starts approximately 8 to 12 hours postinjection and is characterized by well-circumscribed, pruritic, painful, and mildly indurated lesions. The lesions peak at 24 hours and disappear between 48 and 72 hours. Further evidence for cell-mediated immunity involve-

Table 42. IgE/IgG ratio in diabetes

Group	IgE (cpm/ml)	IgG (cpm/ml)	Ratio IgE/IgG × 10^{-3}
Control	ND	ND	—
Insulin dependent	812 ± 117	51,827 ± 6982	20 ± 4
Insulin allergic (systemic)	18,763 ± 6988[a]	135,050 ± 31,403[a]	131 ± 35[a]
Insulin resistant	10,042 ± 3486[a]	179,180 ± 16,088[a]	30 ± 11
	NS[b]	$(p < 0.01)$[b]	$(p < 0.05)$[b]

ND = not detectable; NS = not significant.
[a]$p < 0.01$ when compared with group B.
[b]Compared with group C.
Source: D. Kumar, Anti-insulin IgE in diabetics. *J. Clin. Endocrinol. Metab.* 45:1159–1164, 1977.

ment in these adverse reactions to insulin is the increased lymphocyte stimulation in the standard in vitro lymphocyte stimulation tests to the insulin protein itself or only to an insulin preparation containing zinc.

Sometimes soon after reinstitution of insulin therapy, patients who had been maintained off insulin for an appreciable length of time (often years) may experience *systemic reactions*. They are usually preceded by increasingly large local reactions, and a history of other allergies often is evident. Manifestations of systemic reactions are generalized urticaria, angioneurotic edema, and even anaphylactic shock.

All patients who receive insulin will develop antibodies. However, *resistance* will only develop in those patients whose antibodies have a high affinity for the insulin molecule. The plasma-insulin binding capacity, measured in IU/ml, will be between 47 and 5700 in resistant patients, whereas in nonresistant patients the level will be only 10 to 20 IU/ml.

Resistance is defined as the requirement of more than 200 units insulin per day for more than 2 days in the absence of ketoacidosis, obesity, endocrinopathy, or infection. It occurs in 1 of 1000 insulin-dependent diabetic patients, typically after 45 years of life, within 5 years of the diagnosis, but in the first year of insulin therapy. Antibody-bound insulin is not biologically active, but is available to dissociate from the antibody molecule as the bioavailable pool decreases. Investigators have suggested that IgG antibodies stabilize the control of diabetes. If this should be confirmed, the introduction of highly purified insulins with little to no antigenic properties might produce a generation of unstable diabetics.

The ratio of IgE to IgG insulin-specific antibodies may differentiate patients allergic to insulin from patients resistant to insulin (Table 42). Patients with neither insulin allergy nor resistance had low levels for both antibodies and a low IgE/IgG ratio. Systemic allergy was characterized by significantly higher levels for both antibodies, but a disproportionate increase of IgE and, therefore, a high IgE/IgG ratio. Resistance showed a proportionate increase of both antibody levels with ratios similar to those nonallergic, nonresistant persons. Four patients have been reported who had allergic reactions to insulin with low levels of IgE antibody to insulin, but virtually absent IgG antibody to insulin. These findings raise the question whether IgG antibody protects against allergy but produces resistance, if a critical plasma-binding capacity is exceeded.

Autoimmune anti-insulin receptor antibodies have been detected in 30 to 40 patients with insulin resistance. These antibodies may produce an insulinlike effect for a brief period. Shortly thereafter they produce extreme insulin resistance. It is presently unclear if this resistance represents a receptor-specific blocking mechanism, or a postreceptor event.

Table 43. Species specific differences of insulin molecules

Insulin	Alpha chain		Beta chain
	Position 8	Position 10	Position 30
Human	Threonine	Isoleucine	Threonine
Pork	Threonine	Isoleucine	Alanine
Beef	Alanine	Valine	Alanine

Approach to the Patient with Insulin Allergy

Although approximately 400,000 patients in the United States have adverse reactions to insulin, only a few patients have required drastic changes in their therapy or hyposensitization. In the elderly patient, management with oral agents may be indicated, but the physician should keep in mind that reinstitution of insulin therapy at a later time bears a high risk of systemic reactions. The patient should be informed of this risk in case future care is to be delivered by a different physician.

The first step in dealing with an adverse reaction following the administration of insulin should be to rule out errors in the injection technique or the introduction of foreign materials such as isopropyl alcohol into the injection site. Even in cases where the local reaction is due specifically to insulin, the symptoms are generally mild and will abate during the next few months of insulin therapy. Therefore, in most cases close follow-up to ensure that the reactions are not increasing in severity and reassurance are all that is necessary. In cases that do not resolve, substitution by a less antigenic preparation may be beneficial. Single component insulin reduced the local allergic manifestations in 56% of allergic patients in one study. Pork insulin is closest related to human insulin in its structure and less antigenic (Table 43). If severe local reactions persist despite the above measures, oral antihistamines (hydroxyzine—Atarax, 50 mg orally h.s.) or steroids (dexamethasone, 0.1–0.5 mg added to each injection of insulin) can be used. Severe cases of local lipodystrophy have also successfully been reversed by the use of monocomponent pork insulin.

Incapacitating local reactions and any systemic reactions warrant a trial of desensitization. The choice of the material used for the injection therapy should be guided by the results of prior skin testing. The least antigenic purified insulin will then be used. Two different schedules have been reported to produce adequate tolerance. The more rapid one suggests injection every 15 to 30 minutes until therapeutic doses are achieved (see Table 45). This may be the method of choice in the patient with brittle diabetes who would not tolerate withdrawal of insulin for a longer period of time. More gradual desensitization can be achieved over 7 days when following the second schedule (Table 44). After the patient has achieved tolerance, frequent injections (b.i.d.–q.i.d.) are necessary to maintain the results.

Table 44. Slow, or gradual, desensitization schedule

Day	Hour	Dose (IU)	Route	Type
1	8 A.M.	0.00001	ID	Pure pork
	12 P.M.	0.0001	ID	Pure pork
	5 P.M.	0.001	ID	Pure pork
2	8 A.M.	0.01	ID	Pure pork
	12 P.M.	0.1	ID	Pure pork
	5 P.M.	1.0	ID	Pure pork
3	8 A.M.	2	ID	Pure pork
	12 P.M.	4	SQ	Pure pork
	5 P.M.	6	SQ	Pure pork
4	8 A.M.	8	SQ	Pure pork
	12 P.M.	12	SQ	Pure pork
	5 P.M.	15	SQ	Pure pork
5	8 A.M.	20	SQ	Pure pork
6	8 A.M.	25	SQ	Pure pork
7	8 A.M.	30	SQ	Pure pork

Source: P. Lieberman, R. Patterson, R. Metz, and G. Lucena, Allergic reactions to insulin. *J.A.M.A.* 215:1106–1112, 1971. Copyright 1971, American Medical Association.

Table 45. Suggested desensitization schedule for rapid desensitization

Dose number	Units
1	0.00001
2	0.0001
3	0.001
4	0.005
5	0.01
6	0.05
7	0.1
8	0.2
9	0.5
10	1
11	2
12	4
13	8
14	10

Administration: subcutaneously every 15 to 30 minutes.
Use a diluent containing 0.5% human serum albumin to prevent adsorption to the glass vial of the insulin at the low concentration.
Source: R. M. Elenbaas and P. J. Forni, Management of insulin allergy and resistance. *Am. J. Hosp. Pharm.* 33:491–497, 1976.

Davidson, J. A., et al. The use of purified insulin in insulin allergy (abstr.). *Diabetes* 23(Suppl. I):352, 1974.
Single component insulin reduced local allergic manifestations in 56% of the patients.

deShazo, R. D. Insulin allergy and insulin resistance. *Postgrad. Med.* 63:85–92, 1978.
Excellent review article by an author who has published widely in this field.

deShazo, R. D., et al. Dermal hypersensitivity reactions to insulin: Correlations of three patterns to their histopathology. *J. Allergy Clin. Immunol.* 69:229–237, 1982.
Recurrent local reactions to insulin may be of three types: (1) IgE mediated "late phase" reactions, (2) Arthus local vasculitic reactions, (3) or tuberculin-type delayed hypersensitivity reactions. Specific insulin antibody determination was not helpful in distinguishing these three types of reactions.

Diehm, P. Allergy to insulin. *Br. Med. J.* 281:1068–1069, 1980.
Isopropyl alcohol (Webcol Alcohol Preps) caused skin reactions similar to the immediate type immune response.

Dixon, K., Exon, P. D., and Malins, J. M. Insulin antibodies and the control of diabetes. *Q. J. Med.* 44:543–553, 1975.
Anti-insulin IgG may stabilize diabetic control by creating an insulin pool with delayed bioavailability.

Galloway, J. A. When the patient is resistant or allergic to insulin. *Med. Times* 108:91–101, 1980.
Steroids, either mixed with the insulin or administered systemically, may control adverse reactions.

Galloway, J. A., et al. New Forms of Insulin. In L. J. Kryson and R. A. Shaw (Eds.), *Endocrinology and Diabetes.* New York: Grune & Stratton, 1975. Pp. 329–342.
Approximately 25% of insulin-dependent diabetic patients with adverse reactions to insulin have other concomitant allergies.

Kahn, R. C., and Rosenthal, A. S. Immunologic reactions to insulin: Insulin allergy, insulin resistance, and the autoimmune insulin syndrome. *Diabetes Care* 2:283–295, 1979.
This is an excellent review article with many helpful practical hints for the management of patients with adverse reactions to insulin.

Klein, S. P. Insulin allergy: treatment with histamine antagonists. *Arch. Intern. Med.* 81:316–327, 1948.
Diphenhydramine, either mixed with the insulin or taken orally, may control adverse reactions.

Kumar, D. Insulin allergy: Differences in the binding of porcine, bovine, and human insulins with anti-insulin IgE. *Diabetes Care* 4:104–107, 1981.
Anti-insulin IgE has a higher avidity to the bovine than to the porcine molecule.

Kumar, D. Anti-insulin IgE in diabetics. *J. Clin. Endocrinol. Metab.* 45:1159–64, 1977.
When increased levels of anti-insulin immunoglobulins are present the ratio of IgE/IgG seems to determine if resistance or allergies develop.

Stobo, J. D. Autoimmune antireceptor diseases. *Hosp. Pract.* 16:49–56, 1981.
Stobo has written a good review including myasthenia gravis insulin resistance, Graves' disease, and asthma.

DERMATOLOGIC REACTIONS

Nancy P. Cummings

Atopic dermatitis is a chronic, hereditable, pruritic skin disease associated with flexural lichenification in adults and facial and extensor involvement in infants. Atopic dermatitis is frequently associated with a personal or family history of atopic disease, such as asthma and allergic rhinitis. Initially described by Besnier in 1892, it was noted by early observers that the cutaneous manifestations of atopic dermatitis resulted from the intense pruritus. A prominent dermatologist stated, "It isn't the eruption that itches but the itch that erupts." Atopic dermatitis has been called Besnier's prurigo, atopic eczema, neurodermatitis, and flexural and infantile eczema.

The incidence of atopic dermatitis varies between 1 and 3%. Forty to sixty-five percent of family members of children with atopic dermatitis will have another manifestation of the atopic state. Atopic dermatitis resolves spontaneously in approximately half of children with early childhood eczema; half develop hay fever or allergic rhinitis and 20 to 30% develop asthma. In severe childhood atopic dermatitis, 35% of patients have persistent symptoms for at least 20 years.

Although atopic dermatitis may appear at any age, in the childhood type it usually begins during the fourth through sixth month of life. An erythematous, pruritic, weeping dermatitis occurs on the cheeks, spreading to the forehead and the extensor surfaces of the arms and legs. In older children between the ages of 2 and 4 years, the predilection for antecubital and popliteal spaces becomes more prominent, and the chronic dermatitis is characterized by large areas with confluent papules and prominent lichenification of the flexural regions. Involvement of the forehead, neck, wrist, and feet may occur.

Atopic dermatitis is characterized by intense pruritus. Dry scaly skin frequently develops and may be more susceptible to irritation by rough fibers in clothing. Stigmata of allergy such as Dennie's lines (prominent folds on the lower eyelid), increased palmar creases, buffed nails, allergic "shiners," and an allergic nasal crease are often present in children with atopic dermatitis.

Several types of abnormal vascular reactions occur in the skin of patients with atopic dermatitis. The presence of these reactions is related to the extent of the skin involvement and the reactions may totally regress when the skin goes into remission. In the triple response of Lewis, when normal skin is stroked, an erythematous line is followed by a flare and then edema. White dermatographism occurs in children with atopic dermatitis, and the usual erythematous line is replaced by a larger line of pallor not associated with edema when involved skin is stroked. Intradermal injection of acetylcholine (1:10,000) causes erythema and flare in normal skin, but children with atopic dermatitis develop blanching. Abnormal cutaneous responses also occur following application of nicotinic esters, intradermal injection of histamine, serotonin, and bradykinin. Furthermore, children with atopic dermatitis have abnormally low skin temperatures over their fingers and toes.

In the laboratory evaluation of children with atopic dermatitis, most will have normal or slightly increased levels of IgG, IgM, IgA, and IgD. IgE is elevated in 80 to 90% of patients. Some patients will have a decreased number of T-lymphocytes and an increased number of IgE-carrying B-lymphocytes. Peripheral blood eosinophil counts are frequently elevated and polymorphonuclear leukocyte counts are usually normal. Serum complement levels are usually normal or slightly elevated. The skin of patients with active atopic dermatitis has greater numbers of *Staphylococcus aureus* than does normal skin. Positive immediate hypersensitivity skin tests to common allergens are present in 50 to 80% of children with atopic dermatitis. The role of allergens in the course of the atopic dermatitis is difficult to determine; in order for allergens to play a role in this disease, they must first produce some type of skin reaction that itches. Such reactions can be seen in grass-sensitive persons when the grass contacts the skin directly. A similar situation may occur with animal dander sensitivity. The role of food allergens is more difficult to determine. Careful challenges of atopic dermatitis patients who are sensitive to foods have demonstrated papular, erythematous lesions that are intensely pruritic. It is possible that this type of reaction may initiate scratching and thus exacerbate the disease process. Positive skin tests—especially to foods—in the management of atopic dermatitis must be interpreted with caution, as it is easy to make therapeutic recommendations such as elimination of a food or foods from the diet, which will have no benefit on the disease process and may be difficult for the family to comply with.

The etiology of atopic dermatitis remains unknown. The presence of immunologic abnormalities is suggested by the increased serum concentration of IgE in 80% of patients. In addition, some patients have defective cell-mediated immunity as evidenced by suppression of delayed hypersensitivity reactions. Examples of defective cell-mediated immunity include anergy to *Candida albicans,* depressed responsiveness of lymphocytes to stimulation by concanavalin A, pokeweed, or phytohemagglutinin, and decreased numbers of thymus-derived lymphocytes. Defective neutrophil chemotaxis has been described in a number of children with severe chronic eczema, extremely elevated IgE levels, and recurrent staphylococcal abscesses.

Atopic dermatitis must be differentiated from a number of diseases. The diseases most frequently confused with atopic dermatitis in infancy are seborrheic dermatitis and scabies. Seborrheic dermatitis is generally not pruritic, and is more prominent in the scalp and diaper region with dry or greasy scales over areas of the body where sebaceous glands are plentiful. Scabies is characterized by papules over the palms and soles of infants and burrows with linear excoriations from scratching. Other family members are often affected. Contact dermatitis of the primary irritant or allergic type is also frequently confused with atopic dermatitis. It usually develops in older children, and can be differentiated from atopic dermatitis by appearance and distribution. Other diseases that can be confused with atopic dermatitis include tinea corporis, nummular dermatitis, and Letterer-Siwe disease, which has a maculopapular petechial eruption on the scalp and trunk. Eczematous skin disease occurs in hereditary diseases such as Leiner's disease, familial C5 dysfunction (i.e., generalized seborrheic dermatitis, intract able diarrhea, and recurrent infections), Wiskott-Aldrich syndrome, biotin deficiency, phenylketonuria, Bruton's agammaglobulinemia, severe combined immunodeficiency, and ataxia telangiectasia.

Treatment of the acute phase of atopic dermatitis consists of wet dressings to relieve itching and corticosteroids to reduce inflammation. Topical corticosteroid lotions or creams are tolerated better than ointments because ointments can cause increased warmth and pruritus. Either 1% hydrocortisone or 0.025% triamcinolone can be applied between changes of wet dressings. When secondary bacterial infection is present, a 10-day course of oral erythromycin or penicillin is indicated. Topical antibiotic preparations should be avoided because they are generally ineffective and are potentially sensitizing. The subacute phase is effectively treated by frequent applications of corticosteroid cream, which can be used under occlusive dressings if the disease is resistant to treatment. During the treatment of the subacute phase in children care must be taken to use low-potency corticosteroids such as hydrocortisone, because, when topical corticosteroids are applied over large skin areas in children, systemic side effects can occur.

Chronic treatment is directed at reducing the itching so that scratching is kept to a minimum, and at prompt treatment of minor exacerbations with topical steroids (1% hydrocortisone) so that the acute and subacute phases can be prevented. Contact with irritating fabrics such as wool should be avoided. Allergens that can be clearly implicated should be avoided; skin contact should especially be avoided. There is probably no role for immunotherapy. Baths are given at least once a day to provide hydration of the skin. Emollients, such as Eucerin or 10% urea cream, can be applied following bathing to help seal in moisture and maintain hydration of the skin. The emollients should also be applied frequently during the day to maintain the hydration. Neutragena may be substituted for soap, which should be used as little as possible because it can be drying. An alternate method of treatment is to avoid contact with both bath soap and water as much as possible, and to substitute Cetaphil lotion for cleaning the skin. Coal tar preparations are also effective in treating the subacute chronic atopic dermatitis. Antihistamines, particularly hydroxyzine, are effective antipruritics. Dietary restrictions are of little benefit in the great majority of infants with atopic dermatitis.

Complications of atopic dermatitis include increased susceptibility to both bacterial and viral cutaneous infections. *Staphylococcus aureus* is cultured most frequently, but beta-hemolytic streptococci may also cause superimposed infection. Increased susceptibility occurs to both vaccinia and herpes simplex (i.e., Kaposi's varicelliform eruption), and begins with multiple vesicular-pustular lesions which can be associated with regional lymphadenopathy, fever, and hepatosplenomegaly. Molluscum contagiosum also occurs with increased frequency. Ocular complications include cataracts in 1 to 3% of patients with atopic dermatitis and increased incidence of keratoconus.

Blaylock, W. K. Atopic dermatitis: Diagnosis and pathobiology. *J. Allergy Clin. Immunol.* 57:62–79, 1976.
  Blaylock has written an excellent review of skin pathology and immunologic abnormalities.
Hanifin, J. M. Atopic dermatitis. *J. Am. Acad. Dermatol.* 6:1–13, 1982.
  Reviews atopic dermatitis.
Hanifin, J. M., and Lobitz, W. C. Newer concepts of atopic dermatitis. *Arch. Dermatol.* 113:663–670, 1977.
  This article reviews atopic dermatitis.
Jacobs, A. H. Local management of atopic dermatitis in infants and children. *Clin. Pediatr.* 8:201–203, 1972.
  In 46 children treated with a modification of the Scholtz regimen, 85% had good to excellent treatment results.
McGeady, S. J., and Buckley, R. H. Depression of cell-mediated immunity in atopic eczema. *J. Allergy Clin. Immunol.* 56:393–406, 1975.
  The severity of eczema correlates with skin anergy and serum IgE concentration.
Norins, A. L. Atopic dermatitis. *Pediatr. Clin. North Am.* 18:801–838, 1971.
  Norins reviews atopic dermatitis.
Rasmussen, J. E., and Provost, T. T. Atopic Dermatitis. In E. Middleton Jr., C. E. Reed, and E. F. Ellis (Eds.), *Allergy: Principles and Practice.* St. Louis: Mosby, 1978. Pp. 1039–1054.
  The authors provide an excellent review of atopic dermatitis.
Roth, H. C. Pathophysiology and treatment of atopic dermatitis. *Int. J. Dermatol.* 16:163–178, 1977.
  This article reviews the forms of treatment of atopic dermatitis: diet, environmental control, tars, steroids, psychotherapy, hypnosis, systemic drugs, and immunotherapy.
Sedlis, E. Natural history of infantile eczema: Its incidence and course. *J. Pediatr.* 66:158–163, 1965.
  Thirty percent of children who had severe infantile atopic dermatitis had moderate disease after 5 years.
Sly, R. M., and Heimlich, E. M. Physiologic abnormalities in the atopic state: A review. *Ann. Allergy* 25:192–210, 1967.

Patients with atopic dermatitis have an increased tendency for vasoconstriction and abnormal skin responses to histamine, acetylcholine, serotonin, epinephrine, and norepinephrine.

Snyderman, R., Rogers, E., and Buckley, R. H.   Abnormalities of leukotaxis in atopic dermatitis. *J. Allergy Clin. Immunol.* 60:121–126, 1977.

In 8 of 14 patients with atopic dermatitis, depressed monocyte chemotaxis was present; in 3 of 10 patients, depressed polymorphonuclear chemotaxis was present.

50. CONTACT DERMATITIS
Lela A. Lee

There are two types of contact dermatitis: irritant and allergic. Irritant dermatitis is caused by contact with substances that are directly toxic to the skin. Allergic contact dermatitis is caused by substances that require participation of the immune system to evoke a response.

In **irritant contact dermatitis** the offending substance may be a strong irritant, such as concentrated hydrochloric acid, which produces adverse effects rapidly in most persons exposed, or a weak irritant, such as a detergent, which requires prolonged exposure or individual susceptibility to produce a cutaneous eruption. Persons at particular risk include those with a defective stratum corneum—the protective outer layer of epidermis—such as in persons with dry, macerated, or excoriated skin.

Irritant dermatitis is common and is usually caused by a variety of mild irritants. Examples are diaper dermatitis, which is often the result of the irritant effect of urine and feces on macerated skin, and hand dermatitis, which is frequently caused or exacerbated by a number of mild irritants, particularly detergents. The clinical appearance is that of a nonspecific eczematous dermatitis, varying from mild erythema and scaling to marked erythema, edema, and vesicles or bullae. The palms are often involved in hand dermatitis. The location of the eruption, in addition to a history of exposure to irritants, generally suggests the diagnosis. The histologic appearance is nonspecific.

In **allergic contact dermatitis** the initiating compound, usually a relatively small molecule, acts as a hapten and binds with structures in the skin forming an immunogenic hapten-carrier complex. In order for this binding to occur, the compound must be able to penetrate the stratum corneum. Areas where the stratum corneum is thin, or where it is damaged, are therefore more susceptible. During the sensitization phase of the immune system's reaction, the hapten-carrier complex is presented to T-lymphocytes by a cell of macrophage origin, the epidermal Langerhans' cell. After this sensitization phase the sensitized T-lymphocytes disseminate throughout the body so that reapplication of the antigen will elicit a reaction anywhere the allergen contacts the skin. In this elicitation phase, sensitized T-lymphocytes initiate an inflammatory response that takes place in the portion of the skin where the allergen is found.

Allergic contact dermatitis is common and is often caused by substances listed in Table 46. The clinical appearance may range from erythema and scaling to edema and vesicles. The location may immediately suggest the etiologic agent, such as dermatitis under a necklace, but in many instances the offending agent is not obvious. The thin skin of the eyelids and genitals is most susceptible to contact dermatitis. The palms, soles, and scalp are relatively resistant. Handling of poison ivy, for example, might result in dermatitis only on the eyelids or genitals. Allergy to hair dyes may cause dermatitis on the face and neck but not

Table 46. Common causes of allergic contact dermatitis

Compound	Sources*
Pentadecacatechol	Poison ivy, oak, and sumac
Nickel	Jewelry, belt buckles, zippers
Paraphenylenediamine	Hair dyes, fur dyes, rubber
Tetramethylthiuram	Rubber
Mercaptobenzothiazole (MBT)	Rubber
Ethylenediamine	Antibiotic creams, cosmetics
Dichromates	Cement, tanned leather
Benzocaine	Topical anesthetics
Parabens	Cosmetics, topical medications
Balsam of Peru	Cosmetics, shampoos
Formaldehyde	Wash-and-wear clothing, shampoos
Neomycin	Topical medications
Epoxy resin	Glues
Other fragrant substances	Perfumes, cosmetics

*This list is not intended to be complete. For a comprehensive catalogue, refer to texts cited in the references.

on the scalp. Dermatitis in exposed areas of the skin, especially the eyelids, may be caused by contact with an airborne allergen.

The diagnosis of allergic contact dermatitis is suggested by the eczematous appearance, the location, and the history of exposure. The causative agent need not be a new exposure, though it often is. Because there is a lag time of up to 2 days between the time of exposure and the appearance of the rash, the patient may not readily relate the two events.

Photoallergic contact dermatitis is an allergic dermatitis that requires both direct contact with an offending chemical and the action of ultraviolet light. The light may create a photoproduct of the original substance, which will then act as a hapten; alternatively, light may affect binding of the original substance to the skin.

Photoallergic contact dermatitis is uncommon. Furacoumarins such as psoralen, which is found in certain perfumes, or musk ambrette, an ingredient of some men's colognes, are occasionally implicated. Appearance and diagnostic clues are similar to those of allergic contact dermatitis. By the nature of the reaction, it occurs only in sun-exposed areas. Photo patch testing may be confirmatory.

Patch testing is a method of applying to the skin chemicals that commonly cause contact hypersensitivity. The patches are removed after 48 hours and the reaction of the skin is measured at 72 hours. The chemicals are applied at concentrations dilute enough to minimize irritation; nevertheless, some experience is required to distinguish irritant- from allergic-contact reactions. Patch testing kits containing the more common offending substances are available commercially. Patch tests are occasionally helpful and may be used to document a reaction. Unfortunately, when the causative agent has not been found after a careful history and examination, the patch tests are frequently unproductive. Testing should not be done until the contact dermatitis has subsided because of the possibility of false-positive reactions. Skin biopsies reveal nonspecific findings and are rarely indicated.

Treatment is directed toward avoidance of the offending irritant or allergen. A reference of cross-reacting chemicals may be helpful in identifying additional substances that should be avoided, though not all the substances cited will invariably cause a reaction. Topical corticosteroids are quite helpful in suppressing inflammation and relieving symptoms. Oral corticosteroids may be indicated for severe reactions. Allergic contact dermatitis may persist for about 3 weeks after discontinuing contact with the allergen; thus, oral corticosteroids may be required over a 3-week course. Restoration of the function of the stratum corneum may be facilitated by appropriate use of emollients on dry skin or by drying macerated skin. Desensitization to common contact sensitizers such as poison ivy has been attempted. Both oral and parenteral injections have been used but neither has clearly been shown to be successful or practical.

Adams, R. M.   Patch testing—a recapitulation. *J. Am. Acad. Dermatol.* 5:629–646, 1981.
   Adams has written a guide for interpreting patch-test results.
Andersen, K. E., and Maibach, H. I.   Allergic reaction to drugs used topically. *Clin. Toxicol.* 16:415–465, 1980.
   This is one of the most comprehensive papers ever written on the subject.
Cronin, E.   *Contact Dermatitis.* London: Churchill Livingstone, 1980.
   Cronin provides an up-to-date, comprehensive, and recommended text.
Fisher, A. A.   *Contact Dermatitis* (2nd ed.). Philadelphia: Lea & Febiger, 1973.
   This is the classic text of contact dermatitis.
Fisher, A. A.   New advances in contact dermatitis. *Int. J. Dermatol.* 16:552–568, 1977.
   Presents a complete, authoritative review of the research and clinical aspects of contact dermatitis.
Maibach, H. I., and Epstein, E.   Contact Dermatitis. In E. Middleton, C. E. Reed, and E. F. Ellis (Eds.), *Allergy: Principles and Practice.* St. Louis: Mosby, 1978. Pp. 1055–1079.
   The authors have written a relevant review for the clinical allergist.
Parker, F.   Contact Dermatitis. In C. W. Bierman and D. S. Pearlman (Eds.), *Allergic Diseases of Infancy, Childhood, and Adolescence.* Philadelphia: Saunders, 1980. Pp. 431–439.
   A brief review for the clinical allergist, which is divided into subheadings as to the area of the body affected and the differential diagnosis.
Rudner, E. J., et al.   The frequency of contact sensitivity in North America, 1972–1974. *Contact Dermatitis* 1:277–280, 1975.
   The title is self-explanatory.
Silberberg-Sinakin, I., and Thorbecke, G. J.   Contact hypersensitivity and Langerhans cells. *J. Invest. Dermatol.* 75:61–67, 1980.
   The authors review the evidence linking the Langerhans' cell to contact hypersensitivity.
Streilein, J. W., and Bergstresser, P. R.   Langerhans cell function dictates induction of contact hypersensitivity or unresponsiveness to DNFB in Syrian hamsters. *J. Invest. Dermatol.* 77:272–277, 1981.
   This article provides more details linking the Langerhans' cell to contact hypersensitivity.

51. CHRONIC AND ACUTE URTICARIA
Ray S. Davis

Urticaria (hives) is a common dermatologic disorder that affects at least 20% of the population of the United States at some time in their lives. Urticarial reactions occur when either immunologic or nonimmunologic stimuli trigger the release of mediators of inflammation. The resultant edema in the upper dermis produces a wheal usually associated with erythema and pruritus. Angioedema, a similar reaction in the lower dermis, produces localized swelling.

Urticaria may be classified as either acute or chronic based on the duration of symptoms. Because acute urticaria is transient and usually lasts less than 1 month, patients often fail to seek medical attention. The offending agent is often obvious to the patient because the reaction occurs soon after ingestion of certain foods or drugs, or following insect stings. The patient, therefore, learns to avoid the suspected allergen. Acute urticaria is often reagin, or IgE, mediated.

Urticaria of more than 1 month's duration is considered to be chronic. Urticaria of this duration is usually a vexing problem, and, even after extensive evaluation, a cause can be discovered in only 30% of the cases. The history is paramount, and specific tests other than CBC, erythrocyte sedimentation rate, and a urinalysis, should be dictated by historical leads. Multiple skin and blood tests, combined with the results of roentgenograms to rule out occult infections, have proved costly and rarely lead to a cure.

Although type I allergic reactions rarely cause chronic urticaria, a complete evaluation must include a careful food and drug history, and a determination of whether the reaction has occurred after contact with animals, chemicals, jewelry, or clothing. Common offending foods include seafood, nuts, and eggs. Penicillin, the most common drug involved in allergic reactions, is found in small quantities in many dairy products. Aspirin, tartrazine dye, and benzoic acid derivatives have been known to exacerbate chronic urticaria. The many drugs that are non-specific histamine releasers include amphetamines (i.e., diet pills), thiamine, morphine, atropine, quinine, and polymyxin. Inhalant allergy is rarely a cause of chronic urticaria, although animal danders have been reported to cause urticaria of this duration.

Underlying viral, bacterial, fungal, and parasitic infections can cause chronic urticaria. Infectious mononucleosis and hepatitis should be considered with a history of systemic symptoms (i.e., pharyngitis, lymphadenopathy, fever rash, arthritis). Roentgenograms looking for occult bacterial infections such as sinusitis, dental abscesses, or pneumonia rarely prove useful. One should consider testing stool for parasites only if there is significant peripheral eosinophilia, GI symptoms, and a history of travel to an endemic area. Skin tests to uncover occult candidiasis and treatment with low-yeast diets and nystatin have shown promising results in several studies.

Genetic types of urticaria are rare, but a complete history should include family history. These rare entities include hereditary angioedema (C1 esterase inhibitor deficiency); vibratory angioedema; the syndrome of urticaria, deafness, and amyloidosis; delayed cold urticaria; localized heat urticaria; and C3b inactivator (factor I) deficiency.

The physical urticarias are usually reproducible, and evaluation is simple. Cholinergic urticaria is characterized by multiple 1- to 2-mm papules surrounded by erythematous halos, which occur after exercise, warm baths, or showers, and anxiety. Aquagenic urticaria is very rare, but has similar papular lesions that develop in response to water of any temperature. Cold urticaria can be diagnosed by placing an ice cube on the volar surface of the forearm for 4 to 5 minutes; upon rewarming, the local area will urticate within 5 to 10 minutes. Cold urticaria can rarely be associated with cryoglobulinemia and lymphoreticular malignancies. Solar urticaria can be examined by exposure to various wavelengths of light. Dermatographism is an exaggerated and prolonged wheal-and-flare reaction, which will occur following firm stroking of the skin (usually the back) with a broken tongue blade; rarely, a delayed dermatographic response will occur 3 to 6 hours later. Pressure urticaria is another rare variant, which can occur up to 8 hours after application of prolonged pressure to a local skin area. A multitude of systemic disorders has been associated with chronic urticaria. When there is a history of fever, arthritis, weight loss, or unusual bleeding problems, the lymphomas and leukemias must be considered, as well as autoimmune disorders such as systemic lupus erythematosus and juvenile rheumatoid arthritis. Urticaria pigmentosa is a disorder in which diffuse accumulations of mast cells occur over the body; rubbing a lesion can cause immediate wheal formation. If a thorough history suggests any of the above disorders, routine screening tests may provide invaluable supportive evidence as an aid to confirming the diagnosis. Appropriate specific tests can then be ordered to confirm the diagnosis.

Obviously, the treatment of choice is avoidance if the cause of the urticaria can be discovered. However, since the cause is usually unknown, drug therapy is often required. Antihistamines are the mainstay in the treatment of urticaria. Although H_1 receptor blockers such as chlorphenamiramine and diphenhydramine have been used, hydroxyzine, with its added tranquilizing effects, seems to be more beneficial. Hydroxyzine is often effective in 1 to 2 mg/kg/day doses. When hydroxyzine alone is not effective, it has been used in combination with oral sympathomimetics drugs, such as ephedrine or terbutaline, or H_2 blockers, such as cimetadine. Cromolyn has not proved to be beneficial. Specific treatment of cold urticaria with cyproheptadine and hereditary angioedema with danazol has been well documented. Although induction of tolerance has been attempted in the various forms of physical urticaria, success has been limited.

The prognosis of chronic urticaria is generally good. The goal of therapy is to effectively relieve the symptoms in order to improve the quality of life for these patients until the disorder gradually resolves.

Champion, R. H.   Drug therapy of urticaria. *Br. Med. J.* 4:730–732, 1973.
Champion provides a nice discussion on antihistamines.

Champion, R. H., Roberts, S. O., and Carpenter, R. G.   Urticaria and angio-edema: A review of 554 patients. *Br. J. Dermatol.* 81:588–597, 1969.
This study is the largest series reported in the literature (554 subjects) with a thorough discussion provided.

Commens, C. A., and Greaves, M. W.   Tests to establish the diagnosis in cholinergic urticaria. *Br. J. Dermatol.* 98:47–51, 1978.
Exercise and warm baths were the most sensitive tests to reproduce cholinergic urticaria when suggested by history. Mecholyl skin tests were positive in only half of cases.

Harvey, R. P., and Schocket, A. L.   The effect of H_1 and H_2 blockade on cutaneous histamine response in man. *J. Allergy Clin. Immunol.* 65:136–139, 1980.
The authors suggest that combined hydroxyzine and cimetidine therapy may be efficacious in patients refractory to H_1 antihistamines alone.

Jacobson, K. W., Branch, L. B., and Nelson, H. S.   Laboratory tests in chronic urticaria. *J.A.M.A.* 243:1644–1646, 1980.
This article is an excellent discussion of the cost effectiveness of multiple laboratory studies in search of an etiology in patients with chronic urticaria.

James, J., and Warin, R. P.   An assessment of the role of *Candida albicans* and food yeasts in chronic urticaria. *Br. J. Dermatol.* 84:227–237, 1971.
Antifungal therapy and low yeast diets significantly improved those patients who had positive prick tests to Candida.

Juhlin, L.   Clinical studies on the diagnosis and treatment of urticaria. *Ann. Allergy* 39:356–361, 1977.
Juhlin succinctly covers the multiple etiologies.

Juhlin, L., Michaëlsson, G., and Zetterström, O.   Urticaria and asthma induced by food and drug additives in patients with aspirin hypersensitivity. *J. Allergy Clin. Immunol.* 50:92–98, 1972.
Presentation of seven aspirin-sensitive patients who developed asthma, urticaria, or both when challenged with tartrazine and some benzoic acid derivatives.

Mathews, K. P.   Urticaria and angioedema. *J. Allergy Clin. Immunol.* 72:1–14, 1983.
This is an excellent review of both diagnosis and treatment.

Mathews, K. P.   Management of urticaria and angioedema. *J. Allergy Clin. Immunol.* 66:347–357, 1980.
A current review that stresses mechanisms and mediators, but also includes the myriad etiologies.

Mathison, D. A., et al.   Hypocomplementemia in chronic urticaria. *Ann. Intern. Med.* 86:534–538, 1977.
In this study, 10 of 72 patients with chronic urticaria had low complement levels, suggesting an immunologic defect.

Moore-Robinson, M., and Warin, R. P.   Some clinical aspects of cholinergic urticaria. *Br. J. Dermatol.* 80:794–799, 1968.
A classic paper that includes incidence, course, diagnosis, and treatment of cholinergic urticaria. Hydroxyzine was the preferred medication.

Pasricha, J. S., Pasricha, A., and Prakash, O. M.   Role of gastrointestinal parasites in urticaria. *Ann. Allergy* 30:348–351, 1972.
This study showed that even in India, parasites rarely cause chronic urticaria; therefore, stool examinations for parasites are rarely indicated.

Robinson, H. M., Robinson, R. C. V., and Strahan, J. F.   Hydroxyzine (Atarax) hydrochloride in dermatological therapy. *J.A.M.A.* 161:604–606, 1956.
This article is a good discussion of one of the most commonly used antihistamines.

Sheffer, A. L.   Urticaria and angio-edema. *Pediatr. Clin. North Am.* 22:193–201, 1975.
Presents a pediatric point of view of this disease.

Shelley, W. B., and Rawnsley, H. M.   Aquagenic urticaria. Contact sensitivity reaction to water. *J.A.M.A.* 189:895–898, 1964.
The original report of three cases in which urticaria, similar morphologically to cholinergic urticaria, occurred after local exposure to water to various temperatures.

Thormann, J., Laurberg, G., and Zachariae, H.   Oral sodium cromoglycate in chronic urticaria. *Allergy* 35:139–141, 1980.
No benefit could be demonstrated in this double-blind study of oral cromolyn versus placebo.

Wanderer, A. A., and Ellis, E. F.   Treatment of cold urticaria with cyproheptadine. *J. Allergy Clin. Immunol.* 48:366–371, 1971.
Success is demonstrated in treating eight of nine patients with cyproheptadine.

Warin, R. P., and Champion, R. H.   *Urticaria—Major Problems in Dermatology.* London: Saunders, 1974.
This monograph provides everything you always wanted to know about urticaria, complete with references for each chapter.

SPECIAL PROBLEMS

52. ANAPHYLACTOID REACTIONS TO IODINATED CONTRAST MEDIA
Rajesh G. Bhagat

Since the introduction of radiographic contrast media (RCM) in the 1920s, various untoward reactions have been reported in patients undergoing diagnostic procedures that utilize these materials (see Table 47). The exact incidence of such reactions is difficult to establish, but it is estimated that untoward reactions, regardless of type and severity, occur in 5 to 8% of patients undergoing procedures using RCM. Approximately one-third of these reactions are anaphylactoid in nature. Fortunately the vast majority of the anaphylactoid reactions are mild and require little or no therapy. Nevertheless, fatal reactions to RCM are well recognized and have been reported to occur in 1:40,000 to 1:400,000 patients receiving these agents.

The pathogenesis of these anaphylactoid reactions has not been clearly identified. Several different possible mechanisms have been evaluated, and there are data to support the involvement of each of the mechanisms in some but not all clinical settings. It is therefore likely that RCM may act by more than one mechanism to cause such reactions.

Initially RCM was thought to induce the adverse reactions mimicking allergic symptomatology by an IgE-mediated mechanism; however, most experimental evidence suggests that this mechanism is not operative. RCM reactions can occur following first-time administration of these agents. Repeat reactions have occurred inconsistently suggesting that these reactions are not mediated by an antibody. Immediate skin tests are not helpful in identifying patients at risk of encountering such reactions. For these reasons these reactions are termed *anaphylactoid,* not anaphylactic.

In spite of the lack of evidence of IgE-mediated mechanisms, many in vitro and in vivo studies have demonstrated the evidence of histamine release following administration of RCM. However, anaphylactoid reactions to RCM can occur without detectable levels of histamine in the serum and, at times, elevated serum levels of histamine can be detected in patients who have not had symptoms. Thus, histamine release does not always correlate with clinical symptoms.

The role of complement activation in the pathogenesis of the anaphylactoid reactions to RCM has been studied extensively. Activation of complement components produces the biologically active fragments C3a and C5a that induce mast cells and basophils to release mediators such as histamine and leukotrienes. These mediators could be responsible for the anaphylactoid symptoms. Several studies have shown that RCM can activate the complement components in vitro; however, the relationship between the in vitro activation of complement and the clinical response is tenuous. Nonetheless, patients with anaphylactoid reactions to RCM often exhibit a lower baseline level of CH50 (total hemolytic complement). Thus, the ongoing degree of complement activation prior to the infusion of RCM may be an important variable in determining whether a patient will de-

Table 47. Reactions to intravascular administration of RCM

Immediate	
Anaphylactoid	Urticaria, angioedema, wheezing, hypotension, shock
Cardiac	Cardiac arrhythmias, pulmonary edema, cardiac arrest
Neurologic	Seizures
Miscellaneous	Nausea, vomiting, paresthesias, diaphoresis, bradycardia
Delayed	Renal failure

velop reactions, and may explain the inconsistency of recurrent reactions in susceptible persons.

In some patients RCM may be capable of stimulating mast cells (or basophils) and platelets directly and nonspecifically to induce the release of mediators. This observation, however, is not always correlated with clinical symptoms.

RCM has also been shown to (1) inhibit platelet aggregation in high doses; (2) activate certain enzymes, including B glucuronidase and other lysozomal enzymes; (3) exert its effects on the clotting system by activation of fibrinolytic enzymes; and (4) cause serotonin release from the platelets. The exact role played by these actions of RCM in causing anaphylactoid reactions is not clear at the present time.

Approach to the Patient

Because the first exposure to RCM can induce an anaphylactoid reaction, all patients should be carefully observed by a physician during the procedure. An intravenous line should be placed before the procedure starts and all medications necessary to treat an anaphylactoid reaction must be available. Several investigators have used pretreatment with antihistamines in all patients undergoing studies with RCM and they found that overall incidence of anaphylactoid reactions decreased. Pretreatment with antihistamines did not eliminate the severe reactions. Moreover, the administration of antihistamines in every patient undergoing procedures using RCM is impractical because of the relative infrequency of RCM-induced reactions.

In general, patients with a prior history of anaphylactoid reaction to RCM are at greater risk of having such a reaction on subsequent exposure. It is difficult to predict with certainty which patients will react upon subsequent exposure. Several investigators have tried to develop a reliable pretest procedure that would identify patients who will have recurrent reactions. Tests that have proved to be unsuccessful in predicting reactions have included oral administration, conjunctival instillation, and intradermal injections of RCM. A test that has had some predictive value is intravenous administration of a small amount (0.1 ml) of dilute solution (1:10,000) of RCM, in graded increments (in amount and concentration) every 15 minutes. The lack of adverse reactions after administration of 5 ml of full-strength RCM constitutes a negative test. Although positive intravenous tests identify a majority of patients likely to develop the anaphylactoid reactions, a negative test result does not exclude such reactions. In addition, anaphylactoid reactions can occur during the intravenous test itself. Because the graded administration of dilute solution is time consuming and requires significant physician or technician time, such tests are not routinely employed.

Multicenter studies have shown that a combination of antihistamines and corticosteroid pretreatment is a highly beneficial prophylactic measure in patients with a history of previous anaphylactoid reaction to RCM. The suggested approach to the patient who has experienced a previous reaction is as follows:

1. Inform the patient of the risk involved and document the need for the study using RCM.
2. If the need for the study is clear and the patient is aware of and accepts the risk, pretreat with (a) prednisone, 50 mg orally every 6 hours beginning 19 hours before the study (the third dose is given 1 hour before the study), and (b) diphenhydramine, 50 mg intramuscularly 1 hour before the study.

This protocol requires at least 18 hours of pretreatment with prednisone and diphenhydramine. Recently, several authors have suggested adding cimetidine, 300 mg orally 1 hour before the study, to this regimen.

In situations where high-risk patients require emergency radiographic contrast procedures and where adequate time for pretreatment with oral prednisone and antihistaminics is not available, the following approach is suggested:

1. Document absolute indication for the emergency procedure.
2. Inform the patient of the risk involved.
3. Immediately administer hydrocortisone 200 mg IV and at 4-hour intervals until the procedure is completed.
4. Administer diphenhydramine 50 mg IM before the procedure.
5. Have emergency equipment available.

The efficacy of this regimen needs to be determined.

Arroyave, C. M., Bhat, K. N., and Crown, R.   Activation of the alternate pathway of complement system by radiographic contrast media. *J. Immunol.* 117:1866–1869, 1978.
This article provided the first demonstration of complement activation after RCM infusion in man, through alternate pathway. None of the patients with complement activation had symptoms.

Arroyave, C. M., Schatz, M., and Simon, R. A.   Activation of complement system by radiographic contrast media: Studies in vivo and in vitro. *J. Allergy Clin. Immunol.* 63:276–280, 1979.
The authors showed that in vivo and in vitro complement activation occurs following infusion of RCM in a nonsequential fashion. The changes in complement levels did not correlate with symptoms.

Brasch, R. C., Rockoff, S. D., and Kuhn, C.   Contrast media as histamine liberators. *Invest. Radiol.* 5:510–513, 1970.
This study was the first to show that histamine is released during perfusion of RCM. The study also showed that there was no correlation between the increase in plasma histamine and clinical reactions.

Cho, K. J., and Thornbury, J. R.   Severe reactions to contrast material by three consecutive routes: Intravenous, subcutaneous and intraarterial. *A.J.R.* 131:509–510, 1978.
The authors present a case report of a patient who had anaphylactoid reaction to RCM administered via intravenous, intraarterial, and subcutaneous route.

Cogen, F. C., et al.   Histamine release and complement changes following injection of contrast media in humans. *J. Allergy Clin. Immunol.* 64:299–303, 1979.
The study confirmed that elevated arterial histamine levels are seen following RCM injection, in the absence of clinical reactions.

Gorevic, P., and Kaplan, A. P.   Contrast agents and anaphylactic-like reactions (edit.) *J. Allergy Clin. Immunol.* 63:225–227, 1979.
The article briefly reviews possible mechanisms involved in the adverse reactions to RCM.

Greenberger, P. A., et al.   Pretreatment of high risk patients requiring radiographic contrast media studies. *J. Allergy Clin. Immunol.* 67:185–187, 1981.
A prospective study of 318 patients demonstrating the efficacy of pretreatment program using prednisone and diphenhydramine 18 hours prior to the radiographic procedure.

Liberman, P., and Siegle, R. L.   Complement activation following intravenous contrast material administration. *J. Allergy Clin. Immunol.* 64:13–17, 1979.
This study investigated complement components (C3, C4, C5, and CH50) in patients undergoing studies with RCM. A consistent fall in complement occurred regardless of the presence or absence of anaphylactoid reaction. The patients with clinical reactions had a statistically significant fall in CH50 and lower baseline CH50 than did the nonreactor group.

Liberman, P., Siegle, R. L., Kaplan, R. J., and Hashimoto, K.   Chronic urticaria and intermittent anaphylaxis. Reaction to iophendylate. *J.A.M.A.* 236:1495–1497, 1976.
The authors discussed a case of anaphylaxis following administration of RCM and showed by means of skin test and passive transfer reaction that this was caused by an IgE-mediated mechanism. They further confirmed the mechanism by heating the patients' serum at 56°C for 1 hour and abolishing the passive transfer. (As mentioned before, only a few such case reports confirming IgE-mediated mechanism exist.)

Liberman, P., Siegle, R. L., and Taylor, W. W.   Anaphylactoid reactions to iodinated contrast material. *J. Allergy Clin. Immunol.* 62:174–180, 1978.

A concise review that deals with various aspects of the problem and the developments up to 1978.

Witten, D. M.   Reactions to urographic contrast media. *J.A.M.A.* 231:974–977, 1975.

The cumulative incidence of all adverse reactions, regardless of type and severity is between 5 and 8%, whereas anaphylactoid reactions occurred in 2% studied. The incidence of fatalities was between 1 in 40,000 and 1 in 116,000 of all studies performed.

Yocum, M. W., Heller, A. M., and Abls, R. I.   Efficacy of intravenous pretesting and antihistamine prophylaxis in radio contrast media sensitive patients. *J. Allergy Clin. Immunol.* 62:309–313, 1978.

The authors showed that intravenous pretesting with RCM may not always identify patients likely to develop anaphylactoid reaction to RCM, and that pretreatment of such patients with steroids and antihistaminics may be helpful, but not totally protective against subsequent anaphylactoid reactions to RCM.

53. SULFITE SENSITIVITY
Robert D. Cook

The problem of intermittent, inconsistent, and multiple food sensitivities is all too common, and its evaluation has been dissatisfying for both the patient and the physician. The reaction, be it asthmatic, cutaneous, or anaphylactoid, is usually attributed to either a true IgE-mediated allergic mechanism or to the emotional instability of the patient. Treatment is often a rigid avoidance diet that is determined either empirically or with the aid of immediate hypersensitivity food skin tests and is often not relevant to the clinical history.

As with other clinical problems that suggest an allergic etiology, identification, rigorous documentation, and avoidance of the *specific* agents are the most important elements of management. When considering a history of intermittent and inconsistent food intolerance, the possibility of food-additive sensitivity should be considered. The purpose of this chapter is to review a recently described food additive syndrome: sulfite sensitivity.

Although interest initially focused on anaphylaxislike reactions associated with sulfite ingestion, a much more common **clinical syndrome** resembles that of the respiratory form of aspirin and tartrazine idiosyncrasy. These patients, however, are usually neither aspirin nor tartrazine sensitive. The typical sulfite-sensitive patients are middle-aged women with a history of paroxysmal exacerbations of asthma. These patients are usually steroid-requiring, frequently have perennial rhinitis, and seem to have an increased incidence of sinusitis and nasal polyposis. Acute episodes, which occur more frequently in restaurants, are often accompanied by an upper body flush. The patients have negative or irrelevant immediate hypersensitivity inhalant and food skin tests, and skin tests with sulfite solutions also are usually negative. Although the history can be highly suggestive, documentation requires a positive provocative ingestion challenge.

The typical attack on sulfite sensitivity consists of chest tightness, cough, wheezing, dyspnea, an erythematous or subjective flush, and a sensation of faintness or weakness. It begins rapidly after exposure to the sulfite—often within minutes. Other less common reactions include swelling of the lips or tongue, throat tightness, hypotension, loss of consciousness, and respiratory arrest. Urticaria and angioedema have only been described in conjunction with the generalized anaphylactoid reaction.

Asthmatic reactions are dose-dependent for each patient, but positive provocation challenges are marked by a dramatic decrease in pulmonary function when the threshold dose is reached. Positive challenges have required as little as 5 mg, to as much as 200 mg, of sulfite. Bronchodilator therapy is often required for

Table 48. Sulfites in food, beverages, and pharmaceuticals

Restaurant meals (e.g., salads, avocado dip, potatoes, shrimp)
Foods*
    Dehydrated fruits (e.g., apricots, apples, peaches, pears, and other blanched fruits)
    Fruit products (e.g., concentrates, syrups, purees, jams)
    Dehydrated vegetables (e.g., carrots, potatoes, cabbage, dehydrated meals for campers
    and hikers, soup mixes)
    Raw vegetables (cut potatoes for french fries)
    Shrimp
Beverages
    Wine (especially homemade and foreign wines)
    Beer
    Fruit juices
    Orange drinks
    Milk powder
Pharmaceuticals
    Epinephrine (Adrenalin)
    Lidocaine with epinephrine (Xylocaine with epinephrine)
    Isoproterenol solution (Vapo-Iso, Isuprel)
    Isoetharine solution (Bronkosol)
    Metaproterenol solution (Alupent, Metaprel)
    Dexamethasone injectable (Decadron)
    Amino acid IV hyperalimentation fluids (Travasol)

*Cooking decreases sulfite content of foods by volatilization of sulfur dioxide and nonenzymatic conversion of sulfites to sulfates.

symptom reversal. The incidence of documented sulfite-induced asthma is between 3 and 8% of the asthmatic population. In one study, 56% of asthmatic patients with a history suggestive of sulfite sensitivity had a positive challenge.

Sulfites (i.e., sulfur dioxide and the potassium and sodium salts of sulfite, bisulfite, and metabisulfite) are among the oldest and currently most ubiquitous food additives (Table 48). Used as antibacterials, selective antifungals, antioxidants, and antibrowning agents, sulfites can be found in many foods, beverages, and pharmaceuticals. Section 403K of the Food, Drug and Cosmetic Act requires disclosure of the presence of sulfites only if they are used as preservatives. The FDA regulation dealing with sulfites places no restriction on the amount that may be added to food products except as in accordance with good manufacturing practice and where they are specifically prohibited (e.g., meats, sausage, fish, egg products, and primary thiamine sources).

Sulfur dioxide and sulfites are found in greatest quantity in restaurant meals where it is sprayed in liquid form on salads, shrimp, avocado dip, and potatoes, and, at times, indiscriminately on foods left exposed in buffets. Hospitals and other institutions also make wide use of these solutions to prevent food spoilage and discoloration. Other sulfite-containing foods and beverages include wine, beer, powdered milk, fruit juices and drinks, dehydrated fruits and vegetables, raw vegetables, and shrimp (see Table 48). The average American consumes between 2 and 10 mg of sulfites per day. One restaurant meal may contain 100 mg of sulfite.

Used as preservatives and antioxidants in parenteral medications and solutions for inhalation, ironically sulfites may be found in many of the agents used to treat asthma. The bronchodilating effects of the sympathomimetics usually are sufficiently potent and long acting that adverse reactions to sulfite are overcome by the bronchodilation and thus not observed. However, some of the reports of refractoriness and paradoxical reactions to inhaled isoproterenol may have been caused by sulfite sensitivity, which was manifested over the action of a relatively short-acting bronchodilator. The use of nebulized bronchodilators should not be abandoned because of the fear of sulfite sensitivity. Rather, a paradoxic response to an inhaled bronchodilator solution should alert the physician to the possibility of sulfite idiosyncrasy.

Occupational and atmospheric exposure to sulfur dioxide also occurs. As one would expect, occupational asthma caused by sulfites relates to the food-processing and food-handling industries. Reported cases have included a "fry-cook" who developed bronchospasm after potatoes were placed in boiling oil, liberating sulfur dioxide; a worker in a soft drink plant where sulfur dioxide was used; and a hop-sampler who tasted dried sulfited hops. Industrial and urban exposure also occurs where high sulfur content coal is burned.

Bronchial hyperreactivity to inhaled sulfur dioxide is a characteristic of most asthmatic patients. The majority of sulfite-sensitive patients give a history of sensitivity to pollution. Whether or not they are more sensitive than the asthmatic population to inhaled sulfur dioxide has yet to be studied.

The **pathogenesis** of sulfite intolerance is not currently understood. There is one reported case of anaphylactic sensitivity where an IgE mechanism has been documented by positive direct immediate hypersensitivity skin tests and by Pransnitz-Küstner testing. Speculation about the cause of respiratory sulfite sensitivity has focused on direct bronchial irritation from vapor phase sulfur dioxide in liquids, and on cholinergic parasympathetic reflex activity.

Once sulfite sensitivity has been documented, **therapy** is directed at avoidance. Patients should (1) avoid restaurant meals and wine, (2) be provided with the most current lists of sulfite-containing foods, (3) and consult labels for sulfur dioxide, sulfite, bisulfite, and metabisulfite (although sulfites may still be present even if they are not listed). Processed foods should be cooked thoroughly to decrease the amount of any sulfites present. If possible, a drug regimen should be established that can block the reaction to sulfite with subsequent challenge in the laboratory. Some studies have suggested that cromolyn or antihistamines may be useful in preventing reactions. An anaphylaxis kit should be given to the patient with a history of severe, life-threatening reactions to sulfites, but only after documenting the absence of a paradoxic reaction to epinephrine. A Medic Alert bracelet should also be prescribed.

Chichester, D. F., and Tanner, F. W., Jr. Sulfur Dioxide and Sulfites. In T. E. Furia (Ed.), *Handbook of Food Additives (2nd ed.)*. Cleveland: CRC Press, 1979–1980. Pp. 142.
  Presents a discussion of the types, mechanisms of action, approved uses, and content of sulfite in various products.
Freedman, B. J. Sulphur dioxide in foods and beverages: its use as a preservative and its effect on asthma. *Br. J. Dis. Chest* 74:128–134, 1980.
  Freedman reiterates the data from his 1977 article, reviews the sources and amounts of dietary sulfites, and presents several cases of occupational asthma to sulfites.
Freedman, B. J. Asthma induced by sulphur dioxide, benzoate, and tartrazine contained in orange drinks. *Clin. Allergy* 7:407–415, 1977.
  The author found that 30 of 272 asthmatic patients (11%) had a history of increased bronchospasm after drinking orange drinks. He challenged 14 of these patients; 8 (57%) were sensitive to sulfur dioxide, 4 reacted to benzoate (3 were also sulfur dioxide reactors), and 1 to tartrazine. Four had no reaction. Freedman was able to block the reaction by administering cromoglycate prior to challenge.
Freedman, B. J. A dietary free from additives in the management of allergic disease. *Clin. Allergy* 7:417–421, 1977.
  Because it is often difficult to provide a complete list of foods that must be avoided, Freedman provides a list of foods that are free from sulfur dioxide, benzoates, and azo dyes. The permitted food list is helpful but many are proprietary brands available in the United Kingdom.

Keighley, J. F. Iatrogenic asthma associated with adrenergic aerosols. *Ann. Intern. Med.* 65:985–995, 1966.

This article describes three cases of patients with asthma precipitated by inhaled isoproterenol or epinephrine, but who experienced no adverse effects from sublingual isoproterenol.

Koenig, J. Q., Pierson, W. E., Horike, M., and Frank, R. Bronchoconstrictor responses to sulfur dioxide or sulfur dioxide plus sodium chloride droplets in allergic, nonasthmatic adolescents. *J. Allergy Clin. Immunol.* 69:339–344, 1982.

The title is misleading. The authors studied eight atopic adolescents with documented exercise-induced asthma. Subthreshold exercise challenges plus subprovocative exposure to sulfur dioxide synergistically produced bronchospasm.

Prenner, B. M., and Stevens, J. J. Anaphylaxis after ingestion of sodium bisulfite. *Ann. Allergy* 37:180–182, 1976.

A case of anaphylactic sensitivity to sodium bisulfite documented by positive scratch and intradermal skin tests, passive transfer (Prausnitz-Küstner reaction), and a positive oral provocative challenge. The article also anecdotally mentions contact sensitivity to bisulfite in food handlers.

Schwartz, H. J. Sensitivity to ingested metabisulfite: Variations in clinical presentation. *J. Allergy Clin. Immunol.* 71:487–9, 1983.

This study presents two patients with histories compatible with an anaphylactic reaction temporally related to meals. The reactions in both patients appeared to be due to sensitivity to metabisulfites.

Sheppard, D., et al. Lower threshold and greater bronchomotor responsiveness of asthmatic subjects to sulfur dioxide. *Am. Rev. Respir. Dis.* 122:873–878, 1980.

The authors challenged normal, atopic, and asthmatic subjects with increasing concentrations of inhaled sulfur dioxide, and found that asthmatic patients reacted to as low as 1 PPM SO_2 whereas it required 5 PPM SO_2 to increase airway resistance in normal or atopic subjects. The authors found that the response could be completely blocked in each of the three groups by pretreatment with inhaled atropine.

Simon, R. A., Green, L., and Stevenson, D. D. The incidence of ingested metabisulfite sensitivity in an asthmatic population (abstr.). *J. Allergy Clin. Immunol.* 69 (Suppl.):118, 1982.

Sixty-one asthmatic patients were chosen at random and challenged with a graded amount (10–200 mg) of metabisulfite. Five (8.2%) patients had a positive challenge; reactions were milder and occurred at higher dosages of sulfite than in their prior study of patients with a suggestive history.

Stevenson, D. D., and Simon, R. A. Sensitivity to ingested metabisulfites in asthmatic subjects. *J. Allergy Clin. Immunol.* 68:26–32, 1981.

This article is the definitive and best documented study of sulfite sensitivity. It presents four cases of patients with asthmatic sensitivity to metabisulfite and one with an episode of a generalized systemic reaction as well. Oral challenges were positive in all patients, but skin tests and peripheral basophil histamine release were negative.

54. DIET AND HYPERACTIVITY
Manon Brenner

Reports of behavioral changes related to foods have appeared in the pediatric and allergy literature for 50 years. Even though there has been no association of such symptoms as irritability, hyperactivity, headache, and fatigue with atopic conditions such as eczema, rhinitis, or asthma, the idea of an altered reaction of the central nervous system to food substances initially seemed to fall under the domain of allergy, and terms such as *allergic toxemia* and *allergic tension-fatigue syndrome* were coined in the 1950s.

Many case reports have been published concerning ingestion of foods and hyperactivity. Uncontrolled studies and case reports have cited the improvement of various behavioral and psychological disturbances with elimination of such common foods as milk, corn, wheat, eggs, oranges, chocolate, and sugar.

Further interest and controversy in this general area was stirred by Dr. Benjamin Feingold, who proposed a new hypothesis and popularized his observations in a book in 1975. Dr. Feingold's hypothesis was that hyperactivity was produced not by an allergic mechanism, but by an idiosyncratic, nonimmunologic reaction to food substances in genetically predisposed persons. His hypothesis evolved from observations of persons with intolerance to aspirin and tartrazine (FDSC yellow dye #5), whose urticaria and wheezing disappeared with the elimination of these substances, and whose behavioral and psychiatric problems coincidentally improved. Feingold extended his theory to associate hyperactivity and learning disorders in children with an idiosyncratic reaction to naturally occurring salicylates, artificial dyes, the antioxidant preservatives BHA and BHT, and artificial flavorings. He reported that 50% of the hyperactive children in his practice at the Kaiser-Permanente Clinic in San Francisco had a dramatic remission of symptoms when placed on a diet eliminating these substances. Although only anecdotal data were presented, his book, *Why Your Child Is Hyperactive*, received wide publicity in the lay press and was enthusiastically received by parents anxious for a cure, and by physicians hoping to avoid pharmacologic management.

The original Feingold diet, also known as the K-P (Kaiser-Permanente) diet, restricted foods containing natural salicylates (e.g., apples, apricots, grapes, berries, cherries, oranges, peaches, tomatoes, cucumbers, and so on) and foods containing artificial coloring, artificial flavorings, or preservatives (e.g., all manufactured bakery goods, most breakfast cereals, bologna, ham, salami, frankfurters, manufactured ice creams and candies, oleomargarine, mustard, soft drinks, tea, toothpaste, and so on). Feingold later stated that he believed that salicylates were not the usual cause of difficulty; he then suggested that a "modified Feingold diet"—excluding dyes, artificial flavorings, and additives, but not salicylates—be used for most children. Feingold also stated in his book that "allergy skin tests for foods are not applicable to this problem," and the emphasis of recent behavioral studies has been on either refuting or supporting the Feingold hypothesis, not investigating dietary allergens. Because the controversy about Feingold's hypothesis is still going on, a discussion of the few controlled studies to date is warranted.

Conners and colleagues (1976) at the University of Pittsburgh conducted the earliest experiments to test the Feingold hypothesis. They used a double-blind crossover diet study in 15 children, using a control diet and the Feingold diet for 4 weeks in succession. Teachers and parents were asked to rate improvement using Conners' previously standardized parent-teacher questionnaires on hyperactivity. Ratings by the teachers noted a reduction in symptoms on the Feingold diet, but the parents' ratings did not. There was also a significant order effect: those children who did show improvement did so only when the Feingold diet followed the control diet, implying that other factors than the diet might be playing a part in children who improved. This study has also been criticized because the diets were poorly disguised.

This same group of investigators subsequently performed experiments with specific challenges. They selected a group of 16 hyperactive children who had previously improved on the diet and challenged them in double-blind fashion with chocolate cookies baked with large amounts of dye or containing no dye. Behavior was rated by parents and teachers. They found no statistically significant behavioral changes with ingestion of the cookies containing dye. However, because of a suggestion of deterioration in behavior in three younger children after ingestion of the dye-containing cookies, they performed a third, smaller experiment in eight younger children whose behavior, according to parents, had improved with the diet. The researchers measured performance of a specific task involving attention and distractibility following challenge with cookies containing artificial colors, and found a significant increase in hyperactivity 1 to 3 hours postchallenge as measured by parental ratings. Although their third experiment supported Feingold's hypothesis, the numbers were small, and only one task was measured subjectively by raters. It is important to note that even after extremely large doses of dyes, the children in these studies did not show the dramatic change in behavior that Feingold said would occur after ingestion of even small amounts of additives.

An important study was performed soon afterward by Harley and co-workers (1978b) at the University of Wisconsin. Similar to Conners and colleagues, they used a double-blind crossover design but attempted to overcome the criticisms of Conners' study by using clever means to disguise the two diets and by rearranging the diet order for both groups. In addition to the Conners' questionnaire they used objective classroom observations by independent observers, laboratory observation based on multiple standardized tasks, and a battery of psychological tests. The number of subjects was also much larger. Mothers' ratings on the questionnaire revealed positive improvement for 13 of 36 school-aged children on the behavioral diet, but these were attributable to only one diet sequence—control followed by experimental diet. Teacher ratings were improved for 6 of the 36 children, but did not agree with parent ratings. There was consistent improvement in both teacher and parent ratings in only 4 of 36 children, and there was no difference in laboratory or classroom observations, nor in psychological tests in any of the schoolchildren. Parent ratings in 10 preschool children indicated a positive effect of the diet, but these were not corroborated by laboratory measures.

Harley and colleagues (1978a) then selected nine preschool boys who were believed to be previous diet responders by parents, and gave them multiple placebo and challenge food materials. Using the same multiple outcome measures as in their first study, they found only one child who showed improvement in the direction expected. Harley believed that his studies did not support the efficacy of the Feingold elimination diet, but made the guarded statement that "it is not possible from our data to categorically dismiss the possibility that a small subset of children, especially those of preschool age, may demonstrate hyperkinetic symptoms following the ingestion of synthetic foods and flavors."

Williams and colleagues (1978) at the University of Ontario, conducted double-blind challenge experiments in 26 hyperactive children while they were maintained on the Feingold diet. The researchers compared challenge cookies containing artificial food colors with placebo cookies. They also compared the effect of the challenge versus placebo cookies with stimulant versus placebo medications. Each child participated in the four treatment conditions: (1) stimulant medication/placebo cookie, (2) stimulant medication/challenge cookie, (3) placebo medication/placebo cookie, or (4) placebo medication/challenge cookie. Both parents and teachers noted marked improvement while the children were taking stimulant medication. The effects of the challenges were not as clear; using the criterion that children had to show a one-third reduction in individual hyperactivity scores while eating placebo cookies (compared with challenge cookies) to demonstrate any effect of diet, 3 of 26 children could be identified as improved by parents, and 5 by teachers. There was no agreement between the parents' and teachers' ratings. Williams attributed this latter finding to the effect of additives reaching their peak shortly after ingestion, as Conners had suggested; because the cookies were given in the early morning and at noon, the effects were noted primarily by the teachers during school hours. He thought that there was suggestive evidence of improvement in 3 to 8 children of the 26, depending on the criteria used. When asked to identify whether the child was on the additive-free or control diet, however, neither teachers nor parents could identify the diet correctly, again in contrast to the marked dramatic change in behavior cited in earlier anecdotal reports.

These studies did not substantiate Feingold's findings that a diet free from additives, dyes, and artificial flavorings produces a marked or even moderate remission in symptoms of the hyperactivity syndrome. As Dr. Frederick Stare points out in a recent review, "The fact that most of the children who improve on the Feingold diet do not respond to the additives with an increase in hyperactivity indicates that other factors in the diet regimen, not the artificial colors, are the key variables. This may be a change in family dynamics, increased attention, placebo, a change in nutritional status, or others."

Some positive findings from the challenge phase of these studies need further investigation: (1) preschool children seemed to be the most clearly positive reactors to challenges with artificial colors, (2) effects were most clearly noted 1 to 3 hours after ingestion in these preschoolers, (3) while a global increase in hyperactivity was not shown, there was a deterioration in performance on a specific task, which although subtle, might relate to more generalized behavioral disturbances, and (4) a question of dose response was raised by findings of an effect peaking shortly after ingestion.

Swanson and Kinsbourne (1980) from Toronto studied the effects of food colorings in higher dosages (100–150 mg) than previously reported (26 mg) on a specific task measuring sustained attention. They tested 40 children, classified as hyperactive or nonhyperactive by previous response to stimulant medication as measured by the Conners rating scales. Swanson and Kinsbourne demonstrated a statistically significant difference in the number of errors made on a paired-associate learning test 1½ to 3½ hours after the challenge with the food coloring in the hyperactive group; however, this difference was not associated with a change in the Conners behavioral rating scales. The authors concluded that a statistically significant response to food colorings was demonstrated in a highly selected group of patients with preexisting behavioral disturbances.

Weiss and colleagues (1980) studied 22 preschoolers with previous favorable responses to an additive- and coloring-free diet in informal trials. The children were placed on a strict Feingold diet, including salicylate elimination, and then challenged daily with placebo or a mixture of artificial food colorings in a dose of 35 mg. Parents' observations of previously designated target behaviors served as the measurement of response, with spot checks once weekly by outside observers. The authors found a significant increase in disruptive behaviors on the challenge days in only two children.

Thus, the current controversy centers on the prevalence and threshold of sensitivity of diet-responsive children in the large rather vaguely delineated group of children with the "hyperactivity syndrome," which has recently been reclassified as the "attentional deficit disorder syndrome." The following conclusions may be drawn from the studies to date:

1. There is no direct relation between behavioral disorders and IgE-mediated disorders, although children with true allergic disorders may exhibit behavioral and emotional consequences of their diseases.
2. The Feingold diet has not proved to be a cure for the vast majority of hyperactive children.
3. Environmental changes surrounding a change in dietary regimen and family habits do seem to produce an improvement in some hyperactive children, which is likely from increased attention, increased structure, altered family dynamics, or different familial perception of the child.
4. Challenge experiments with artificial food colors produced a deterioration in behavior only in small groups of preschool children.

5. Challenge experiments with artificial food colors, when given in high dosages, produced a deterioration in performance on a specific learning task.
6. Transient deterioration in behavior or in performance of a learning task occurred 1 to 3 hours after ingestion of artificial food colors in the groups who responded.

The primary physician is left with the frustrating problem of how best to treat the child with "hyperactivity" or the "attentional deficit disorder syndrome." If the history suggests diet as a precipitating factor of behavioral problems, or the parents are eager to try an elimination diet because of previous publicity about the Feingold diet and the current attraction to "natural foods," there seems to be no harm in concurring with their attempts as long as adequate nutritional status is maintained. More traditional treatments, however, such as behavioral modification, special education classes, family therapy, and medication, should not be ignored. More importantly, as Dr. Stare points out in his review, "the potential benefits [of diet] must be weighed against the harmful long-term educational impact of communicating to a child that his or her behavior is controlled by what he or she eats."

Augustine, G. J., and Levitan, H.   Neurotransmitter release from a vertebrate neuromuscular synapse affected by a food dye. *Science* 207:1489–1490, 1980.
FD&C dye #3 significantly increased transmitter release in isolated frog neuromuscular junctions.
Conners, C. K., et al.   Food additives and hyperkinesis: A controlled double-blind experiment. *Pediatrics* 58:154–165, 1976.
First crossover diet experiment that seemed to refute Feingold diet theory. Some children improved on Feingold diet by teacher ratings especially, but only when the Feingold diet followed control diet, leading to a question of order effect.
Crook, W. G., Harrison, W. W., and Crawford, S. E.   Systemic manifestations due to allergy. *Pediatrics* 27:790–799, 1961.
This article contains a report of 50 patients, as well as a review of literature on the subject.
Feingold, B.   *Why Your Child Is Hyperactive.* New York: Random House, 1975.
This book includes case reports from personal experience and parent testimonials; states 50 to 75% hyperactive children improved with diet free of salicylates and additives. The book received widespread attention from the media and lay public, and was widely quoted.
Goyette, C. H., Conners, C. K., Petti, T. A., and Curtis, L. E.   Effects of artificial colors on hyperkinetic children: A double blind challenge study. *Psychopharmacol. Bull.* 14:39–40, 1978.
The authors challenged 16 diet-responsive children and found no change in parent or teacher ratings after challenges. In fact children tended to be worse not better on a visual motor task 1 hour postchallenge. In younger children, there was a significant effect on parent ratings 3 hours postchallenge.
Harley, J. P., et al.   Hyperkinesis and food additives: Testing the Feingold hypothesis. *Pediatrics* 61:818–828, 1978.
This was an ingenious double-blind crossover study in which the investigators supplied all foods. Parents were never able to identify the sequence or timing of diet changes. There was a diet effect on the scores of parents of only a few preschoolers. The overall effect of food additives was negative.
Harley, J. P., Matthews, C. G., and Eichman, P.   Synthetic food colors and hyperactivity in children: A double-blind challenge experiment. *Pediatrics* 62:975–983, 1978.
This was a double-blind challenge experiment with dye-filled cookies in 9 preschoolers. The challenges were negative in all but one child.
Lockey, S. D.   Reactions to hidden agents in foods, beverages, and drugs. *Ann. Allergy* 29:461–466, 1971.
Lockey reports case histories of persons reacting to dyes and flavorings. Individual dose response is stressed.
Randolph, T. G.   Allergy as a causative factor of fatigue, irritability, and behavior problems in children. *J. Pediatr.* 31:560–572, 1947.

This article is the original published description attributing behavioral problems in children to a possible allergic etiology.

Shaywitz, B. A., Goldenring, J. R., and Wool, R. S.   The effects of chronic administration of food colorings on activity levels and cognitive performance in normal and hyperactive developing rat pups. *Ann. Neurol.* 4:196, 1978.
The authors suggest that cognitive function, as well as behavior, is affected by large doses of food colorings in rats.

Speer, F.   The allergic tension fatigue syndrome. *Pediatr. Clin. North Am.* 1:1029–1037, 1954.
This article is the first description of this syndrome and is an attempt to characterize the vague symptoms thought to be associated with "behavioral" reactions to foods. Case reports are presented.

Stare, F. J., Whelan, E. M., and Sheridan, M.   Diet and hyperactivity: Is there a relationship? *Pediatrics* 66:521–525, 1980.
This article gives an essentially negative review of controlled studies.

Swanson, J. M., and Kinsbourne, M.   Food dyes impair performance of hyperactive children on a laboratory learning test. *Science* 207:1485–1487, 1980.
The authors found a significantly decreased performance in a specific learning task after challenge with high dose of additives. They believe that dose response is more important than previously recognized.

Taylor, E.   Food additives, allergy and hyperkinesis. *J. Child. Psychol. Psychiatry* 20:357–363, 1979.
This article is a good review of literature from a psychodynamic point of view.

Weiss, B.   In rebuttal. *Am. J. Dis. Child.* 134:1126–1127, 1980.
Weiss offers rebuttals to a critique of his studies by Wender.

Weiss, B., et al.   Behavioral responses to artificial food colors. *Science* 204:1487–1488, 1980.
In double-blind challenges in 22 children reported to have responded to diet, 20 of 22 patients showed no effect and 1 showed a partial effect. One 3-year-old, however, had consistent dramatic behavioral changes.

Wender, E. H.   New evidence on food additives and hyperkinesis. *Am. J. Dis. Child.* 134:1122–1124, 1980.
Wender offers a critical analysis of the studies of Swanson and Kinsbourne, and of Weiss, with rebuttals by the authors.

Wender, E. H.   New findings on food additives and hyperkinesis. *Am. J. Dis. Child.* 132:1149, 1978.
This article is an editorial comment, an addendum to Wender's (1977) report.

Wender, E. H.   Food additives and hyperkinesis. *Am. J. Dis. Child.* 131:1204–1206, 1977.
This article reports on the three major controlled studies by Conners, Harley, and Williams, which were all essentially negative.

Williams, J. I., Cram, D. M., Tausig, F. T., and Webster, E.   Relative effects of drugs and diet on hyperactive behaviors: An experimental study. *Pediatrics* 61:811–817, 1978.
The authors found stimulant medications were clearly more effective than diet in reducing hyperactive behavior. There was evidence to suggest that three to eight children were diet responsive depending on criteria used.

55. ADVERSE REACTIONS TO IMMUNIZING AGENTS
Karl M. Altenburger

The use of specific immunizing agents has been a major advance in reducing the morbidity and mortality of a variety of infectious diseases. Adverse reactions to immunizations do occur occasionally, although they are uncommon. Unfortunately, the fear that such reactions may occur sometimes prevents appropriate use of immunizing agents in susceptible persons. Many such reactions are termed *allergic* although the immunologic mechanism involved is most often obscure. Critical evaluation is required to determine whether the patient can be safely immunized or whether he or she must be denied protection. Commercially available bacterial and viral vaccines and recommendations for their use are reviewed in the latest addition of the "Red Book" published by the American Academy of Pediatrics. Reactions to vaccines may be either allergic (IgE or reagin, mediated) or nonallergic. This chapter will be limited to a discussion of IgE-mediated reactions.

IgE-mediated reactions to live viral vaccines prepared in eggs (e.g., influenza, yellow fever, rabies) or chick embryo cell cultures (e.g., measles) have been described. Although the incidence is difficult to determine such reactions appear to be rare. In the two decades since the introduction of measles vaccine, over one hundred million doses have been administered and only five allergic reactions have been described. All these reactions occurred in persons who had a history of anaphylactoid reactions after egg ingestion. Many persons claim to be "allergic" to eggs although they are able to ingest varying amounts of egg protein without difficulty. These persons are not at risk for allergic reactions to the viral vaccines prepared in eggs. Another group of patients to be considered are those with skin-test reactivity to egg protein. The great majority of these persons ($\geq$75 percent) are asymptomatic after challenge and thus are not at risk for allergic reactions.

Recently Herman and colleagues (1983) evaluated two children with allergy to ovalbumin (egg-white protein) who had generalized urticaria, angioedema, and respiratory difficulty after immunization with live rubeola vaccine. Serum IgE antibodies against ovalbumin-related antigens in the vaccine were present in sera of both patients. In subsequent studies they demonstrated that children with ovalbumin allergy (positive ovalbumin skin tests) but no clinical reaction to egg white, had negative skin tests (prick and intradermal) to measles vaccine and were safely immunized. These children had no IgE antibody against the vaccine, although IgE directed at ovalbumin was present. Six patients who had severe allergic hypersensitivity reactions on exposure to ovalbumin had IgE antimeasles vaccine antibody and had positive reactions after intradermal testing with the vaccine. These patients were safely immunized with increasing volumes of measles vaccine (0.05 ml increments every 20 min) until the full dose was administered.

Mumps vaccine, like measles vaccine, is grown in a chick embryo cell culture and could be a problem in egg-sensitive persons. To date, no adverse reactions are reported. Rubella, rabies, and oral polio vaccines are prepared in human cell cultures and IgE-mediated reactions have not been described.

In evaluating a patient with a history of egg sensitivity for vaccine administration, the following guidelines may be helpful:

Chick embryo tissue culture vaccines
    1. Vaccines prepared in chick embryo tissue culture (live measles virus vaccine or live mumps virus vaccine) are virtually devoid of allergenic substances derived from chick embryo cell cultures used for growth of live vaccine viruses. However, there is a potential risk of hypersensitivity reaction in patients allergic to eggs, chicken, or chicken feathers.
    2. Patients with a history of egg sensitivity (with or without positive skin tests), but who can ingest eggs without difficulty, can be safely vaccinated with these vaccines.
    3. Patients with a positive skin test to ovalbumin and clinical egg sensitivity should receive an intradermal skin test with the vaccine. If the vaccine skin test is negative, the patient can receive the vaccine in a setting where adverse reactions can be treated (the patient should wait at least 20–30 min in that setting after receiving the vaccine).
    4. Patients with a positive intradermal skin test to the vaccine can probably be safely immunized with increasing small volumes of the vaccine until the full dose

has been given, as described by Herman and co-workers (1983). This procedure should be done only if severe reactions can be treated immediately. The risks and benefits of immunization should be thoroughly reviewed with the patient, the parents, or both.

Egg vaccines

1. Egg vaccine recommendations are similar to those for chick embryo tissue culture vaccines: patients with a history of egg sensitivity, but who can ingest eggs without difficulty, can be safely vaccinated.

2. Patients with a definite history of allergy to egg should receive skin tests with the undiluted vaccine (prick or puncture followed by intradermal). A positive skin test is considered an absolute contraindication to vaccination.

3. Patients with a negative vaccine skin test, but with a large skin prick or puncture test to egg or high levels of specific IgE to egg extracts, should be considered at risk for vaccination.

Some live virus vaccines contain trace amounts of antibiotics to which patients may be allergic. Causal relationships are difficult—usually impossible—to confirm. Prior to administering vaccines, the label information should be carefully reviewed before deciding whether patients with known allergies to antibiotics can be vaccinated safely.

Live measles, mumps, and rubella virus vaccine contain an extremely small amount of neomycin. Some persons allergic to neomycin may rarely experience a delayed-type local reaction consisting of an erythematous, pruritic papule 48 to 72 hours postimmunization. This possible minor reaction is of little importance when weighed against the benefits of immunization. As with other antibiotics, if the person has a documented history of anaphylactoid reaction to neomycin, these vaccines should not be used.

Local and systemic reactions to purified diphtheria and tetanus toxoids occur in 10% of recipients although such reactions are generally mild. Systemic anaphylactic (presumably IgE-mediated) reactions to tetanus toxoid have been described but are extremely rare. If reactions occur, further immunization is usually not needed because most of these patients have high levels of IgG antibodies to tetanus. Reactions to diphtheria toxoid are difficult to quantitate because it is now used in combination with tetanus toxoid and pertussis vaccine. From early experience with diphtheria and tetanus toxoids, systemic reactions rarely occur and do not appear to be IgE mediated. The addition of pertussis vaccine (a suspension of killed bacteria) greatly increases the incidence and severity of reactions. Serious reactions (e.g., seizures, encephalopathy) do occur rarely but they are not believed to be IgE mediated. The benefits of pertussis immunizations definitely continue to outweigh the risks.

Anaphylactoid reactions to pneumococcal vaccine have been reported (5 cases per 1 million doses administered). Hepatitis B, live-attenuated varicella, meningococcal, and *Haemophilus influenzae* vaccines are in various stages of investigation and use. Reports of adverse reactions to these vaccines should soon follow.

As a general rule the use of many vaccines carries a risk, although small, of allergic—even anaphylactic—reactions. Their use is recommended only in settings where such allergic reactions can be immediately diagnosed and treated. The morbidity and mortality of infectious diseases remains high; therefore, the decision to withhold immunization from a susceptible "allergic" person should not be made unless the results of a thorough evaluation indicate that the risks of immunization outweigh the estimated benefits.

Committee on Infectious Diseases.   Revised recommendations on rubella vaccine. *Pediatrics* 65:1182–1184, 1980.
The importance of vaccine use and rare adverse reactions are discussed.

Davies, R., and Pepys, J.   Egg allergy, influenza vaccine, and immunoglobulin E antibody. *J. Allergy Clin. Immunol.* 57:373–383, 1976.
The authors' advice: when in doubt take a history.

Fulginiti, V. A.   Immunizations: Current controversies. *J. Pediatr.* 101:487–494, 1982.
This review weighs risks and benefits of immunizations.

Fulginiti, V. A., et al.   "Red Book" update. *Pediatrics* 70:819, 1982.
This article is a supplement to the "Red Book."

Harrison, H. R., and Fulginiti, V. A.   Bacterial immunizations. *Am. J. Dis. Child.* 134:184–193, 1980.
This article is an excellent review of commonly used vaccines and other less well-known vaccines.

Herman, J. J., Radin, R., and Schneiderman, R.   Allergic reactions to measles (rubeola) vaccine in patients hypersensitive to egg protein. *J. Pediatr.* 102:196–198, 1983.
The authors provide case reports, literature review, and recommendations for management.

Hirtz, D. G., Nelson, K. B., and Ellenberg, J. H.   Seizures following childhood immunizations. *J. Pediatr.* 102:14–18, 1983.
Seizures following DPT and rubeola vaccination resemble febrile seizures and are rarely associated with long-term neurologic deficits.

Immunization Practices Advisory Committee. Centers for Disease Control. Pneumococcal polysaccharide vaccine. *Ann. Intern. Med.* 96:203–205, 1983.
Available vaccines, recommendation for use, and adverse reactions are discussed.

Klein, J. D. (Ed.).   Report of the Committee on Infectious Diseases (19th ed.). Evanston, Ill.: American Academy of Pediatrics, 1982.
This is the "Red Book." It includes a good review of current immunization practices.

Miller, J. R., Orgel, H. A., and Meltzer, E. O.   The safety of egg-containing vaccines for egg-allergic patients. *J. Allergy Clin. Immunol.* 71:568–73, 1983.
The authors studied 42 patients. The results of an intradermal skin test using a 1:100 dilution of the vaccine may predict those patients who are likely to get a severe reaction.

Patterson, R., and Anderson, J.   Allergic reactions to drugs and biologic agents. *J.A.M.A.* 248:2637, 1982.
The entire issue (No. 20) is a "Primer on Allergic and Immunologic Diseases."

Ratner, B., and Untracht, S.   Egg allergy in children. *Am. J. Dis. Child.* 83:309–316, 1952.
The authors provide skin test and challenge results to egg allergy in children.

Zaloga, G. P., and Chernow, B.   Life-threatening anaphylactic reaction to tetanus toxoid. *Ann. Allergy* 49:107–108, 1982.
A case report and literature review are discussed.

56. CONTROVERSIAL DIAGNOSTIC AND THERAPEUTIC TECHNIQUES EMPLOYED IN ALLERGY

Don A. Bukstein

During the past 80 years, the practice of allergy has changed dramatically. Our current practices have been dictated by astute clinical observation combined with increasing knowledge of basic immunologic principles. The concepts and methods accepted today should be based on reproducible laboratory and clinical studies meeting the standards of modern scientific investigation, and not based just on empiric observation. The intent of this chapter is to briefly describe some of the more controversial diagnostic and therapeutic procedures used by some physicians practicing allergy today. This author will give his opinion on whether their rationale or their effectiveness is supported by controlled studies and by current scientific knowledge of known immunologic mechanisms of allergic disease.

Leukocytotoxic testing (Bryan's test) is based on the claim that the addition of an allergen to which the patient is sensitive to the patient's whole blood or purified leukocyte suspension in vitro will result in a reduction in the white count or death of the leukocytes. This result is not supposed to occur when an antigen to which the patient is not sensitive is used. A buffy coat of leukocytes is suspended in one drop of water, and four to eight drops are placed on a slide with the dried antigen under a cover slip. After 2 hours, the leukocytes are examined for lytic changes and antigen sensitivity assessed.

Leukocytotoxic testing has been claimed to be useful for the diagnosis of both food and inhalant allergy, but this claim has never been proved by controlled studies. Furthermore, no scientific explanation for its use has ever been demonstrated. A number of controlled trials have shown leukocytotoxic testing to be ineffective in making the diagnosis of food or inhalant allergy.

Although no immunologic rationale has ever been given for **urine autoinjection** (autogenous urine immunization), it has been popularized as a treatment for allergic disease. In Plesch's technique, fresh urine is collected and sterilized by filtration or by boiling. Patients are then injected with their own urine. It is said that urine must be collected at a time when the patient is symptomatic because of exposure to the antigens to which desensitization will occur.

Plesch presented no evidence from suitable controlled studies as to the efficacy of this treatment and he provided no scientific basis for this treatment. No rationale or immunologic basis for this treatment has ever been proposed, nor have any further studies concerning its efficacy been published. In addition, this method has not been proved safe. It is potentially dangerous in that injections of kidney protein in the urine might induce nephritis.

Some allergists use **titration of intracutaneous tests** to determine the starting concentration of an antigen for hyposensitization. Selection of a concentration of antigen that gives a small wheal size on intradermal injection will reduce the incidence of side effects during early immunotherapy. This concept was modified and its rationale expanded by Rinkel and Willoughby. Their approach has been called the **Rinkel method.** An end-point dilution is determined by using intradermal injections of 0.01 ml of serial fivefold dilutions of allergenic extracts of both inhalants and foods. The end point is defined as the most dilute solution that produces a positive skin test. Rinkel claimed that the end-point dilution was useful in determining not only the starting dose for immunotherapy, but also the therapeutic dose. A safe starting dose was 0.01 to 0.15 ml of end-point dilution and the optimal therapeutic dose was close to 0.5 ml of end-point dilution. Rinkel stated that the specified starting dose rarely, if ever, caused untoward reactions, and that the specified optimal therapeutic dose rarely, if ever, caused untoward reactions and in many cases promptly relieved symptoms.

The end-point skin titration method of Rinkel provides essentially the same information as that provided by other well-studied skin-test end-point titration methods. Suitably controlled studies show that it is a satisfactory method for quantifying skin sensitivity to ragweed pollen extract and for obtaining information about sensitivity of patients who are highly sensitive to ragweed, and that the method is a rough guide to a safe starting dose. For the highly sensitive patient, the dose predicted by the Rinkel method would be less than the starting dose that has been proved to be tolerated by most patients. However, the Rinkel method would predict a starting dose too low for up to 80 percent of patients and result in a waste of time.

The controlled studies provide no support for Rinkel's claim that the usual optimal dose for providing relief from hay fever symptoms is 0.5 ml of the end-point dilution. In the patient highly sensitive to ragweed, 0.5 ml of the end-point dilution of ragweed pollen extract has been shown to be no more effective than placebo for relieving symptoms of hay fever or for producing immunologic effects. It has also been shown to be much less effective than larger doses, which were about 1000 times larger and produced a significant reduction in symptom-medication scores, an increase in serum levels of antiragweed IgG, and a decrease in the expected seasonal rise in serum levels of antiragweed IgE. These studies indicate that some measurement of patient sensitivity, such as skin-test end-point titration (by Rinkel or other standard methods), may be useful at the onset of immunotherapy to provide a guide to initial dose. Thereafter, costly repetitive end-point titrations are usually unnecessary because, regardless of what the titration indicates, the dose will be advanced either until the patient can tolerate no more or until a dose is reached that produces satisfactory results.

In the **subcutaneous provocational testing** technique, allergen is injected subcutaneously in increasing amounts until the patient's complaints are elicited. This is followed by the immediate injection of another dilution of the same antigen to relieve the provoked symptoms. Depending on the circumstances, either a weaker or stronger dilution of the antigen may be used. These dilutions are the provocational and neutralizational dose used then for the patient's immunotherapy.

Four well-controlled clinical studies have shown this method of diagnosis and treatment to be ineffective. Advocates of the subcutaneous provocational testing believe that their methods are effective in the diagnosis of food allergy, but conventional methods of food allergy diagnosis using oral challenges and blinded techniques have been shown to be more cost effective and efficacious.

The principle of the **sublingual provocational testing** technique is the same as in subcutaneous provocational testing. Advocates of this technique claim that it can be used for diagnosis and treatment of food-induced allergic symptoms including respiratory, gastrointestinal, and other systemic symptoms. The method consists of placing three drops of $1:100$ weight/volume of an aqueous glycerinated allergenic extract under the tongue of the patient and waiting 10 minutes for the appearance of symptoms such as rhinorrhea, sneezing, wheezing, GI reactions, skin eruptions, headache, generalized aches, drowsiness, or anxiety. When an allergen is identified as the cause of the patient's symptoms, the patient is given a neutralizing dose of the same extract (which is usually 3 drops of a very dilute solution, such as $1:300,000$ wt/vol). If an offending food so identified cannot be eliminated from the diet completely, desensitization is carried out with either sublingual drops or subcutaneous injections of antigens administered just before a meal containing the offending food.

Controlled studies indicate that this method is ineffective. Only anecdotal reports have suggested the effectiveness of sublingual antigen administration in the diagnosis or treatment of food allergy. Furthermore, there are no known immunologic mechanisms that could account for the "neutralizing" effect of dilute solutions of allergenic extracts of foods.

Since 1916, several observers including Hoobler, Shannon, Rowe, Rinkel, Randolph-Speer, Deamer, Gerrard, and Alvarez have described persons with systemic and nervous reactions that they believe are caused by specific hypersensitivity to foods. Symptoms are often low grade or subclinical and, thus, can often only be recognized after the offending food has been eliminated from the diet. The term *allergic tension-fatigue syndrome* was coined by Speer in 1954 to describe similar symptoms in allergic children. The symptoms described by Speer include alternating periods of tension and excessive fatigue, restlessness, sleeplessness, allergic rhinitis, abdominal pain, headache, vague muscular aches and pains, and enuresis. These reactions are reported to be delayed in onset, often not occurring until 24 to 48 hours after the ingestion of the food. Elimination of foods from the diet (usually including milk, chocolate, cola, corn, wheat, and egg) resulted in improvement in symptoms. Rechallenge of these foods in a nonblinded manner resulted in exacerbation of the symptoms.

No double-blind studies have been conducted in children or adults with this type of delayed onset of food reactions. Immunologic mechanisms have not been defined for this reaction. Although late-phase IgE reactions have been demonstrated in the skin and respiratory tract, they have not been investigated in these patients.

Vitamin or **nutrient-type** (orthomolecular) **therapies** have been used to treat many different illnesses and have been widely publicized in the lay press. High doses of vitamins including C and D complexes as well as minerals, calcium, and zinc have been used to treat asthma and allergy.

No studies have consistently documented that vitamin C can, as hypothesized, antagonize the mediators of immediate hypersensitivity. Several studies show that vitamin C is not efficacious in improving asthma or other allergic conditions. If minerals and vitamins are useful in an individual patient, it is likely that the placebo effect is responsible. Since improvement is a goal of therapy, physicians should not ignore the benefits of a placebo effect. However, one must be certain that the placebo effect is not being achieved at the expense of possible harm. High doses of vitamins can be harmful; thus, this type of therapy should be used only in moderation. The physician must also confirm the remaining diet is complete and not compromised by zeal for a subset of nutrients.

In this author's opinion, most of the data favoring these controversial approaches for diagnosis and treatment of allergic disease are the result of uncontrolled, anecdotal reports. Prospective double-blind, well-controlled protocols have not demonstrated unequivocally the effectiveness of any of these approaches. Demonstration of the effectiveness of these unconventional methods for diagnosis and therapy of allergic diseases is the responsibility of the proponents of these methods. Until such studies are performed, these unconventional methods should be considered unproved and their use confined only to well-designed clinical trials.

American Academy of Allergy.   Position statements—controversial techniques. *J. Allergy Clin. Immunol.* 67:333–338, 1981.
   The article is a short but thorough review of the scientific merit of many of the controversial techniques used in allergy.
Benson, T. E., and Arkins, J. A.   Cytotoxic testing for food allergy: Evaluations of reproducibility and correlation. *J. Allergy Clin. Immunol.* 58:471–476, 1976.
   This article is one of several studies demonstrating the inability of leukocytotoxic testing to be useful for diagnosis of food allergy.
Bryan, W. T. K., and Bryan, M. P.   Cytotoxic reactions in the diagnosis of food allergy. *Otolaryngol. Clin. North Am.* 4:523–534, 1971.
   The theory and supportive data for leukocytotoxic testing are presented.
Golbert, T. M.   A review of controversial diagnostic and therapeutic techniques employed in allergy. *J. Allergy Clin. Immunol.* 56:170–190, 1975.
   Golbert has written the best and the most comprehensive review on this subject.
Grieco, M. H.   Controversial practices in allergy. *J.A.M.A.* 247:3106–11, 1982.
   This review has a critical discussion of controversial practices in the diagnosis and treatment of allergic disease.
Kailin, E. W., and Collier, R.   "Relieving" therapy for antigen exposure. *J.A.M.A.* 217:78, 1971.
   In this double-blind trial comparing the relieving effect of subcutaneous or sublingual administration of saline versus dose of food extract, saline and aqueous food extracts were both judged by patients to be an active extract 70% of the time.
Lehman, C. W.   A double-blind study of sublingual provocative food testing: A study of its efficacy. *Ann. Allergy* 45:144–149, 1980.
   This report states that changes of symptoms or signs occurred as frequently after sublingual provocation with placebo as with food extract.
Miller, J. B.   A double-blind study of food extract injection therapy: A preliminary report. *Ann. Allergy* 38:185–191, 1977.
   The only controlled double-blind study that supports a favorable result from food injection therapy in eight patients.
Morris, D. L.   Use of sublingual antigen in diagnosis and treatment of food allergy. *Ann. Allergy* 27:289–294, 1969.

Anecdotal report that supports the clinical effectiveness of sublingual antigen administration in diagnosis and treatment of food allergy. No objective data are given in the study.

Plesch, J.   Urine therapy. *Medical Press* 218:128, 1947.
This method of urine autoinjections in the treatment of allergic disease is outlined.

Randolph, T. G.   Ecologic orientation in medicine: Comprehensive environmental control in diagnosis and treatment. *Ann. Allergy* 23:7–22, 1965.
The article details the approach of the clinical ecologists.

Rea, W. J., Bell, I. R., Suits, C. W., and Smiley, R. E.   Food and chemical susceptibility after environmental chemical overexposure: Case histories. *Ann. Allergy* 41:101–110, 1978.
The authors provide an outline of the theory and practice of medical ecology. The use of environmental control units in the diagnosis and treatment of presumed chemical sensitivities and for allergic disease is explained.

Rinkel, H. J.   Inhalant allergy. *Ann. Allergy* 7:625–630, 1949.
This article is the original description of the Rinkel method of skin titration.

VanMetre, T. E., et al.   A comparative study of the effectiveness of the Rinkel method and the current standard method of immunotherapy for ragweed pollen hayfever. *J. Allergy Clin. Immunol.* 66:500–513, 1980.
One of several controlled studies that demonstrates that the Rinkel method of skin titration is not an effective guide in choosing a therapeutic dose of immunotherapy.

Willoughby, J. W.   Provocative food test technique. *Ann. Allergy* 23:543–554, 1965.
The article provides a description of the technique and anecdotal reports of its efficacy.

Willoughby, J. W.   Serial dilution titration skin tests in inhalant allergy: A clinical quantitative assessment of biologic skin reactivity to allergenic extracts. *Otolaryngol Clin. North Am.* 7:579–615, 1974.
A summary of case histories supporting the use of the Rinkel method as an effective guide for choosing a starting and therapeutic dose for immunotherapy.

INDEX

Mast cells—*Continued*
  in rhinitis
    allergic, 70
    nonallergic, 74
Maximal midexpiratory flow rate, 39, 40,
    41, 42
Measles vaccine, 269, 270
Mechanical ventilation
  in infant wheezing, 94
  in respiratory failure, 16, 17–18
Mediators. *See also specific substances*
  in anaphylaxis, 3
  in penicillin allergy, 222
  in radiocontrast media reactions, 257
  in rhinitis, allergic, 70
Medical history, in asthma, 89, 90
Medrol, with troleandomycin, 177, 178,
    179, 180
Meningoceles, vs. polyps, 81
Meningococcal vaccine, 270
Mepivacaine, 231
Mepyramine, 182
Metabisulfate, 262
Metabolic acidosis, and wheezing, 93, 96
Metabolites, of theophylline, 147
Metaproterenol, 155
  in asthma
    exercise-induced, prophylaxis, 104
    mild, 98, 99
  dosages, 156
  in pregnancy, 131
  sulfites in, 261
  with theophylline, 150
Metaraminol, in anaphylaxis, 4
Metered-dose aerosols
  in asthma
    mild, 98, 99
    moderate, 99
  atropine, 165
Meterologic conditions, and asthma, 112
Methacholine. *See* Bronchial challenge
    testing
Methyldopa, lupus-like syndrome, 234
Methylparathion, 96
Methylprednisolone
  in insect sting reaction, 199
  with troleandomycin, 177, 178, 179, 180
Metyrapone, steroid therapy and, 135
Milk
  breast, 24–25, 63, 132–133
  hypersensitivity reactions, 205, 206
Minnesota Multi-Phasic Personality Inven-
    tory, 138
Mites, 110–111
  and hypersensitivity pneumonitis, 210
  pulmonary response patterns, 125
MMEFR, 39, 40, 41, 42
Molds, 111, 115. *See also* Fungal infections
Molluscum contagiosum, 247
Monoamine oxidase, 154
Morphine, 21, 96

Mortality rates, asthma 61–62
Mouth breathing, in rhinitis, 70
Mouth, in asthma, 89, 91
Mucociliary defense mechanisms, asthma
    and, 118
Mucolytics, in conjunctivitis, 68
Mucormycosis, and sinusitis, 79
Mumps vaccine, 269, 270
Muscle
  beta$_2$ receptors, 154
  theophylline and, 147
Myasthenia gravis, 58
Mycoplasma, 97, 177
Mycostatin, 174
Myringectomy, in otitis media 85

Naphazoline, in conjunctivitis, 67
Narcotic analgesics, in labor and delivery,
    132
NARES, 71
Nasal obstruction, and otitis media, 84
Nasal polyps, 80–81
  and sulfite sensitivity, 260
  in aspirin idiosyncrasy, 227, 228, 229
  cromolyn sodium with, 162
Nasalcrom, 72, 163
Nasalide, 173
Nasopharyngeal angiofibromas, vs. polyps,
    81
Nasopharyngeal pressure, and otitis media,
    84
Nausea, radiocontrast media reactions, 257
Nebulization
  of adrenergic agents, 158–159
  of anticholinergic agents, 165
  cromolyn sodium, 161–163
Neomycin, eye reactions, 68
Neurectomy, in sinusitis, 80
Neurodermatitis, 245
Neurologic symptoms, in asthma, 89, 91
Neuromuscular blocking agents, for me-
    chanical ventilation, 17
Neuromuscular diseases, and wheezing, 96
Neutral protamine Hageman, 236
Neutrophil chemotactic factor of anaphy-
    laxis, 128
Neutrophils, in contact dermatoconjunc-
    tivitis, 68
Nitrofurantoin, lupus-like syndrome, 234
Nitrogen dioxide, occupational exposure,
    107
Nocturnal asthma, gastroesophageal reflux
    in, 122
Nonallergic rhinitis with eosinophilia syn-
    drome, 71
Nonreaginic sensitivity, food allergy, 204
Nonsteroidal anti-inflammatory drugs
  in aspirin idiosyncrasy, 229
  in lupus, drug-induced, 235
Nose, in asthma, 89, 91. *See also* Rhinitis